ESSENTIALS OF
# Athletic Training

# ESSENTIALS OF
# Athletic Training

## Fifth Edition

### Daniel D. Arnheim, D.P.E., A.T.C., Deceased
Former Fellow, American College of Sports Medicine

Former Professor Emeritus of Physical Education
California State University
Long Beach, California

### William E. Prentice, Ph.D., P.T., A.T.C.
Professor, Coordinator of the Sports Medicine Specialization,
Department of Exercise and Sports Science
Clinical Professor, Division of Physical Therapy,
Department of Medical Allied Health Professions,
Associate Professor, Department of Orthopaedics
School of Medicine
The University of North Carolina
Chapel Hill, North Carolina

Boston   Burr Ridge, IL   Dubuque, IA   Madison, WI   New York   San Francisco   St. Louis
Bangkok   Bogotá   Caracas   Kuala Lumpur   Lisbon   London   Madrid   Mexico City
Milan   Montreal   New Delhi   Santiago   Seoul   Singapore   Sydney   Taipei   Toronto

# McGraw-Hill Higher Education

*A Division of The* **McGraw-Hill** *Companies*

ESSENTIALS OF ATHLETIC TRAINING, FIFTH EDITION

Published by McGraw-Hill, a business unit of The McGraw-Hill Companies, Inc., 1221 Avenue of the Americas, New York, NY 10020. Copyright © 2002, 1999, 1995, 1991, 1987 by The McGraw-Hill Companies, Inc. All rights reserved. No part of this publication may be reproduced or distributed in any form or by any means, or stored in a database or retrieval system, without the prior written consent of The McGraw-Hill Companies, Inc., including, but not limited to, in any network or other electronic storage or transmission, or broadcast for distance learning.

Some ancillaries, including electronic and print components, may not be available to customers outside the United States.

This book is printed on acid-free paper.

4 5 6 7 8 9 0 QPF/QPF 0 9 8 7 6 5 4 3

ISBN 0–07–244810–5 (softcover)
ISBN 0–07–244854–7 (hardcover)

Executive editor: *Vicki Malinee*
Senior developmental editor: *Michelle Turenne*
Senior marketing manager: *Pamela S. Cooper*
Project manager: *Christine Walker*
Senior production supervisor: *Sandy Ludovissy*
Designer: *Rick D. Noel*
Cover designer: *Rebecca Lloyd Lemna/Lloyd Lemna Design*
Cover image: *SuperStock Inc. Football # 106-5516*
Supplement producer: *Tammy Juran*
Media technology producer: *Judi David*
Compositor: *ElectraGraphics, Inc.*
Typeface: *10/12 Meridien*
Printer: *Quebecor World Fairfield, PA*

The credits section for this book begins on page C-1 and is considered an extension of the copyright page.

This text was based on the most up-to-date research and suggestions made by individuals knowledgeable in the field of athletic training. The authors and publisher disclaim any responsibility for any adverse effects or consequences from the misapplication or injudicious use of information contained within this text. It is also accepted as judicious that the coach and/or athletic trainer performing his or her duties is, at all times, working under the guidance of a licensed physician.

## Library of Congress Cataloging-in-Publication Data

Arnheim, Daniel D.
    Essentials of athletic training / Daniel D. Arnheim, William E. Prentice. — 5th ed.
      p.    cm.
    Includes bibliographical references and index.
    ISBN 0–07–244810–5
    1. Physical education and training.   I. Prentice, William E.   II. Title.

RC1210 .A749     2002
617.1'027—dc21

2001018747
CIP

www.mhhe.com

# *Remembering a Legacy*

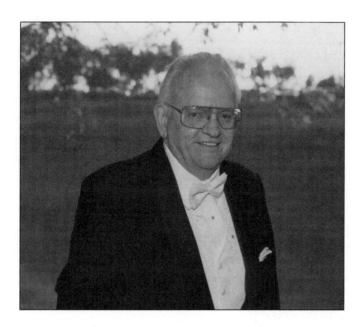

Our longtime author and friend, Daniel D. Arnheim, passed away April 11, 2000. Dr. Arnheim authored numerous textbooks in athletic training including *Essentials of Athletic Training,* as well as in elementary physical education, motor development, and adapted physical education. Among his most recognizable titles is *Principles of Athletic Training,* which is used by most students going into the field of athletic training.

Today, Dr. Arnheim is a legend among men and women who call themselves athletic trainers. For nearly 40 years, anyone who has taken an athletic training course has used one of his textbooks at one time or another. Any of the athletic trainers in the United States as well as throughout the world will recognize his name. He always focused on the needs of students and instructors who would use his books. He cared very much about the professional growth of students, as they hold the keys to the future of his chosen professions—education and athletic training. Dr. Arnheim touched the lives of the thousands of students and athletic trainers through the words in his books, and helped to shape the growth and the direction of athletic training as a profession. His impact as an athletic training educator will be missed. 🙠

*William E. Prentice*
*The Publishers*

# Contents in Brief

# Contents

# Preface

## WHO SHOULD USE THIS TEXT?

The majority of students who take courses about the prevention and management of injuries which typically occur in an athletic population have little or no intention of pursuing athletic training as a career. However, it is also true that a large percentage of those students who are taking these courses are doing so because they intend to pursue careers in coaching, fitness, physical education, or other areas related to exercise and sport science. For these individuals, some knowledge and understanding of the many aspects of health care for both recreational and competitive athletes is "essential" for them to effectively perform the associated responsibilities of their job.

Other students who are personally involved in fitness, or training and conditioning, may be interested in taking a course that will provide them with guidelines and recommendations for preventing injuries, recognizing injuries, and learning how to correctly manage a specific injury. Thus, *Essentials of Athletic Training* has been designed to provide basic information on a variety of topics, all of which relate in one way or another to health care for the athlete.

*Essentials of Athletic Training* was created from the foundations established by another well recognized textbook, *Principles of Athletic Training*, currently in its tenth edition. Whereas *Principles of Athletic Training* serves as a major text for professional athletic trainers and those individuals interested in sports medicine, *Essentials of Athletic Training* is written at a level more appropriate for the coach, fitness professional, and physical educator. It provides guidance, suggestions and recommendations for handling athletic health care situations when an athletic trainer or physician is not available.

## ORGANIZATION AND COVERAGE

The fifth edition of *Essentials of Athletic Training* provides the reader with the most current information possible on the subject of prevention and basic care of sports injuries. The general philosophy of the text is that adverse effects of physical activity arising from participation in sport should be prevented to the greatest extent possible. However, the nature of participation in physical activity dictates that sooner or later injury may occur. In these situations, providing immediate and correct care can minimize the seriousness of an injury.

Overall, this text is designed to take the beginning student from general to more specific concepts. Each chapter focuses on promoting an understanding of the prevention and care of athletic injuries.

*Essentials of Athletic Training* is divided into three parts: *Organizing and Establishing an Effective Athletic Health Care System, Techniques for Preventing or Minimizing Sport-Related Injuries,* and *Recognition and Management of Specific Injuries and Conditions.*

Part One, *Organizing and Establishing an Effective Athletic Health Care System,* begins in Chapter 1 with a discussion of the roles and responsibilities of all of the individuals on the "sports medicine team" who in some way impact the delivery of health care to the athlete. Chapter 2 provides guidelines and recommendations for setting up a system for providing athletic health care in situations where an athletic trainer is not available to oversee that process. In today's society, and in particular for anyone who is remotely involved with providing athletic heath care, the issue of legal responsibility and, perhaps more importantly, legal liability is of utmost concern. Chapter 3 discusses ways to minimize the chances of litigation and also to make certain that both the athlete and the coach are protected by appropriate insurance coverage.

Part Two, *Techniques for Preventing or Minimizing Sport-Related Injuries,* discusses a variety of topics which both individually and collectively can reduce the chances for injury to occur. Chapter 4 emphasizes the importance of making certain that the athlete is fit to prevent injuries. Chapter 5 discusses the importance of a healthy diet and giving attention to sound nutritional practices. Chapter 6 provides guidelines for selecting and using protective equipment. Chapter 7 details how to assess the severity of an injury and then provides specific steps which should be taken to handle emergency situations. Chapter 8 provides guidelines that can help reduce the chances of spreading infectious diseases by taking universal precautions dealing with bloodborne pathogens. Chapter 9 discusses the psychology of preparing to compete and proposes recommendations for how a coach should manage an injury. Chapter 10 looks at ways to minimize the potentially negative threats of various environmental conditions on the health of the athlete. Chapter 11 discusses the more common taping techniques which can be used to prevent new injuries from ocurring and old ones from becoming worse. Chapter 12 includes a brief discussion of the general techniques which may be used in rehabilitation following injury.

Part Three, *Recognition and Management of Specific Injuries and Conditions,* begins with Chapter 13 which defines and classifies the various types of injuries which are most commonly seen in the physically active population.

Chapters 14 through 22 discuss injuries which occur in specific regions of the body including the foot; the ankle and lower leg; the knee; the hip, thigh, and groin; the shoulder; the elbow, wrist, forearm, and hand; the spine; the thorax and abdomen; and, the head and face. Injuries are discussed individually in terms of their most common causes, the signs of injury you would expect to see, and a basic plan of care for that injury. Chapter 23 provides guidelines and suggestions for managing various illnesses and other health conditions that may affect athletes and their ability to play and compete. Chapter 24 provides special considerations for injuries which may occur in young athletes.

## NEW TO THIS EDITION

- New! *Coach's Corner:* The Coach's Corner has been added in Chapters 1 through 12 and 24 to provide a checklist prepared specifically for the coach to help organize the details for a specific procedure discussed in that chapter.

- New! *Dynamic Human 2.0 CD-ROM:* New with this edition, the *Dynamic Human CD* is packaged with each new text purchased. References to the *Dynamic Human CD* appear in Chapters 14 through 22, and help to clarify the student's understanding of the anatomy for a particular body part.

- An expanded discussion of the relationship between the coach, athletic trainer, physician and the athlete's family.

- Changes in the roles and responsibilities of an athletic trainer as defined by the *National Athletic Trainers' Association.*

- Complete lists of supplies and equipment for the athletic training room, and for a field kit.

- Reorganized discussion of the potential legal liabilities of a coach overseeing the administration of an athletic health care program.

- An expanded discussion of the concept of periodization in a training and conditioning program.

- Updated information on the use of sport drinks for fluid replacement during physical activity.

- Significantly updated information of the use of various types of protective equipment.

- Updated information on new CPR techniques.

- A focused discussion about what the coach needs to know for off-the-field injury evaluation.

- Chapter 9, *Psychological Aspects of Sports Injury,* has been completely revised to offer practical suggestions when managing the psychology of the injured athlete.

- Managing bloodborne pathogens and taking universal precautions is given increased emphasis throughout the entire text.

- Updated information about lightning during an electrical storm.

- A scaled-down discussion of bandaging and taping focuses only on those specific techniques that a coach should know about and be able to perform.

- An example of a functional progression for returning an injured athlete to running is presented.

- A consistent presentation format covers the pertinent anatomy and assessment techniques throughout Chapters 14 to 22.

- New line drawings of human anatomical art is presented in Chapters 14 through 22.

- A significant revision and reorganization of Chapter 17, *The Thigh, Hip, Groin, and Pelvis.*

- A significant revision and expansion of information, particularly of finger injuries, is included in Chapter 19, The Elbow, Forearm, Wrist, and Hand.

- Chapter 22, *The Head, Face, Eyes, Ears, Nose, and Throat,* has been completely rewritten to reflect the most current information available, and includes an updated discussion of concussion and mild head injury.

- A discussion of creatine and androstenodione supplementation for performance enhancement has been added to Chapter 23.

- The latest statistics on youth sports injuries have been included in Chapter 24, *Young Athletes.*

- More *Critical Thinking Exercises* have been included throughout the text, enabling the coach to make practical applications to clinical settings.

- Chapter references have been updated and expanded.

- The websites recommended at the end of the chapters have been increased to reflect the expanding scope of the internet.

## PEDAGOGICAL FEATURES

- *Chapter objectives.* Objectives are presented at the beginning of each chapter to reinforce learning goals.

- *Focus Boxes.* Important information is highlighted to provide additional content that supplements the main text.

- *Margin information.* Key concepts, selected definitions and pronunciation guides, helpful training tips, and illustrations are placed in margins throughout the text for added emphasis, and ease of reading and studying.

- *Illustrations and photographs.* These crucial tools are presented to facilitate the student's comprehension of athletic training.

- *Critical Thinking Exercises.* Included in every chapter, these brief case studies correspond with the accompanying text and help students apply the content just learned. Solutions for each exercise are located at the end of the chapters.

- *Coach's Corner.* New checklists prepared specifically for the coach to help organize the details of a specific procedure when managing athletic health care.

- *Chapter summaries.* Chapter content is summarized and bulleted to reinforce key concepts and aid in test preparation.

- *Review questions and class activities.* A list of questions and suggested class activities follows each chapter for review and application of the concepts learned.

- *Dynamic Human 2.0 CD-ROM.* Provides instructions on how to access relevant sections of the *Dynamic Human CD-ROM* for each chapter in Part 3.

- *References.* All chapters have a bibliography of pertinent references that includes the most complete and up-to-date resources available.
- *Annotated bibliography.* To further aid in learning, relevant and timely articles, books, and topics from the current literature have been annotated to provide additional resources.
- *Websites.* A list of useful websites is included to direct the student to additional relevant information that can be found on the internet.
- *Color throughout the text.* A second color appears throughout the text to enhance the overall appearance, and accentuate and clarify illustrations.
- *Glossary.* A comprehensive list of key terms and their definitions are presented at the end of the text.
- *Appendixes.* For those students interested in learning more about athletic training, Appendixes A through C provide information about recognition of the athletic trainer as an allied health professional, employment settings for the athletic trainer, and the requirements for certification as an athletic trainer.
- *Back cover.* Helpful charts for metric and celsius conversions are found inside the back cover.

## ANCILLARIES

### Instructor's Manual and Test Bank

Developed for the fifth edition, the *Instructor's Manual and Test Bank* was prepared by Meredith Petschauer, M.A., A.T.C. Practical features include the following:

- Brief chapter overviews
- Learning objectives
- Key terminology
- Discussion questions
- Class activities
- Worksheets
- Worksheet answer keys
- Test bank
- Appendix of additional resources
- Transparency masters
- Perforated format, ready for immediate use

### Computerized Test Bank

A computerized version of the Test Bank, MicroTest 3, is available to qualified adopters. This software enables the instructor to select, edit, add, or delete questions, and to develop tests and answer keys. Each chapter contains multiple-choice, true-false, and short essay questions, keyed according to level of difficulty.

### Dynamic Human CD

With each purchase of a new text, the *Dynamic Human 2.0 CD-ROM* is included providing an excellent reference that enables students to comprehend the anatomy within the text through the use of its graphics and animation.

### Web Resources

*McGraw-Hill's Human Performance Supersite.* The human performance supersite provides a wide variety of information for instructors and students, from text information to the latest technology. It includes professional organization, convention, and career information. Link to the on-line catalog to find the perfect text or ancillary for your course. Additionally, web links are also provided here for all our course offerings. Visit the website at www.mhhe.com/hper/physed/humanperformance

Additional features of the supersite include:

- *This Just In.* This link provides featured articles, related publications, web resources, and more updated monthly.
- *Faculty Support.* This links to PageOut, online supplements, Online Learning Centers, PowerWeb, and much more.
- *Student Success Center.* This helps students to locate new study skills, job hunting tips, and web links to assist in preparing for the job search and career development.
- *Author Arena.* Contact our authors, visit their websites, and see our featured *Author of the Month* here.

*Essentials of Athletic Training homepage.* Developed specifically for the fifth edition of *Essentials of Athletic Training*, a PowerPoint presentation has been prepared, and can be downloaded from the Instructor Center. Additionally, a link to PageOut, our web-based program which can be used to help create your own website, is included here. Visit the *Essentials of Athletic Training* homepage at www.mhhe.com/hper/physed/arnheim_ess

## ACKNOWLEDGMENTS

Special thanks are extended to Michelle Turenne, with whom I have enjoyed a long-standing relationship as my Development Editor on this and several other projects. As always she has provided invaluable guidance in the preparation of the fifth edition of *Essentials of Athletic Training*.

Meredith Petschauer from the University of North Carolina has been responsible for preparing the Instructor's Manual and Test Bank which accompanies this text. Her efforts have provided a much needed educational resource for individuals teaching a course in athletic injuries and I certainly appreciate the manner in which she has completed her part of this project. I would also like to thank Dr. Elizabeth Hedgpeth from the University of North Carolina for her contribution of the *Psychological Aspects of Sports Injury* chapter. Her input on the project is greatly appreciated.

I would also like to thank the following individuals who served as reviewers for their input into the revision of this text:

*Diane Bartholomew*
**Neosho County Community College**

*John Bartholomew*
**Neosho County Community College**

*Toby J. Brooks*
**University of Arizona**

*Matthew Comeau*
**Arkansas State University**

*Doris E. Flores*
**California State University at Sacramento**

*Larry J. Leverenz*
**Purdue University**

*Ronda Peterson*
**Moorhead State University**

*Mark Stutz*
**Fort Hays State University**

*Steve Condon*
**Iowa State University**

I also want to thank our survey respondents who provided valuable information to improve the accompanying website for *Essentials of Athletic Training,* as well as their other helpful suggestions about media and technology:

*Diane Bartholomew*
**Neosho Community College**

*Shari D. Bartz*
**Grand Valley State University**

*Brian Czajka*
**Millikin University**

*Jean M. Fruh*
**West Virginia Wesleyan College**

*Bonnie Goodwin*
**Capital University**

*Olana Hedrick-Sheaffer*
**Penn State University at Altoona**

*Tisha Hess*
**Millikin University**

*David A. Kaiser*
**Brigham Young University**

*Thomas W. Kaminiski*
**University of Florida**

*William N. Miller*
**Westfield State College**

*Bobby Patton*
**Southwest Texas State University**

*James R. Scifers*
**Salisbury State University**

*Ronald Stefancin*
**James Madison University**

*Catherine L. Stemmans*
**Indiana State University**

*Sue Stanley-Greene*
**Florida Southern College**

*Jeffrey W. Wimer*
**Wilmington College**

Finally, I would like to thank my family, Tena, Brian, and Zach, for always being an important part of everything I do.

*William E. Prentice*

# Applications at a Glance

# PART

# 1

# ORGANIZING AND ESTABLISHING AN EFFECTIVE ATHLETIC HEALTH CARE SYSTEM

# The Sports Medicine Team and Their Roles

*When you finish this chapter you will be able to:*

- Define the umbrella term *sports medicine*.
- Identify various sports medicine organizations.
- Explain how the sports medicine team should interact with the athlete.
- Describe the role of the coach in injury prevention, emergency care, and injury management.
- Identify the responsibilities of the athletic trainer in dealing with the injured athlete.
- Describe the role of the team physician and his or her interaction with the athletic trainer.
- Identify other members of the sports medicine team and describe their roles.

**M**illions of individuals participate on a regular basis in both organized and recreational sport activities. Ironically, participation in sports places the athlete in situations in which injury is likely to occur. Fortunately most injuries are not serious and lend themselves to rapid rehabilitation. Athletes who engage in organized sports have every right to expect their health and safety to be kept as the highest of priorities. Both coaches and athletic trainers must be concerned with the well-being of the athlete and in those roles assume responsibility for overseeing the total health care of the athlete (Figure 1-1).

In an ideal world, specific responsibilities of both the coach and the athletic trainer would be clearly defined. Coaches could concentrate their efforts on coaching, and athletic trainers could assume total responsibility for the health needs of the athlete. Unfortunately, because of budget constraints at institutions or within organizations that offer organized athletic programs, every coach does not have access to an athletic trainer.[3] Even if your school or organization employs an athletic trainer, there is no chance that that single athletic trainer can be available to cover every practice and game of all the teams that compete at your school or within your organization. In these less-than-ideal situations,

**Figure 1-1**

The field of athletic training
is a major link between the
sports program and the
medical community.

coaches are forced not only to be coaches but also to assume more responsibility for providing health care to their athletes. This situation dictates that the coach have some knowledge about injury prevention,
emergency care, and injury management.[10]

## WHAT IS SPORTS MEDICINE?

The term *sports medicine* has many connotations, depending on which
group is using it. The term encompasses many different areas of sports related to both performance and injury. Among the areas of specialization
within sports medicine are athletic training, physical therapy, biomechanics, exercise physiology, the practice of medicine relative to the athlete, sports nutrition, and sports psychology.

### Sports Medicine Organizations

A number of professional organizations are dedicated to athletic training and sports medicine. Professional organizations have many goals:
(1) to upgrade the field by devising and maintaining a set of professional
standards, including a code of ethics; (2) to bring together professionally
competent individuals to exchange ideas, stimulate research, and promote critical thinking; and (3) to give individuals an opportunity to
work as a group with a singleness of purpose, thereby making it possible
for them to achieve objectives that, separately, they could not accomplish. Addresses and Websites for these organizations are listed in Focus
Box 1-1.

    Many of the national organizations interested in athletic health and
safety have state and local associations that are extensions of the larger
bodies. National, state, and local sports organizations have all provided
extensive support to the reduction of illness and injury risk to the athlete.

Sports medicine encompasses
many different fields of study
related to sports, including:
* athletic training
* biomechanics
* exercise physiology
* the practice of medicine
  relative to the athlete
* physical therapy
* sports nutrition
* sports psychology

As a professional, the athletic
trainer must be a member of
and be active in professional
organizations.

---

⟨ 1-1 ⟩  **Focus Box**

---

**List of Professional Sports Medicine Organizations**

American Academy of Pediatrics, Sports Committee, 1801 Hinman Ave., Evanston, IL 60204 http://www.aap.org

American Board of Physical Therapy Specialists, American Physical Therapy Association, 1111 North Fairfax St., Alexandria, VA 22314 apta.edoc.com

American College of Sports Medicine, 401 W. Michigan St., Indianapolis, IN 46202-3233 http://www.acsm.org

American Orthopaedic Society for Sports Medicine, Suite 202, 70 West Hubbard, Chicago, IL 60610 http://www.sportsmed.org

National Athletic Trainers' Association, 2952 Stemmons Freeway, Dallas, TX 75247 http://www.nata.org

National Collegiate Athletic Association, Competitive Safeguards and Medical Aspects of Sports Committee, P.O. Box 1906, Mission, KS 66201 http://www.ncaa.org

The National Federation of State High School Athletic Associations, 11724 Plaza Circle, P.O. Box 20626, Kansas City, MO 64195 http://www.nfsha.org

National Strength and Conditioning Association, P.O. Box 38909, Colorado Springs, CO 80937-8909 http://www.nsca-lift.org

---

Many professional organizations are dedicated to achieving health and safety in sports.

### The National Athletic Trainers' Association

The professional organization to which most athletic trainers belong is the National Athletic Trainers' Association (NATA). Before the formation of the NATA in 1950, athletic trainers occupied a somewhat insecure place in the athletic program. Since that time, as a result of the raising of professional standards and the establishment of a code of ethics, the field has experienced considerable professional advancement. The NATA accepts as members only those athletic trainers who are properly qualified and who are prepared to subscribe to a code of ethics and to uphold the standards of the association.[4] The NATA is constantly working to improve both the quality and the status of athletic training. Through the efforts of the membership of the NATA, the profession of athletic training is now recognized as an allied health profession and is accredited by the Commission on Accreditation of Allied Health Education Programs (CAAHEP) (see Appendix A).

## THE PLAYERS ON THE SPORTS MEDICINE TEAM

The primary athletic training team consists of the coach, the athletic trainer, and the team physician.

The provision of health care to the athlete requires a group effort to be most effective.[2,9] The sports medicine team involves a number of individuals, each of whom must perform specific functions relative to caring for the injured athlete. Those people having the closest relationship with the injured athlete are the coach, the athletic trainer, and the team physician.

## The Relationship Among the Coach, Athletic Trainer, Physician, and Athlete

The major concern of everyone on the sports medicine team should always be the athlete. If not for the athlete, the coach, athletic trainer, and team physician would have nothing to do in sports. All decisions made by the physician, coach, and athletic trainer ultimately affect the athlete. It should be clear that the physician working in cooperation with the athletic trainer assumes the responsibility of making the final decisions relative to the course of health care for the athlete from the time of injury until full return to activity. The coach must defer and should support the decisions of the medical staff in any matter regarding health care for the athlete.

**Critical Thinking** Exercise

What are some things that a coach working in cooperation with an athletic trainer can do to help minimize the chances of injury?

This is not to say, however, that the coach should not be involved with the decision-making process. For example, during the time the athlete is rehabilitating an injury, there may be drills or technical instruction sessions that the athlete can participate in that will not exacerbate the existing problem. Thus the coach, the athletic trainer, and the team physician should be able to negotiate what the athlete can and cannot do safely in the course of a practice.

Athletes are frequently caught in the middle between coaches who tell them to do one thing and medical staff who tell them something else. Close communication between the coach and athletic trainer is essential so that everyone is on the same page.

Any personal relationship takes some time to grow and develop. The relationship between the coach and the athletic trainer is no different. The athletic trainer must demonstrate to the coach his or her capability to correctly manage an injury and guide the course of a rehabilitation program. It will take some time for the coach to develop trust and confidence in the athletic trainer. The coach must understand that what the athletic trainer wants for the athlete is exactly the same as what the coach wants—to get an athlete healthy and back to practice as quickly and safely as possible.

On the other hand, the athletic trainer must respect the job that the coach has to do and should do whatever can be done to support the coach.

The injured athlete must always be informed and made aware of the why, how, and when factors that collectively dictate the course of an injury rehabilitation program. Both the coach and the athletic trainer should make it a priority to educate student-athletes about injury prevention and management. Athletes should learn about techniques of training and conditioning that may reduce the likelihood of injury. They should be well informed about their injuries and about listening to what their bodies are telling them to prevent reinjury.

## The Importance of the Family in the Sports Medicine Team

In a high school or junior high school setting, the coach, the athletic trainer, and the physician must also take the time to explain to and inform the parents about injury management and prevention.[3] With an athlete of secondary school age, the parents' decisions regarding health care must be of primary consideration.

In certain situations, particularly at the high school and junior high levels, many parents will insist that their child be seen by their family physician rather than by the individual who may be designated as the team physician. This creates a situation in which the athletic trainer must work and communicate with many different "team physicians." The opinion of the family physician must be respected even if the individual has little or no experience with injuries related to sports.

### Responsibilities of the Coach

The coach is directly responsible for preventing injuries by seeing that athletes have undergone a preventive injury conditioning program. The coach must ensure that sports equipment, especially protective equipment, is of the highest quality and is properly fitted. The coach must also make sure that protective equipment is properly maintained.[9] A coach must be keenly aware of what produces injuries in his or her particular sport and what measures must be taken to avoid them (Figure 1-2). A coach should be able, when called on to do so, to apply proper first aid. This knowledge is especially important in serious head and spinal injuries. **All coaches (both head and assistants) should be certified in cardiopulmonary resuscitation** (CPR) by either the American Red Cross, the American Heart Association, or the National Safety Council. **Coaches should also be certified in first aid** by the American Red Cross or the National Safety Council.[10]

All head and assistant coaches should be certified in CPR and first aid.

**Figure 1-2**

The coach is directly responsible for preventing injuries in his or her sport.

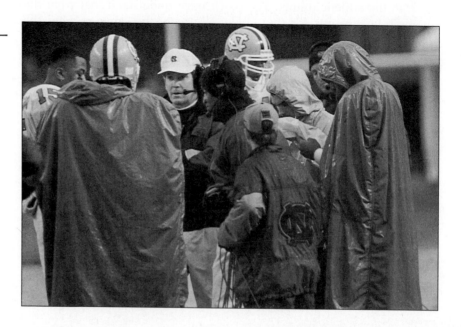

It is essential that a coach have a thorough understanding of the skill techniques and environmental factors that may adversely affect the athlete. Poor biomechanics in skill areas such as throwing and running can lead to overuse injuries of the arms and legs, whereas overexposure to heat and humidity may cause death. Just because a coach is experienced in coaching does not mean that he or she knows proper skill techniques. Coaches must engage in a continual process of education to further their knowledge in their particular sport. When a sports program or specific sport is without an athletic trainer, the coach very often takes over this role.

Coaches work closely with athletic trainers; therefore both must develop an awareness and an insight into each other's problems so that they can function effectively. The athletic trainer must develop patience and must earn the respect of the coaches so that his or her judgment in all training matters is fully accepted. In turn, the athletic trainer must avoid questioning the abilities of the coaches in their particular fields and must restrict opinions to athletic training matters. To avoid frustration and hard feelings, the coach must coach, and the athletic trainer must conduct athletic training matters. In terms of the health and well-being of the athlete, the physician and the athletic trainer have the last word. This position must be backed at all times by the athletic director.

## Roles and Responsibilities of the Athletic Trainer

Of all the professionals charged with injury prevention and health care provision for the athlete, perhaps none is more intimately involved with the athlete than the athletic trainer.[9] The athletic trainer is the one individual who deals with the athlete from the time of the initial injury, throughout the period of rehabilitation, until the athlete's complete, unrestricted return to practice or competition.[12] The athletic trainer is most directly responsible for all phases of health care in an athletic environment, including preventing injuries from occurring, providing initial first aid and injury management, evaluating injuries, and designing and supervising a timely and effective program of rehabilitation that can facilitate the safe and expeditious return of the athlete to activity.[6] Athletic trainers are employed by schools and school systems, colleges and universities, professional athletic teams, sports medicine clinics, and by corporations in industry (see Appendix B).

Employment settings for athletic trainers:
- schools
- school systems
- colleges and universities
- professional teams
- clinics
- corporations

If no athletic trainer is available, the coach should assume the responsibility for the health care of the athlete.

### Qualifications for an Athletic Trainer

The athletic trainer must be knowledgeable and competent in a variety of sports medicine specialities if he or she is to be effective in preventing and treating injuries to the athlete.[1,7] The NATA has established specific requirements that must be met for an individual to become certified as an athletic trainer.[7] These requirements include a combination of both academic coursework and clinical experience in athletic training settings (see Appendix C). (*In this text all references to athletic trainers imply that this individual has met the requirements for certification set forth by the NATA.*) The

Organizing and Establishing
an Effective Athletic Health
Care System

Athletic training must be
considered as a specialization
under the broad field of
sports medicine.

Roles and responsibilities of
the athletic trainer:
(1) athletic injury prevention
    and risk management
(2) recognition, evaluation,
    and assessment of
    injuries
(3) immediate care of injury
    and illness
(4) rehabilitation and
    reconditioning of athletic
    injuries
(5) health care organization
    and administration
(6) professional
    development and
    responsibility

specific roles and responsibilities of the athletic trainer will differ and, to a certain extent, will be defined by the situation in which he or she works.[6]

### Athletic Injury Prevention and Risk Management

Participation in competitive sports places the athlete in a situation in which injuries are possible at any time. One major responsibility of the athletic trainer is to make the competitive environment as safe as possible to reduce the likelihood of injury. If injury can be prevented initially, then there is no need for first aid and subsequent rehabilitation.

Injury prevention includes (1) ensuring appropriate training and conditioning of the athlete (see Chapter 4), (2) monitoring environmental conditions to ensure safe participation (see Chapter 10), (3) selecting, properly fitting, and maintaining protective equipment (see Chapter 6), (4) explaining the importance of proper nutrition (see Chapter 5), and (5) using medications appropriately.

### Recognition, Evaluation, and Assessment of Injuries

The athletic trainer is responsible for conducting physical examinations and preparticipation screenings to identify conditions that predispose an athlete to injury (see Chapter 2), and educating parents, coaches, and athletes about the risks inherent to sport participation.

Frequently, the athletic trainer is the first person to see an athlete who has sustained an injury. The athletic trainer must be skilled in recognizing the nature and extent of an injury through competency in injury evaluation. The athletic trainer must be able to efficiently and accurately evaluate that injury (see Chapter 7). Information obtained in this initial evaluation may be critical later on when swelling, pain, and guarding mask some of the functional signs of this injury.

### Immediate Care of Injuries and Illnesses

Once the initial on-the-field assessment is done the athletic trainer then must assume responsibility for administering appropriate first aid to the injured athlete and for making correct decisions in the management of acute injury (see Chapter 7). Thus the athletic trainer must possess sound skills not only in the initial recognition and evaluation of potentially serious or life-threatening injuries but also in emergency care.

The athletic trainer should be certified in CPR and first aid by the American Red Cross or the National Safety Council. Many athletic trainers have gone beyond these essential basic certifications and have completed requirements for emergency medical technician (EMT).

### Treatment, Rehabilitation, and Reconditioning

An athletic trainer must work closely with and under the supervision of the team physician with respect to designing rehabilitation and reconditioning protocols that make use of appropriate rehabilitative equipment, manual therapy techniques, or therapeutic modalities. The athletic trainer should then assume the responsibility of overseeing the rehabilitative process ultimating returning the athlete to full activity (see Chapter 12). In certain settings the athletic trainer may work closely with physical therapists and/or strength and conditioning specialists in designing functional return to play activities.

### Health Care Organization and Administration

The athletic trainer is responsible for the organization and administration of the athletic training program, including the maintenance of health and injury records for each athlete, the requisition and inventory of necessary supplies and equipment, the submission of insurance information to third-party payers, the supervision of assistant or student athletic trainers, and the establishment of policies and procedures for day-to-day operation of the athletic training program (see Chapter 2).

### Professional Development and Responsibility

The athletic trainer must educate the general public, in addition to a large segment of the various allied medical health care professions, as to exactly what athletic trainers are and what their roles and responsibilities are. This education is perhaps best accomplished by holding professional seminars, publishing research in scholarly journals, meeting with local and community organizations, and most important, doing a good and professional job of providing health care to the injured athlete.

The athletic trainer must act at all times with the highest standards of conduct and integrity.[4] To ensure this behavior, the NATA has developed a code of ethics[8] that includes the following:

1. Athletic trainers shall respect the rights, welfare, and dignity of all individuals.
2. Athletic trainers shall comply with the laws and regulations governing the practice of athletic training.
3. Athletic trainers shall accept the responsibility for the exercise of sound judgment.
4. Athletic trainers shall maintain and promote high standards in the provision of services.
5. Athletic trainers shall not engage in conduct that constitutes a conflict of interest or that adversely reflects on the profession.

Athletic trainers who act in a manner that is unethical or unbecoming to the profession can ultimately lose their certification.

## Responsibilities of the Team Physician

The athletic trainer works primarily under the supervision of the team physician, who is ultimately responsible for directing the total health care of the athlete (Figure 1-3). In cooperation with the team physician, the athletic trainer must make decisions that ultimately have a direct effect on the athlete who has sustained an injury.

1-2

***Critical Thinking*** Exercise

A basketball player suffers a grade 2 ankle sprain during midseason of the competitive schedule. After a 3-week course of rehabilitation, most of the athlete's pain and swelling have been eliminated. The athlete is anxious to get back into practice and competitive games as soon as possible and subsequent injuries to other players have put pressure on the coach to force this player's return. Unfortunately the athlete is still unable to perform functional tasks (cutting and jumping) essential in basketball.

**?** Who is responsible for making the decision regarding when the athlete can fully return to practice and game situations?

**Figure 1-3**

In treating the athlete, the athletic trainer carries out the directions of the physician.

The team physician assumes a number of roles and responsibilities with regard to injury prevention and the health care of the athlete.[5,11]

The physician should be a supervisor and an advisor to the athletic trainer and coach. However, the athletic trainer must be given flexibility to function independently in the decision-making process and must often act without the advice or direction of the physician. Therefore it is critical that the team physician and the athletic trainer share philosophical opinions regarding injury management and rehabilitation programs so as to minimize any discrepancies or inconsistencies that may exist. Most athletic trainers prefer to work with rather than for a team physician.

### Compiling Medical Histories

The team physician should be responsible for compiling medical histories and conducting physical examinations for each athlete, both of which can provide critical information that may reduce the possibility of injury. Preparticipation screening done by both the athletic trainer and physician is important in establishing baseline information to be used for comparison should injury occur during the season.

### Diagnosing Injury

Team physicians must have absolute authority in determining the health status of an athlete who wishes to participate in the sports program.

The team physician should assume responsibility for diagnosing an injury and should be keenly aware of the program of rehabilitation as designed by the athletic trainer following the diagnosis. Athletic trainers should be capable of doing an accurate initial evaluation following acute injury. Input from that evaluation may be essential to the physician, who may not see the patient for several hours or perhaps days following the injury. However, the physician has been trained specifically to diagnose injuries and to make recommendations to the athletic trainer for treatment based on that diagnosis. The athletic trainer should have a sound background in injury rehabilitation and must be the one to design and supervise an effective rehabilitation scheme. These roles are closely related yet very distinct and require both cooperation and close communication if they are to be optimized.

### Deciding on Disqualification

The physician should determine when an athlete should be disqualified from competition on medical grounds and must have the final say in when an injured athlete may return to activity. Any decision to allow an athlete to resume activity should be based on recommendations from the athletic trainer. An athletic trainer most often has the advantage of knowing the injured athletes well, how they respond to injury, how they move, and how hard to push to return them safely to activity. The physician's judgment must be based not only on medical knowledge but also on knowledge of the psychophysiological demands of a particular sport.[1]

### Attending Practices and Games

A team physician should make an effort to attend as many practices, scrimmages, and competitions as possible. This attendance obviously becomes very difficult at an institution with twenty or more athletic teams. Thus the physician must make himself or herself readily available should the athletic trainer (who generally is at most practices and games) require consultation or advice.

### Commitment to Sports and the Athlete

Most important, the team physician must have a strong love of sports and must be generally interested in and concerned for the young people who compete. Colleges and universities typically employ a full-time team physician. But high schools most often rely on local physicians who volunteer their time. Serving as a team physician for the purpose of enhancing social standing in the community can be a frustrating and potentially dangerous situation for everyone involved in the athletic program.

It is essential that the team physician promote and maintain consistently high quality care for the athlete in all phases of the sports medicine program.

## Other Members of the Sports Medicine Team

A number of support health services may be used by a sports program. Those people may include a nurse, physicians in specialties such as orthopedics, dentist, podiatrist, physician's assistants, strength and conditioning coaches, nutritionist, sport psychologists, exercise physiologists, physical therapists, equipment personnel, and referees.

Support personnel concerned with athletes' health and safety:
- nurse
- school health services
- orthopedist
- dentist
- podiatrist
- physician's assistant
- biomechanist
- strength and conditioning coach
- sport psychologist
- physical therapist
- exercise physiologist
- nutritionist
- equipment personnel
- referees

### Nurse

As a rule, the nurse is not usually responsible for the recognition of sports injuries. Education and background, however, render the nurse quite capable in the recognition of skin disease, infections, and minor irritations. The nurse works under the direction of the physician and in liaison with the athletic trainer and the school health services.

### Physicians

A number of physicians with a variety of specializations can aid the sports medicine team in treating the athlete.

**Orthopedist**   The orthopedist is responsible for treating injuries and disorders of the musculoskeletal system. Many colleges and universities have a team orthopedist on their staff.

**Neurologist**   A neurologist specializes in treating disorders of and injuries to the nervous system. There are common situations in athletics in which consultation with a neurologist is warranted, such as cases of head injury or peripheral nerve injury.

**Internist**   An internist is a physician who specializes in the practice of internal medicine. An internist treats diseases of the internal organs by using measures other than surgery.

**Family medicine physician**   A physician who specializes in family medicine is concerned with supervising or providing medical care to all members of a family. Many team physicians in colleges and universities and particularly at the high school level are engaged in family practice.

**Ophthalmologist**   Physicians who manage and treat injuries to the eye are ophthalmologists. An optometrist is an individual who evaluates and fits patients with glasses or contact lens.

**Pediatrician**   A pediatrician is concerned with the practice of caring for or treating injuries and illnesses that occur in young physically active children and adolescents.

**Psychiatrist**   Psychiatry is a medical practice that deals with the diagnosis, treatment, and prevention of mental illness.

**Dentist**   The role of team dentist is somewhat analogous to that of team physician. He or she serves as a dental consultant for the team and should be available for first aid and emergency care. Good communication between the dentist and the coach or athletic trainer should ensure a good dental program. The team dentist has three areas of responsibility:

1. Organizing and performing the preseason dental examination
2. Being available to provide emergency care when needed
3. Conducting the fitting of mouth protectors

**Podiatrist**   Podiatry, the specialized field dealing with the study and care of the foot, has become an integral part of sports health care. Many podiatrists are trained in surgical procedures, foot biomechanics, and the fitting and construction of orthotic devices for the shoe. Like the team dentist, a podiatrist should be available on a consulting basis.

### Physician's Assistants

Physician's assistants (PAs) are trained to assume some of the responsibilities for patient care traditionally done by the physician. They assist the physician by conducting preliminary patient evaluations, arranging for various hospital-based diagnostic tests, and dispensing appropriate medications. A number of athletic trainers have also become PAs in recent years.

### Strength and Conditioning Coach

Many colleges and universities and some high schools employ full-time strength coaches to advise athletes on training and conditioning programs. Athletic trainers should routinely consult with these individuals to advise them about injuries to a particular athlete and exercises that should be avoided or modified relative to a specific injury.

### Sports Psychologists

The sports psychologist can advise the athletic trainer on matters related to the psychological aspects of the rehabilitation process. The way the athlete feels about his or her injury and how it affects his or her social, emotional, intellectual, and physical dimensions can have a substantial effect on the course of a treatment program and how quickly the athlete may return to competition. The sports psychologist uses different intervention strategies to help the athlete cope with injury.

### Physical Therapists

Some athletic trainers use physical therapists to supervise the rehabilitation programs for injured athletes while the athletic trainer concentrates primarily on getting a player ready to practice or compete. A number of athletic trainers are also physical therapists.

The individual who achieves both certification as an athletic trainer and licensure as a physical therapist is extremely well qualified to function in various sports medicine settings, including both the private clinic and the colleges and universities.

### Exercise Physiologists

The exercise physiologist can significantly influence the athletic training program by giving input to the trainer regarding training and conditioning techniques, body composition analysis, and nutritional considerations.

### Nutritionists

Increasingly, individuals in the field of nutrition are becoming interested in athletics. Some large athletic training programs engage a nutritionist as a consultant who plans eating programs that are geared to the needs of a particular sport. He or she also assists individual athletes who need special nutritional counseling.

**_Critical Thinking_** Exercise

A new high school has hired a coach to establish and develop the football program. Unfortunately, the school does not have enough funds to also hire an athletic trainer. Thus the coach must assume the responsibility of creating a safe playing environment for the athletes.

**?** What considerations should the coach make to ensure that his athletes will be competing under the safest possible conditions?

### Equipment Personnel

Sports equipment personnel are becoming specialists in the purchase and proper fitting of protective equipment. They work closely with the coach and the athletic trainer.

### Referees

Referees must be highly knowledgeable regarding rules and regulations, especially those that relate to the health and welfare of the athlete. They work cooperatively with the coach and the athletic trainer. They must be capable of checking the playing facility for dangerous situations and equipment that may predispose the athlete to injury. They must routinely check athletes to ensure that they are wearing adequate protective pads.

## COACH'S CORNER

The following checklist contains things the coach can do to minimize the chance of injury.

☐ Arrange for physical examinations and preparticipation screening
☐ Ensure appropriate training and conditioning of the athlete
☐ Monitor environmental conditions to ensure safe participation
☐ Select and maintain properly fitting protective equipment
☐ Educate parents, coaches, and athletes about the risks inherent to sports participation
☐ Teach proper techniques
☐ Be certified in CPR
☐ Be certified in first aid

## SUMMARY

- The sports medicine team consists of the coach, the athletic trainer, and the team physician.
- The term *sports medicine* has many connotations, depending on which group is using it. The term encompasses many different areas of sports related to both performance and injury.
- The provision of health care to the athlete requires a group effort to be most effective.
- The coach must ensure that the environment and the equipment that is worn are the safest possible, that all injuries and illnesses are properly cared for, that skills are properly taught, and that conditioning is at the highest level.
- The athletic trainer is responsible for preventing injuries from occurring, for providing initial first aid and injury management, for evaluating injuries, and for designing and supervising a program of rehabilitation that can facilitate the safe return to activity.
- The team physician is responsible for preparticipation health examinations, for diagnosing and treating illnesses and injuries, for advising

and teaching the athletic training staff, for attending games, scrimmages, and practices, and for counseling the athlete about health matters.

- Other members of the sports medicine team may include a nurse, physicians in specializations such as orthopedics, dentist, podiatrist, physician's assistants, strength and conditioning coaches, nutritionist, sport psychologists, exercise physiologists, physical therapists, equipment personnel, and referees.

---

*Solutions to Critical Thinking* Exercises

**1-1** To help prevent injury the athletic trainer should (1) arrange for physical examinations and preparticipation screenings to identify conditions that predispose an athlete to injury, (2) ensure appropriate training and conditioning of the athlete, (3) monitor environmental conditions to ensure safe participation, (4) select and maintain properly fitting protective equipment, and (5) educate parents, coaches, and athletes about the risks inherent to sports participation.

**1-2** Ultimately the team physician is responsible for making that decision. However, that decision must be based on collective input from the coach, the athletic trainer, and the athlete. Remember that everyone in the sports medicine team has the same ultimate goal—returning the athlete to full competitive levels as quickly and safely as possible.

**1-3** The coach should be responsible for designing an effective conditioning program; be responsible for ensuring that protective equipment is of the highest quality, properly fitted, and properly maintained; be able to apply proper first aid; be certified in CPR and first aid; and be aware of the environmental factors that may adversely affect the athlete.

## REVIEW QUESTIONS AND CLASS ACTIVITIES

1. What areas of specialization are encompassed under the general heading of sports medicine?
2. List some of the professional sports medicine organizations.
3. How should the sports medicine team work together to provide optimal health care for the athlete?
4. What are the responsibilities of a coach who must assume the role of a health care provider when an athletic trainer is not available?
5. What are the specific roles of the athletic trainer in overseeing the total health care of the athlete?
6. Discuss the role of the team physician as an important member of the sports medicine team.
7. What special impact can other members of the sports medicine team have in providing health care for the athlete?

## REFERENCES

1. Arnold B, Gansneder B, VanLunen B: Importance of selected athletic trainer employment characteristics in collegiate, sports medicine clinic and high school settings, *J Ath Train* 33(3):254, 1998.

2. Barefield S, McCallister S: Social supports in the athletic training room: athletes' expectations of staff and student athletic trainers, *J Ath Train* 32(4):333, 1997.

3. Lyznicki J, Riggs J, Champion H: Certified athletic trainers in secondary schools: report of the council on scientific affairs, American Medical Association, *J Ath Train* 34(3):272, 1999.

4. Mangus BC, Ingersoll CD: Approaches to ethical decision making in athletic training, *J Ath Train* 25(4):340, 1990.

5. Mellion MB, Walsh WM: The team physician. In Mellion MB, editor: *Sports medicine secrets*, Philadelphia, 1999, Henly-Belfus.

6. National Athletic Trainers Association Board of Certification, Inc: *Role delineation study*, Raleigh, NC, 1995, Columbia Assessment Services.

7. National Athletic Trainers Association: *Athletic training educational competencies*, Dallas, 1999, National Athletic Trainers Association.

8. National Athletic Trainers Association: New NATA code of ethics approved, *NATA News* 4(7):15, 1992.

9. Prentice W: The athletic trainer. In Mueller F, Ryan A, editors: *Prevention of athletic injuries: the role of the sports medicine team*, Philadelphia, 1991, Davis.

10. Ransone J, Dunn-Bennett L: Assessment of first-aid knowledge and decision making of high school athletic coaches, *J Ath Train* 34(3):267, 1999.

11. Rich BS: All physicians are not created equal; understanding the educational background of the sports medicine physician, *J Ath Train* 28(2):177, 1993.

12. Winterstein A: Organizational commitment among intercollegiate head athletic trainers: examining our work environment, *J Ath Train* 33(1):54, 1998.

**ANNOTATED BIBLIOGRAPHY**

Arnheim D, Prentice W: *Principles of athletic training*, ed 10, St. Louis, 2000, McGraw-Hill.

*Discusses the sports medicine team approach paying particular attention to the role of the athletic trainer in providing health care to the athlete.*

Cartwright L, Pittney W: *Athletic training for student assistants*, Champaign, Ill, 1999, Human Kinetics.

*A practical guide for student athletic training assistants including their roles and responsibilities within the sports medicine team.*

Hannum S: *Professional behaviors in athletic training*, Thorofare, NJ, 2000, Slack.

*Focuses on essentials of effective career development. Addresses many skills students will require to build their image as health care professionals, such as communication, critical thinking, networking, interpersonal skills, and recognition of cultural differences.*

Mueller F, Ryan A: *Prevention of athletic injuries: the role of the sports medicine team*, Philadelphia, 1991, Davis.

*Provides an in-depth discussion of the various members of the sports medicine team.*

Van Ost L, Manfre K: *Athletic training student guide to success*, Thorofare, NJ, 2000, Slack.

*This text emphasizes the roles and responsibilities of the student athletic trainer necessary to make them successful as health care professionals.*

**WEBSITES**

National Athletic Trainers' Association: http://www.nata.org

*Presents a description of the athletic training profession, the role of an athletic trainer, and how to become involved in athletic training.*

American Sports Medicine Institute:
http://www.asmi.org

*The American Sports Medicine Institute's mission is to improve the understanding, prevention, and treatment of sports-related injuries through research and education. In addition to stating this mission, the site provides access to current research and journal articles.*

American Academy of Orthopaedic
Surgeons: http://www.aaos.org

*Presents general public information and information to its members. The public information is in the form of patient education brochures and a description of the organization and a definition of orthopedics.*

The American Orthopaedic Society for
Sports Medicine: http://www.sports-med.org

*Dedicated to educating health care professionals and the general public about sports medicine; access is provided to the* American Journal of Sports Medicine *and a wide variety of links to related sites.*

Athletic Trainer.com: http://athletic-trainer.com

*Specifically designed to give information to athletic trainers, including students and those interested in athletic training; provides access to interesting journal articles and links to several additional informative Websites.*

NCAA: http://www.ncaa.org

*Provides general information about the NCAA and the publications that the NCAA circulates; is useful for those working in the collegiate setting.*

# Organizing and Administering an Athletic Health Care Program

*When you finish this chapter you will be able to:*

- Describe a well-designed athletic training facility.
- Identify the rules of operation that should be enforced in an athletic training program.
- Explain budgetary concerns for ordering supplies and equipment.
- Explain the importance of the preparticipation physical examination.
- Identify the records that must be maintained by the athletic trainer.

Operating an effective athletic health care program requires careful organization and administration regardless of whether the setting is a high school, college or university, or at the professional level. If no athletic trainer is available to oversee the athletic health care program, the coach must also be an administrator who performs both managerial and supervisory duties in organizing such a program.[5] This chapter looks at the administrative tasks required of the coach for successful operation of an athletic health care program, including facility design, policies and procedures, budget considerations, administration of physical examinations, and record keeping.

## CONSIDERATIONS IN PLANNING AN ATHLETIC TRAINING FACILITY

For a coach who may have to assume responsibility for planning an athletic training room facility in the absence of an athletic trainer, some guidance in and understanding of what should be included in that facility is necessary.

Essential to any sports program is the maximum use of facilities and the most effective use of equipment and supplies. The athletic training facility must be specially designed to meet the many requirements of the sports athletic training program (Figure 2-1).[7] The size and the layout of the athletic training facility are dependent on the scope of the athletic program, including the size and number of teams and athletes and what

**Figure 2-1**

The ideal training room facility should be well designed to maximize its use.

sports are offered. To accommodate the various functions of an athletic program, it must serve as a health care center for athletes.[12]

An athletic training area of less than 1,000 square feet is impractical. An athletic training facility 1,000 to 1,200 square feet in size is satisfactory for most schools. The 1,200-square-foot area (40 feet by 30 feet) permits the handling of a number of athletes at one time and allows ample room for the bulky equipment needed. A facility of this size is well suited for pregame preparation. Careful planning will determine whether a larger area is needed or is desirable.[2]

The athletic training facility should be located immediately adjacent to the locker rooms. The facility should have an outside entrance from the field or court, making it unnecessary to bring injured athletes in through the building. This door also permits access when the rest of the building is not in use.

The training room should be organized to provide distinct areas for (1) taping and bandaging; (2) injury treatment using rehabilitative

**Figure 2-2**

An effective athletic training program must have appropriate storage facilities that are highly organized.

The training facility is a multipurpose area used for first aid, therapy and exercise rehabilitation, injury prevention, medical procedures such as the physical examination, and athletic training administration.

It is essential to have sufficient storage space for supplies and equipment.

Every athletic training program must develop policies and procedures that carefully delineate the daily routine of the program.

equipment and/or therapeutic modalities; and (3) a wet area for whirl-pools, a refrigerator, and an ice machine.

### Storage Facilities

Many athletic training facilities lack adequate storage space (Figure 2-2). Often storage facilities are located a considerable distance away, which is extremely inconvenient. Each of the three special service areas should contain storage cabinets and shelves for storing general supplies and the small specialized equipment used in the respective areas. A large walk-in closet is a necessity for storing bulky equipment, medical supplies, adhesive tape, bandages, and protective devices. Another important piece of equipment is a refrigerator for storing frozen water in styrofoam cups for ice massage, and other necessities.

## ESTABLISHING RULES OF OPERATION FOR AN ATHLETIC TRAINING PROGRAM

Every athletic training program must develop policies and procedures that carefully delineate the daily routine of the program. This is imperative for handling health problems and injuries.

It is first necessary to decide exactly who will be taken care of in the athletic training room. The coach must decide the extent to which the athlete will be served. For example, will prevention and care activities be extended to athletes for the entire year, including summer and other vacations, or only during the competitive season? A policy should clarify whether students other than athletes, athletes from other schools, faculty, and staff are to receive care.[6] Often legal concerns and the school liability insurance dictate who, other than the athlete, is to be served.

### Providing Coverage

A major concern of any athletic department is to try to provide the most qualified health care possible to the athlete. Unfortunately, as indicated

2-1 *Focus Box*

**Rules and Policies of the Athletic Training Room**

- *No cleated shoes are allowed.* Dirt and debris tend to cling to cleated shoes; therefore cleated shoes should be removed before athletes enter the athletic training facility.

- *Game equipment is kept outside.* Because game equipment such as balls and bats adds to the sanitation problem, it should be kept out of the athletic training room. Athletes must be continually reminded that the athletic training room is not a storage room for sports equipment.

- *Shoes must be kept off treatment tables.* Because shoes tend to contaminate treatment tables, they must be removed before any care is given to the athlete.

- *Athletes must shower before receiving treatment.* The athlete should make it a habit to shower before being treated if the treatment is not an emergency. This procedure helps keep tables and therapeutic modalities sanitary.

- *Roughhousing and profanity are not allowed.* Athletes must be continually reminded that the athletic training facility is for injury care and prevention. Horseplay and foul language lower the basic purpose of the athletic training room.

- *No food or smokeless tobacco is allowed.*

in Chapter 1, budgetary limitations often dictate who is responsible for overseeing the health care program for the athletes. Ideally an institution hires a certified athletic trainer who is primarily responsible. In some cases, schools rely on a nurse to provide care. And in other situations in which there are no athletic trainers or nurses, health care responsibility usually falls on the coach. Regardless of who is in charge of the health care program, policies must be established concerning how to best provide coverage to various athletic teams. High schools with limited available supervision may only be able to provide athletic training facility coverage in the afternoons and during vacation periods. Ideally, high-risk sports should have a certified athletic trainer and physician present at all practices and contests.

## Athletic Training Room Policies

The athletic training room should be used only for the prevention and care of sports injuries. Too often the athletic training facility becomes a meeting or club room for teams and athletes. Unless definite rules are established and practiced, room cleanliness and sanitation become an impossible chore. Focus Box 2-1 lists some important athletic training room policies.

## Keeping Facilities Clean

The practice of good hygiene and sanitation is of the utmost importance in an athletic training program. The prevention of infectious diseases is a

2-1
**Critical Thinking** Exercise

The members of the school board at All-American High School voted to allocate $25,000 to renovate a 25 foot by 40 foot storage space and to purchase new equipment for an athletic training room. The coach has been asked to provide the school principal with a wish list of what should be included in this facility. It has been estimated that the physical renovation will cost approximately $17,000.

**?** How may this space be best used, and what type of equipment should be purchased to maximize the effectiveness of this new facility?

2-2   *Focus Box*

**Suggestions for Maintaining a Sanitary Environment**

- Sweep the gymnasium floors daily.
- Clean and disinfect drinking fountains, showers, sinks, urinals, and toilets daily.
- Air out and sanitize lockers frequently.
- Clean wrestling mats and wall mats daily.
- Provide clean dry towels each day for each individual athlete.
- Issue individual equipment and clothing to each athlete to avoid skin irritations.
- Do not allow swapping of equipment and clothing.
- Launder and change clothing frequently.
- Allow wet clothing to dry thoroughly before the athlete wears it again.

Good hygiene and sanitation
are essential for an athletic
training program.

direct responsibility of the coach, whose duty it is to see that all athletes are surrounded by as hygienic an environment as is possible and that each individual is practicing sound health habits. Chapter 8 discusses the management of bloodborne pathogens. The coach must be aware of and adhere to guidelines for the operation of an athletic care facility as dictated by the Occupational Safety and Health Administration (OSHA).

Focus Box 2-2 lists guidelines to help maintain a sanitary environment.

Cleaning responsibilities in most schools are divided between the athletic training or coaching staff and the maintenance crew. Care of permanent building structures and trash disposal are usually the responsibilities of maintenance, whereas upkeep of specialized equipment falls within the province of the coaches or athletic trainers. Division of routine cleaning responsibilities may be organized as suggested in Focus Box 2-3.

## Establishing Health Habits for the Athlete

To promote good health among the athletes, the coach or the athletic trainer should encourage sound health habits. Focus Box 2-4 provides a checklist that may be a useful guide for coaches, athletic trainers, and athletes.

## Providing Emergency Phones

The installation of an emergency telephone adjacent to all major activity areas or the availability of a wireless phone is a must. It should be possible to use this phone to call outside for emergency aid or to contact the athletic training facilities when additional assistance is required. Walkie-talkies are also useful when practices or games occur at several different facilities simultaneously. These devices can greatly enhance communication without incurring a tremendous expense.

---

**2-3** **Focus Box**

**Cleaning Responsibilities**

The maintenance crew should:

- Sweep floors daily.
- Clean and disinfect sinks and built-in tubs daily.
- Mop and disinfect hydrotherapy area twice a week.
- Refill paper towel and drinking cup dispensers as needed.
- Empty wastebaskets and dispose of trash daily.

The athletic training staff should:

- Clean and disinfect treatment tables daily.
- Clean and disinfect hydrotherapy modalities daily.
- Clean and polish other therapeutic modalities weekly.

---

## RECORD KEEPING

Record keeping is a major responsibility in an athletic training program. Some coaches and athletic trainers object to keeping records and filling out forms, stating they have neither the time nor the inclination to be bookkeepers. Nevertheless, in a time in which lawsuits are the rule rather than the exception, accurate and up-to-date records are an absolute necessity. In addition to keeping medical records, the coach or athletic trainer should maintain injury reports, treatment logs, personal

*Keeping adequate records is of major importance in the athletic training program.*

---

**2-4** **Focus Box**

**Recommended Health Practices Checklist**

- Are the athletes medically cleared to participate?
- Is each athlete insured?
- Do the athletes promptly report injuries, illnesses, and skin disorders to the coach or the athletic trainer?
- Do the athletes practice good daily living habits of resting, sleeping, and proper nutrition?
- Do they shower after practice?
- Do they dry thoroughly and cool off before departing from the gymnasium?
- Do they avoid drinking from a common water dispenser?
- Do they avoid using a common towel?
- Do they avoid exchanging gym clothes with teammates?
- Do they practice good foot hygiene?
- Do they avoid contact with teammates who have a contagious disease or infection?

Preparticipation health
examination:
Medical history
Physical examination
Maturity assessment
Orthopedic screening

information cards, injury evaluations and progress notes, supply and equipment inventories, and annual reports.

## Administering Preparticipation Health Examinations

The primary purpose of the preseason health examination is to identify whether an athlete is at risk before he or she participates in a specific sport.[3] The preparticipation examination should consist of a medical history, a physical examination, and a brief orthopedic screening. Information obtained during this examination will establish a baseline to which comparisons may be made following injury. The examination may reveal conditions that could warrant disqualification from certain sports. The examination will also satisfy insurance and liability issues (see Chapter 3).

The preparticipation physical may be administered on an individual basis by a personal physician, or it may be done using a station examination system with a team of examiners.[4] Examination by a personal physician has the advantage of yielding an in-depth history and an ideal physician-patient relationship. A disadvantage of this type of examination is that it may not be directed to detection of factors that predispose the athlete to a sports injury.[13]

The most thorough and sport-specific type of preparticipation examination is the station examination.[4] This method can provide the athlete with a detailed examination in a short time. A team of nine people is needed to examine thirty or more athletes. The team should include two physicians, two medically trained nonphysicians (nurse, athletic trainer, physical therapist, or physician's assistant), and five managers, student athletic trainers, or assistant coaches.

A preparticipation exam should include all of the following items.

### Medical History

A medical history form should be completed before the physical examination and orthopedic screening; its purpose is to identify any past or existing medical problems. This form should be updated for each athlete every year. Medical histories should be closely reviewed by the physician, the coach, and the athletic trainer so that they will be prepared should some medical emergency arise. Necessary participation release forms and insurance information should be collected along with the medical history (Figure 2-3).

### Physical Examination

The physical examination should include assessment of height, weight, body composition, blood pressure, pulse, vision, skin, teeth, ears, nose, throat, heart and lung function, abdomen, lymphatics, genitalia, maturation index, urinalysis, and blood work (Figure 2-4).

### Maturity Assessment

Maturity assessment should be part of the physical examination as a means of protecting the young athlete.[1] Most commonly used methods are the circumpubertal (sexual maturity), skeletal, and dental assess-

**2–2**

***Critical Thinking*** Exercise

All-American High School offers eighteen sports, which are divided into six fall, six winter, and six spring sports. The school has a total of approximately 500 athletes, and approximately 200 of them are involved in the fall sports. The coach is charged with the responsibility of arranging and administering preparticipation examinations so that each athlete can be cleared for competition.

**?** How can the coach most efficiently set up the preparticipation exams to clear 200 athletes for competition in the fall sports?

**MEDICAL HISTORY FORM**

**HEAD**
1. Do you experience headaches? _____
   If yes, how frequently do they appear? _____
   Where are they located? _____
   Do you take any medicine to relieve them? _____
   If yes, what do you use? _____
2. Do you have any episodes of dizziness, seizures, or
   convulsions? _____
3. Have you ever fainted? _____
4. Have you ever had a head or neck injury? _____
   If yes, did you lose consciousness? _____
   If yes, how long? _____
   Were you under the care of a doctor? _____
   Were you hospitalized? _____
   Paralysis? _____ Numbness, tingling, or weakness of any extremity?
   _____
   How long before you resumed normal activity? _____

**EYES**
1. Have you ever had a problem with your eyes? Trauma?_____
   Loss of vision? _____ Pink eye? _____ Pain? _____

**EARS**
1. Have you ever had a problem with your ears? _____
   Infection? _____ Swimmer's ear? _____ Pain? _____
   Drainage? _____ Loss of hearing? _____

**NOSE**
1. Have you ever had a problem with your nose? _____
   Broken? _____ Sneezing? _____ Nosebleeds? _____

**THROAT**
1. How often do you have colds or sore throats? _____

**SKIN**
1. Do you ever have a skin rash? _____
   If yes, explain. _____

**CHEST**
1. Do you ever have chest pain? _____
   If yes, explain. _____
2. Do you have chronic cough? _____ Asthma? _____
   Hay fever? _____ Have you ever coughed up blood? _____

**HEART**
1. Have you ever been told you had a heart murmur? _____
   If yes, explain. _____
2. Have you ever been told you had elevated blood pressure?
   If yes, explain. _____
3. Is heart disease present in your family? _____
   If yes, explain. _____
4. Have you ever been told that a member of your family died suddenly or had a heart attack at a young age? _____

**GI**
1. Do you have trouble with heartburn? _____ Indigestion _____
   Nausea? _____ Vomiting? _____ Constipation? _____
   Diarrhea? _____ Have you ever vomited blood? _____
   If yes, explain. _____
2. Have you ever passed blood in your stools? _____
   If yes, explain. _____

**GU**
1. Have you ever noted burning on urination? _____
   Urgency? _____ Frequency? _____ Wake up at night to
   pass urine? _____ Penile discharge? _____ Passed blood
   on urination? _____ Kidney stone? _____

**SKELETAL**
1. Have you ever had arthritis? _____
   Sprained ankle? _____ If yes, explain. _____
   Knee injury? _____ If yes, explain. _____
   Shoulder injury? _____ If yes, explain. _____
   Broken bone? _____ If yes, explain. _____
   Neck injury? _____ If yes, explain. _____
   Back trouble? _____ If yes, explain. _____
   Have you ever had surgery? _____ If yes, explain. _____
   Have you ever had a dislocation? If yes, explain. _____
2. Does any joint feel as if it is slipping? _____
3. Do you have a pin, plate, screw, or anything metal in your
   body? _____ If yes, explain. _____

**GENERAL**
1. Do you have any drug allergies? _____
2. Are you allergic to insect bites? _____
3. Are you allergic to anything? _____
4. Have you ever had hepatitis? _____ Mononucleosis? _____
   Diabetes? _____ Does any family member have diabetes? _____
5. Have you ever had any serious disease? _____ If yes, explain. _____
6. Have you ever had heat exhaustion or heat stroke? _____
   If yes, explain. _____
7. Has any member of your family ever had head exhaustion or heat
   stroke? _____
8. Has any member of your family been told they were allergic to
   medication used as anesthesia? _____
9. Have you ever been allergic to local anesthetics used by doctors
   or dentists? _____
10. Has your weight changed in the last three months? _____
    If yes, explain. _____

**Figure 2-3**

Sample medical history examination form

ments. Of the three, Tanner's five stages of assessment, indicating maturity of secondary sexual characteristics, is the most expedient for use in the station method of examination. The Tanner approach evaluates pubic hair and genitalia development in boys and pubic hair and breast development in girls. Other indicators that may be noted are facial and axillary hair. Stage one indicates that puberty is not evident, whereas stage five indicates full development. The crucial stage in terms of collision and high-intensity noncontact sports is stage three, in which there is the fastest bone growth. In this stage the growth plates are two to five times weaker than the joint capsule and tendon attachments.[14] Young athletes in grades seven to twelve must be matched by maturity, not age.

### Orthopedic Screening

Orthopedic screening may be done as part of the physical examination or separately by the athletic trainer. An example of a very quick

Name _____ SS# _____ Date _____
Height _____ Weight _____ Percent body fat _____

Check if negative

1. Blood pressure _____ / _____
2. Pulse _____
3. Vision
   Without glasses R 20/_____ L 20/_____
   With glasses R 20/_____ L 20/_____
4. Skin _____
5. Dental/mouth _____
6. Ears _____
7. Nose _____
8. Throat _____
9. Chest
   Heart rhythm _____
   Lungs _____
   Breasts _____
10. Abdomen
    Liver _____
    Spleen _____
    Kidneys _____
    Stomach _____
    Bowel _____
11. Lymphatics
    Cervical _____
    Axillary _____
    Femoral _____
12. Genitalia _____
13. Maturation Index _____
14. Urinalysis
    Protein _____
    Sugar _____
15. Blood
    Hematocrit _____
16. Other _____
Disposition
    No participation
    Limited participation
    Clearance withheld
    Cleared for participation
Comments _____
_____
_____

_____
Physician's signature
_____
Date

**Figure 2-4**

Sample physical examination
form

orthopedic screening examination appears in Table 2-1; it usually takes about 90 seconds. A more detailed orthopedic examination may be conducted to assess strength, range of motion, and stability at various joints.

### Sport Disqualification

As discussed previously, sports participation involves risks. Most conditions that warrant a recommendation for disqualification can be identified during a preparticipation health evaluation and should be noted in the medical history.[13] Because of the Americans with Disabilities Act, a physician cannot legally disqualify athletes from competing because of an

**TABLE 2-1** Orthopedic Screening Examination

| Activity and Instruction | To Determine |
| --- | --- |
| Stand facing examiner | Acromioclavicular joints; general habitus |
| Look at ceiling, floor, over both shoulders; touch ears to shoulders | Cervical spine motion |
| Shrug shoulders (examiner resists) | Trapezius strength |
| Abduct shoulders 90 degrees (examiner resists at 90 degrees) | Deltoid strength |
| Full external rotation of arms | Shoulder motion |
| Flex and extend elbows | Elbow motion |
| Arms at sides, elbows 90 degrees flexed; pronate and supinate wrists | Elbow and wrist motion |
| Spread fingers; make fist | Hand or finger motion and deformities |
| Tighten (contract) quadriceps; relax quadriceps | Symmetry and knee effusion; ankle effusion |
| Duckwalk four steps (away from examiner with buttocks on heels) | Hip, knee, and ankle motion |
| Stand with back to examiner | Shoulder symmetry; scoliosis |
| Knees straight, touch toes | Scoliosis, hip motion, hamstring tightness |
| Raise up on toes, raise heels | Calf symmetry, leg strength |

existing medical problem. They can only recommend that the athlete voluntarily choose not to participate. In general, the athlete who has lost one of two paired organs such as eyes or kidneys is cautioned against playing a collision or contact sport.[13] Such an athlete should be counseled into participating in a noncontact sport. The athlete with one testicle, or one or both that are undescended, must be apprised that there is a small risk, which is substantially minimized with the use of an athletic supporter and a protective device.

## Injury Reports

An injury report serves as a record for future reference (Figure 2-5). If the emergency procedures followed are questioned at a later date, a person's memory of the details may be somewhat hazy, but a report completed on the spot provides specific information. In a litigation situation, an athletic trainer may be asked questions about an injury that occurred 3 years in the past. All injury reports should be filed in the athletic trainer's office. The reports should be made out in triplicate, with one copy sent to the school health office, one to the physician, and one retained.

## Treatment Log

Each athletic facility should have a sign-in log available for the athlete who receives any service. Emphasis is placed on recording treatments for

**Figure 2-5**

Athletic injury record form

Name _____ Sport _____ Date: ___ / ___ / ___ Time: _____ Injury number: _____

Player I.D. _____ Age: _____ Location: _____ Intercollegiate-nonintercollegiate

Initial injury        Recheck        Reinjury                              Preseason—Practice—Game                          Incurred while participating in sport: yes ___ no ___

Description: How did it happen? _____
_____

Initial impression: _____
_____
_____
_____

| Site of injury | Body part | | Structure | Treatment |
|---|---|---|---|---|
| 1 Right | 1 Head | 25 MP joint | 1 Skin | |
| 2 Left | 2 Face | 26 PIP joint | 2 Muscle | |
| 3 Proximal | 3 Eye | 27 Abdomen | 3 Fascia | |
| 4 Distal | 4 Nose | 28 Hip | 4 Bone | |
| 5 Anterior | 5 Ear | 29 Thigh | 5 Nerve | |
| 6 Posterior | 6 Mouth | 30 Knee | 6 Fat pad | |
| 7 Medial | 7 Neck | 31 Patella | 7 Tendon | |
| 8 Lateral | 8 Thorax | 32 Lower leg | 8 Ligament | |
| 9 Other | 9 Ribs | 33 Ankle | 9 Cartilage | |
| | 10 Sternum | 34 Achilles tendon | 10 Capsule | |
| | 11 Upper back | 35 Foot | 11 Compartment | |
| Site of evaluation | 12 Lower back | 36 Toes | 12 Dental | |
| 1 SHS | 13 Shoulder | 37 Other | 13 _____ | |
| 2 Athletic Trn Rm. | 14 Rotator cuff | | | |
| 3 Site-Competition | 15 AC joint | | | Medication |
| 4 _____ | 16 Glenohumeral | | | |
| | 17 Sternoclavicular | Nontraumatic | Nature of injury | |
| Procedures | 18 Upper arm | 1 Dermatological | 1 Contusion | |
| 1 Physical exam | 19 Elbow | 2 Allergy | 2 Strain | |
| 2 X-ray | 20 Forearm | 3 Influenza | 3 Sprain | |
| 3 Splint | 21 Wrist | 4 URI | 4 Fracture | |
| 4 Wrap | 22 Hand | 5 GU | 5 Rupture | |
| 5 Cast | 23 Thumb | 6 Systemic infect. | 6 Tendonitis | |
| 6 Aspiration | 24 Finger | 7 Local infect. | 7 Bursitis | |
| 7 Other | | 8 Other | 8 Myositis | Prescription dispensed |
| | | | 9 Laceration | 1 Antibiotics    5 Muscle relaxant |
| | | | 10 Concussion | 2 Antiinflammatory  6 Enzyme |
| | | | 11 Avulsion | 3 Decongestant   7 _____ |
| | | | 12 Abrasion | 4 Analgesic |
| Disposition | Referral | Disposition of injury | 13 _____ | Injections |
| 1 SHS | 1 Arthrogram | 1 No part. | | |
| 2 Trainer | 2 Neurological | 2 Part part. | | 1 Steroids |
| 3 Hospital | 3 Int. Med. | 3 Full part. | Degree | 2 Antibiotics |
| 4 H.D. | 4 Orthopedic | | 1°   2°   3° | 3 Steroids-xylo |
| 5 Other | 5 EENT | | | 4 _____ |
| | 6 Dentist | | | |
| | 7 Other | | | |

Previous injury _____
_____

the athlete who is receiving daily therapy for an injury. As with injury records, treatment logs often have the status of legal documents and are used to establish certain facts in a civil litigation, an insurance action, or a criminal action following injury.

## Personal Information Card

The coach or athletic trainer should maintain on file an athlete's personal information card. This card is completed by the athlete at the time of the health examination and serves as a means of contacting the family, personal physician, and insurance company in case of emergency.

## Injury Evaluation and Progress Notes

Injuries should be evaluated by the coach, who must record this information in some consistent format. The SOAP format is a concise method of recording the evaluation and the treatment plan for the injured athlete (see Chapter 7). The *subjective* portion of the SOAP note refers to what the athlete tells the athletic trainer about the injury relative to the history or what he or she felt. The *objective* portion documents information that the athletic trainer gathers during the evaluation, such as range of motion, strength levels, patterns of pain, and so forth. The *assessment* records the athletic trainer's professional opinion about the injury based on information obtained during the subjective and objective portions. The *plan* for treatment indicates how the injury will be managed and includes short- and long-term goals for rehabilitation.

SOAP format:
• Subjective
• Objective
• Assessment
• Plan

## Supply and Equipment Inventory

A major responsibility of the coach is to manage a budget, most of which is spent on equipment and supplies. Every year an inventory must be conducted and recorded on such items as new equipment that is needed, equipment that needs to be replaced or repaired, and expendable supplies that need replenishing.

## Annual Reports

Most athletic departments require an annual report on the functions of the athletic training program. This report serves as a means for making program changes and improvements. It commonly includes the number of athletes served, a survey of the number and types of injuries, an analysis of the program, and recommendations for future improvements.

## Release of Medical Records

The coach may not release an athlete's medical records to anyone without written consent. If the athlete wishes to have medical records released to colleges or universities, professional sports organizations, insurance companies, the news media, or any other group or individual, he, she, the parent, or the guardian must sign a waiver that specifies which information is to be released.

2–3

***Critical Thinking*** Exercise

One of the responsibilities of overseeing an athletic health care program is maintaining accurate records for every athlete.

**?** What kinds of records or types of information should be included in these records?

A major problem often facing
athletic trainers is obtaining a
budget of sufficient size.

# DEVELOPING A BUDGET

One of the major problems faced by coaches is to obtain a budget of sufficient size to permit them to perform a creditable job of providing health care to the athlete. Many high schools fail to make any budgetary provisions for athletic training except for the purchase of tape, ankle wraps, and a training bag that contains a minimum amount of equipment.[9] Many schools fail to provide a room and any of the special facilities that are needed to establish an effective athletic training program. Some school boards and administrators fail to recognize that the functions performed in the athletic training facility are an essential component of the athletic program and that even if no specialist is used, the facilities are nonetheless necessary.[8] Colleges and universities do not usually face this problem to the extent that high schools do. By and large, athletic training is recognized as an important aspect of the college athletic program.

Budgetary needs vary considerably within programs; some require only a few thousand dollars, whereas others spend hundreds of thousands of dollars. The amount spent on building and equipping a training facility, of course, is entirely a matter of local option. In purchasing equipment, immediate needs as well as availability of personnel to operate specialized equipment should be kept in mind.[11]

Budget records should be kept on file so that they are available for use in projecting the following year's budgetary needs. They present a picture of the distribution of current funds and serve to substantiate future budgetary requests. Expenditures for individual items vary in accordance with different training philosophies. Some coaches may spend much of their budget on expendable supplies such as adhesive tape. An annual inventory must be conducted at the end of the year or before replenishing supplies and equipment. Accurate records must be kept to justify future requests.[10]

## Ordering Supplies and Equipment

Equipment may be fixed or
nonfixed.

Purchasing may be done
through direct buy or
competitive bid.

Supplies are expendable and usually are for injury prevention, first aid, and management. Examples of supplies are athletic training tape, germicides, and massage lotion. The term *equipment* refers to those items that are not expendable. Equipment may be further divided into fixed and nonfixed. Fixed equipment does not necessarily mean that it cannot be moved but that it is not usually removed from the athletic training facility. Examples of fixed equipment are icemakers, weight equipment, and electrical therapeutic modalities. Nonfixed equipment refers to nonexpendable items that are less fixed, that may be part of an athletic trainer's kit, or that may be at the sport site. Examples are blankets, scissors, and training kits. Focus Boxes 2-5 and 2-6 provide a list of supplies for the athletic training room and for a field kit.

## Additional Budget Considerations

In addition to supplies and equipment, the coach must also consider other costs that may be included in the operation of an athletic training program; these costs include telephone and postage, contracts with

**Recommended Basic Athletic Training Room Supplies**

**Tape**
White adhesive, $1^1/_2$ inch
White adhesive, 1 inch
Liteguard, 2 inch
Elastic, 2 inch
Elastic, 1 inch
Prewrap

**Bandages**
Coverlet, $1^1/_2$ by 2
Coverlet strips
Telfa, 2 by 3
Band-Aid Clear Patches
Gauze, 4 by 4 (sterile)
Ace Wraps, 3, 4, 6 inch
Steri Strips, $1/_4$ inch

**Foam and Felt**
1-inch felt
$1/_8$-inch adhesive foam
Moleskin

**Braces and Splints**
Finger splints
Air splint, leg
Velcro, 1 inch (both sides)
Knee immobilizer
Aircast, left
Aircast, right
Hexalite, 4 inch
Cervical collar (small, medium, large)
Heel cups (medium, large)
Patella strap, large
Wrist immobilizer (left, right, universal)
Ankle braces (xx-small, x-small, small, medium, large, x-large)

Triangular bandage
Slings
Nose guard
Elbow sleeves
Thigh sleeves
Back support (x-small, small, medium, large, x-large)
Knee sleeves
Stockinet, 3 inch

**Modalities**
Flex All, 1 gallon
Cramergesic, 5 lb tub
Skin lube, 5 lb tub
Gray T-band
Black T-band
Heat packs (medium, large)
Ice bags
Flexi-wrap (small, large)
Lotion, 1 gallon

**First Aid**
Cotton rolls (nose plugs)
Tongue depressors
Cotton tip applicators
Latex gloves (medium, large)
Cotton balls
Skin-preps
Save-A-Tooth
Penlights
Biohazard bags
Safety goggles

**Taping Accessories**
Heel and lace pads
Tape adherent spray
Tape remover

**Sharps**
Scissors
Tweezers
Nail clippers (large, small)
Tape cutters
Shark refill blades

**Antiseptics**
Peroxide
Rubbing alcohol

**Skin Treatments**
Polysporin
Second Skin
Baby powder

**Eye Treatment**
Eye wash
Penlights

**Crutches**
Large
Medium
Small
Large aluminum

**Water**
Bottle carriers
Water bottles
Coolers (3, 7, 10 gallon)
Chest

**Other**
Stools
Spray bottles
Bucket
Cloth towels

**2-6**    *Focus Box*

### Recommended Basic Field Kit Supplies

| | |
|---|---|
| Adhesive bandages | Flex All |
| Tape cutters | Lotion |
| Scissors | Sunscreen |
| Eye cover | Tape supplies: |
| Save-A-Tooth |   white adhesive, stretch, heel and |
| Petroleum jelly |   lace pads |
| Razor blades |   prewrap, 3 inch, 2 inch, 1 inch |
| Dacriose sterile eye irrigating |   brown |
| solution |   1 inch white, blood tape |
| Latex gloves | Elastic wraps: |
| QDA spray |   2 inch, 3 inch, 4 inch, 6 inch |
| Skin lube |   double 4 inch, double 6 inch |
| Gauze pads: 2 by 2, 3 by 3, or | Alcohol |
| 4 by 4 | Cramergesic |
| Heel cup | Flex-wrap |
| Sling | Adhesive foam |
| Hydrogen peroxide | Adhesive felt |
| Finger splints | Penlight |
| Cotton-tipped applicators | Contact lens cases |
| Tongue depressors | Contact lens wetting solution |

physicians or clinics for services, professional liability insurance, memberships in professional organizations, the purchase of professional journals or textbooks, travel and expenses for attending professional meetings, and clothing to be worn in the training room.

## COACH'S CORNER

The following is a checklist of things the coach should do in organizing and administering an athletic health care program.

☐ Find a space of reasonable proportions that can be used for an athletic training room

☐ Establish rules and policies for the athletic training room

☐ Arrange for the facilities to be cleaned and maintained in cooperation with the maintenance staff

☐ Establish health habits for the athletes

☐ Arrange for the availability or purchase of emergency phones

☐ Arrange for preparticipation exams for all athletes

☐ Maintain appropriate and necessary injury records (injury reports, medical history, etc.)

☐ Develop a budget for purchasing supplies and equipment

☐ Put together a field kit with the appropriate supplies

## SUMMARY

- Organization of the athletic program demands a significant portion of the coach's time and effort.

- The athletic training program can be enhanced by designing or renovating a facility to maximize the potential use of the space available.

- The athletic training program best serves the athlete by establishing specific policies and regulations governing the use of available services.

- Preparticipation exams must be given to athletes and should include a medical history, a general physical examination, and an orthopedic screening.

- The coach must maintain accurate and up-to-date medical records in addition to the other paperwork necessary for the operation of the athletic training program.

- Budgets should allow for the purchase of equipment and supplies essential for providing appropriate preventive and rehabilitative care for the athlete.

*Solutions to Critical Thinking* Exercises

**2-1** The training room should have specific areas designated for taping and preparation, treatment and rehabilitation, and hydrotherapy, and should have adequate storage facilities that are positioned within the space to allow for an efficient traffic flow. Equipment purchases might include four to five treatment tables and two to three taping tables (these could be made in-house if possible), a large-capacity ice machine, a combination ultrasound/electrical simulating unit, a whirlpool, and various free weights and exercise tubing.

**2-2** The preparticipation examination should consist of a medical history, a physical examination, and a brief orthopedic screening. The preparticipation physical may be effectively administered using a station examination system with a team of examiners. A station examination can provide the athlete with a detailed examination in a short time. A team of people is needed to examine this many athletes. The team should include physicians, medically trained nonphysicians (nurses, athletic trainers, physical therapists, or physician's assistants), and managers, student coaches, or assistant coaches.

**2-3** The coach should keep a record of the medical history, injury reports, a personal individual information card, treatment logs, injury evaluations and progress notes, and a form for release of medical records.

# REVIEW QUESTIONS AND CLASS ACTIVITIES

1. What major administrative functions must a coach in an athletic training setting perform?
2. Design two athletic training facilities—one for a medium-sized university and one for a large university.
3. Observe the activities in the athletic training facility. Pick both a slow time and a busy time to observe.
4. Why do hygiene and sanitation play an important role in athletic training? How should the athletic training facility be maintained?
5. Fully equip a new medium-sized high school or college athletic training facility or a clinical facility. Pick equipment from current catalogs.
6. Establish a reasonable health care budget for a small high school, a large high school, and a large college or university.
7. Identify the groups of individuals to be served in the athletic training facility.
8. Organize a preparticipation health examination for ninety football players.
9. Record keeping is a major function in athletic training. What records are necessary to keep?
10. Debate what conditions constitute good grounds for medical disqualification from a sport.

## REFERENCES

1. American Academy of Pediatrics: *Sports medicine: health care for young athletes,* Elk Grove Village, Ill, 1991, American Academy of Pediatrics.
2. Ashley FB, Courtney S, Hicks VL: Fitness and health-related areas. In Walker ML, Stotlar DK, editors: *Sports facility management,* Sudbury, Mass, 1997, Jones & Bartlett.
3. Herbert D: Professional considerations related to conduct of preparticipation exams, *Sports Med Stand Malpract Report* 6(4):49, 1994.
4. Johnson MD, Kibler B, Smith D: Keys to successful preparticipation exams, *Physician Sportsmed* 21(9):108, 1993.
5. Knells S: Leadership and management techniques and principles for athletic training, *Ath Train* 29(4):328, 1994.
6. Konin J, Donley P: The athletic trainer as a personnel manager. In Konin J: *The clinical athletic trainer,* Gaithersburg, MD, 1997, Slack.
7. Moyer-Knowles J: Planning a new athletic facility. In Konin J: *The clinical athletic trainer,* Gaithersburg, MD, 1997, Slack.
8. Peterson E: Insult to injury: feeling understaffed, underequipped and undervalued, athletic trainers say a minimum of space and equipment will yield extensive benefits, *Ath Bus* 23(1):57, 1999.
9. Rankin J: Financial resources for conducting athletic training programs in the collegiate and high school settings, *J Ath Train* 27(4):344, 1992.
10. Rankin J, Ingersoll C: *Athletic training management: concepts and applications,* St Louis, 2000, McGraw-Hill.
11. Ray R: *Management strategies in athletic training,* Champaign, Ill, 2000, Human Kinetics.
12. Sabo J: Athletic training room design and layout, Proceedings of National Athletic Trainers' Association fiftieth annual meeting and clinical symposia, June 16–19, 1999, Kansas City, MO, 1999, Human Kinetics.
13. Swander H: *Preparticipation physical examination,* Kansas City, 1992, American Academy of Family Physicians, American Academy of Pediatrics, American Orthopedic

Society for Sports Medicine, American Osteopathic Academy for Sports Medicine.

14. Tanner M: *Growth of adolescence,* ed 2, Oxford, England, 1962, Blackwell Scientific.

**ANNOTATED BIBLIOGRAPHY**

Rankin J, Ingersoll C: *Athletic training management: concepts and applications,* ed 2, St Louis, 2000, McGraw-Hill.

*This text is designed for upper-division undergraduate or graduate students interested in all aspects of organization and administration of an athletic training program. The second edition has been expanded to include coverage of sports medicine clinics, industrial athletic training, the process of seeking employment, third-party reimbursement, financial management, risk management, and information technology, including distance learning and the Web.*

Ray R: *Management strategies in athletic training,* ed 2, Champaign, Ill, 2000, Human Kinetics.

*This was the first text available to cover the principles of organization and administration as they apply to many different employment settings in athletic training. The second edition contains many examples and case studies based on principles of administration presented in the text.*

# Legal Liability and Insurance

*When you finish this chapter you will be able to:*

- Explain legal considerations for the coach acting as a health care provider.
- Define the legal concepts of liability, negligence, torts, assumption of risk.
- Identify measures that can be taken by both the coach and athletic trainer to minimize chances of litigation.
- Describe product liability.
- Identify the essential insurance requirements for protection of the athlete.
- Describe the types of insurance necessary to protect the coach acting as a health care provider.

## LEGAL CONCERNS OF THE COACH AND ATHLETIC TRAINER

In recent years negligence suits against teachers, coaches, athletic trainers, school officials, and physicians arising out of sports injuries have increased both in frequency and in the amount of damages awarded.[3] An increasing awareness of the many risk factors present in physical activities has had a major effect on the athletic trainer in particular. **Liability** means being legally responsible for the harm one causes another person.[4] A great deal of care must be taken in following athletic training procedures to reduce the risk of being sued by an athlete and being found liable for negligence.

### The Standard of Reasonable Care

**Negligence** is the failure to use ordinary or reasonable care—care that persons would normally exercise to avoid injury to themselves or to others under similar circumstances. The **standard of reasonable care** assumes that an individual is neither exceptionally skillful nor extraordinarily cautious, but is a person of reasonable and ordinary prudence. Put another way, it is expected that an individual will bring a commonsense approach to the situation at hand and will exercise due care in its handling. In most cases in which someone has been sued for negligence, the actions of a hypothetical, reasonably prudent person are compared with

**liability**
The state of being legally responsible for the harm one causes another person.

**negligence**
The failure to use ordinary or reasonable care.

**standard of reasonable care**
Assumes that an individual is a person of reasonable and ordinary prudence.

**Figure 3-1**

The coach can minimize the
chances of litigation by
providing reasonable and
prudent care to an injured
athlete.

the actions of the defendant to ascertain whether the course of action followed by the defendant was in conformity with the judgment exercised
by such a reasonably prudent person.

The standard of reasonable care requires that a coach or athletic
trainer act according to the standard of care of an individual with similar
educational background or training.[10] A coach or athletic trainer who has
many years of experience, who is well educated in his or her field, and
who is certified or licensed must act in accordance with those qualifica-
tions (Figure 3-1).

## Torts

(liability results)

**Torts** are legal wrongs committed against the person or property of another.[4] Such wrongs may emanate from an **act of omission,** wherein
the individual fails to perform a legal duty, or from an **act of commission,** wherein he or she commits an act that is not legally his or hers to
perform. In either instance, if injury results, the person can be held liable.
In the case of omission a coach or an athletic trainer may fail to refer a
seriously injured athlete for the proper medical attention. In the case of
commission, the coach may perform a medical treatment not within his
or her experience, training, or education from which serious medical
complications develop.

## Negligence

When a coach or an athletic trainer is sued by an athlete, the complaint
typically is for the tort of negligence. Negligence is alleged when an individual (1) does something that a reasonably prudent person would not
do or (2) fails to do something that a reasonably prudent person would
do under circumstances similar to those shown by the evidence.[4] To be
successful in a suit for negligence, an athlete must prove that the athletic
trainer had a duty to exercise reasonable care, breached that duty by

---

**torts**
Legal wrongs committed
against a person.

---

**act of omission**
When an individual fails to
perform a legal duty.

(fail to refer)

---

**act of commission**
When an individual commits
an act that is not legally his
to perform.

(advanced treatment
leading to complications)

A.T. has a duty to provide
coverage to athletes (obligation)

A baseball batter was struck with a pitched ball directly in the orbit of the right eye and fell immediately to the ground. The coach ran to the player to examine the eye. There was some immediate swelling and discoloration around the orbit; however, the eye appeared to be normal. The player insisted that he was fine and told the coach that he could continue to bat. After the game, the coach told the athlete to go back to his room, put ice on his eye, and check in tomorrow. That night the baseball player began to hemorrhage into the anterior chamber of the eye and suffered irreparable damage to his eye.

**?** An ophthalmologist stated that if the athlete's eye had been examined immediately after injury, the bleeding could have been controlled and the athlete would not have suffered any damage to his vision. If the athlete brings a lawsuit against the coach, what must he prove to win a judgment?

**statute of limitation**
A specific length of time to sue for damages from negligence.

failing to use reasonable care, and that there is a reasonable connection between the failure to use reasonable care and the injury suffered by the athlete or that the athletic trainer's action made the injury worse. If the coach breaches a duty to exercise reasonable care, but there is no reasonable connection between the failure to use reasonable care and the injury suffered by the athlete, the athlete's suit for negligence will not succeed.

An example of negligence that occurs all too often in sports is when a coach or an athletic trainer moves a possibly seriously injured athlete from the field of play to permit competition or practice to continue and does so either in an improper manner or before consulting those qualified to know the proper course of action. Should a serious or disabling injury result, the coach or the athletic trainer may be found liable.

It is expected that a person possessing more training in a given field or area will possess a correspondingly higher level of competence than, for example, a student. An individual will therefore be judged in terms of his or her performance in any situation in which legal liability may be assessed. It must be recognized that liability per se in all of its various aspects is not assessed at the same level nationally but varies in interpretation from state to state and from area to area. It is therefore good to know and to acquire the level of competence expected in a particular area. In essence, negligence is conduct that results in the creation of an "unreasonable risk of harm to others."[7]

## Statute of Limitations

A **statute of limitation** sets a specific length of time that individuals may sue for damages from negligence. The length of time to bring suit varies from state to state, but in general, plaintiffs have between 1 and 3 years to file suit for negligence. The statute of limitations begins to run on a plaintiff's time to file a lawsuit for negligence either from the time of the negligent act or omission that gives rise to the suit, or the discovery of an injury caused by the negligent act or omission. Some states permit an injured minor to file suit up to 3 years after the minor reaches the age of eighteen. Therefore, an injured minor athlete's cause of action for negligence remains valid for many years after the negligent act or omission occurred or the discovery of an injury caused by the negligent act or omission.

*minors have generally have an extension*

## Assumption of Risk

An athlete assumes the risk of participating in an activity when he or she knows of and understands the dangers of that activity, and voluntarily chooses to be exposed to those dangers.[1] An **assumption of risk** can be expressed in the form of a waiver signed by an athlete or his or her parents or guardian, or implied from the conduct of an athlete under the circumstances of his or her participation in an activity.[6]

Assumption of risk may be asserted as a defense to a negligence suit brought by an injured athlete. The coach or athletic trainer bears the burden of proving that an athlete assumed the risk by producing the document signed by the athlete or his or her parents or guardian, or proving that the athlete knew the risk of the activity, understood, and voluntarily accepted those risks.

Assumption of risk, however, is subject to many and varied interpretations by courts, especially when a minor is involved, because he or she is not considered able to render a mature judgment about the risks inherent in the situation. Although athletes participating in a sports program are considered to assume a normal risk, this in no way excuses those in charge from exercising reasonable care and prudence in the conduct of such activities or from foreseeing and taking precautionary measures against accident-provoking circumstances. In general, courts have been fairly consistent in upholding waivers and releases of liability for adults unless there is evidence of fraud, misrepresentation, or duress.[4]

## COACH'S CORNER

Coaches can significantly decrease risk of litigation by paying attention to several key points.[7] The following is a checklist of things the coach can do to decrease the risk of litigation.

☐ Warn the athlete of the potential dangers inherent in the sport.

☐ Supervise constantly and attentively.

☐ Properly prepare and condition the athlete.

☐ Properly instruct the athlete in the skills of the sport.

☐ Ensure that proper and safe equipment and facilities are used by the athlete at all times.

☐ Work to establish good personal relationships with the athletes, parents, and coworkers.

☐ Establish specific policies and guidelines for the operation of an athletic training facility and maintain qualified and adequate supervision of the training room, its environs, facilities, and equipment at all times.[4]

☐ Develop and carefully follow an emergency plan.

☐ Make it a point to become familiar with the health status and medical history of the athletes under his or her care so as to be aware of any problems that could present a need for additional care or caution and keep a file that contains medical history, preparticipation exams, and any injury records.

☐ Keep good records that document all injuries and rehabilitation steps.

☐ Document efforts to create a safe playing environment.

☐ Have a detailed job description in writing.

☐ Obtain written consent for providing health care, particularly when minors are involved.

☐ Maintain confidentiality of medical records.

☐ Don't dispense prescription drugs, and if allowed by law, exercise extreme caution in the administration of nonprescription medications.

3–2

*Critical Thinking* Exercise

A coach is cleaning out a filing cabinet with records from past teams and decides to throw some older medical files away. Concern is expressed about how long these files should be maintained for legal purposes.

**?** What is the statute of limitations for a minor to file suit?

**assumption of risk**
The individual, through expressed or implied agreement, assumes that some risk or danger will be involved in the particular undertaking. In other words, a person takes his or her own chances.

□ Use only those therapeutic methods that he or she is qualified to use and that the law states may be used.

□ Don't use or permit the presence of faulty or hazardous equipment.

□ Work cooperatively with the team physician in the selection and use of sports protective equipment, and insist that the best equipment be obtained, properly fitted, and properly maintained.

□ Don't permit injured players to participate unless cleared by the team physician. Players suffering a head injury should not be permitted to reenter the game. In some states a player who has suffered a concussion may not continue in the sport for the balance of the season.

□ Develop an understanding that an injured athlete will not be allowed to reenter competition until, in the opinion of the team physician or the athletic trainer, he or she is psychologically and physically able. Coaches should not allow themselves to be pressured to clear an athlete until he or she is fully cleared by the physician.

□ Follow the express orders of the team physician at all times.

□ Purchase liability insurance to protect against litigation and be aware of the limitations of the policy.

□ Know the limitations of his or her expertise and the applicable state regulations and restrictions limiting his or her scope of practice.

□ Use common sense in making decisions about the athlete's health and safety.

> **managed care**
> Costs of health care are
> monitored closely by insur-
> ance carriers.

*In the case of an injury, a coach must use reasonable care to prevent further injury until medical care is obtained.*

### Product Liability

Manufacturers of athletic equipment have a duty to design and produce equipment that will not cause injury as long as it is used as intended. An express warranty is the manufacturer's written guarantee that a product is safe. Warning labels placed on football helmets inform the player of possible dangers inherent in using the product. Athletes must read and sign a form indicating that they have read and understand the warning. The National Operating Committee on Standards for Athletic Equipment (NOCSAE) establishes minimum standards for equipment that must be met to ensure its safety.

### WHAT TYPES OF INSURANCE ARE NECESSARY TO PROTECT THE ATHLETE?

Because of the high cost of medical care, every athlete should be covered by appropriate insurance policies that maximize the benefits should injury occur. During the past 40 years the insurance industry has undergone a significant evolutionary process. Health care reform initiated in the 1990s has focused on the concept of **managed care** in which costs of a health care provider's medical care are closely monitored and scruti-

---

3–3

**Critical Thinking** Exercise

During a high school gymnastics meet, a gymnast fell off the uneven parallel bars, landing on her forearm. The coach suspected a fracture and decided an x ray was needed. The gymnast's parents have general health insurance through a PPO but because the gymnast was in severe pain she was sent to the nearest emergency room to be treated. Unfortunately the emergency facility was not on the list of preferred providers so the insurance company denied the claim. The coach assured the parents that the school would take care of whatever medical costs were not covered by their insurance policy.

? Because the PPO denied the claim, what type of insurance policy should the school carry to cover the medical costs?

nized by insurance carriers. Often preapproval is required before health care delivery. Since 1971 there has been a significant increase in the number of lawsuits filed, caused in part by the steady increase in individuals who have become active in sports. The costs of insurance have also significantly increased during this period. More lawsuits and much higher medical costs are creating a crisis in the insurance industry.[5] Medical insurance is a contract between an insurance company and a policyholder in which the insurance company agrees to reimburse a portion of the total medical bill after some deductible has been paid by the policyholder. The major types of insurance that coaches should be familiar with are general health insurance, catastrophic insurance, accident insurance, and liability insurance, as well as insurance for errors and omissions. All sports health and safety personnel need to be adequately insured.

## General Health Insurance

Every athlete should have a general health insurance policy that covers illness, hospitalization, and emergency care. Some institutions offer primary insurance coverage in which all medical expenses are paid for by the athletic department. The institutions pay an extremely high premium for this type of coverage. Most institutions offer secondary insurance coverage that pays the athlete's remaining medical bills once the athlete's personal insurance company has made its payment. Secondary insurance always includes a deductible that will not be covered by the plan.

Many athletes are covered under some type of family health insurance policy. However, the school must make certain that personal health insurance is arranged for or purchased by athletes not covered under family policies.[8] A form letter directed to the parents of all athletes should be completed and returned to the institution to make certain that appropriate coverage is provided (Figure 3-2). Some so-called comprehensive

Every athlete should have a general health insurance policy that covers illness, hospitalization, and emergency care.

**Figure 3-2**

Sample insurance information form

---

Insurance Information on Student Athletes

Student's Name _____ Date of Birth _____

Address _____

Social Security Number _____ Sex: M _____ F _____

Names of Insurance Companies _____

Address of Insurance Company _____

Certificate Number _____ Group _____ Type _____

Policy Holder _____ Relationship to Student _____

Employer or Policyholder _____

Should my son/daughter require services beyond those covered by the Sports Medicine Program, I give permission to the Division of Sports Medicine to file a claim for such services with the above health care insurer.

According to NCAA regulations, I understand that any insurance payments I receive must be returned to be placed on my child's account.

Date _____     _____
                                  Parent's Signature

plans do not cover every health need. For example, such plans may cover physicians' care but not hospital charges. Many of these plans require large prepayments before the insurance takes effect. Supplemental policies such as accident insurance and catastrophic insurance are designed to take over where general health insurance stops.

### Third-Party Reimbursement

Third-party reimbursement is the primary mechanism of payment for medical services in the United States.[9] Health care professionals are reimbursed by the policyholder's insurance company for services performed. Medical insurance companies may provide group and individual coverage for employees and dependents. To cut payout costs, many insurance companies have begun to pay for preventive care (to reduce the need for hospitalization) and to limit where the individual can go for care. Managed care involves a prearranged system for delivering health care that is designed to control costs while continuing to provide quality care. A number of different health care systems have been developed to contain costs.[2]

**Health maintenance organizations**   Health maintenance organizations (HMOs) provide preventive measures and limit where the individual can receive care. With the exception of an emergency, permission must be obtained before the individual can go to another provider. HMOs generally pay 100 percent of medical costs as long as care is rendered at an HMO facility. Many supplemental policies will not cover medical costs that would normally be paid by the general policy. Therefore an athlete treated outside the HMO may be ineligible for any insurance benefits. Many HMOs determine fees using a capitation system that limits the amount that is reimbursed for a specific service. Athletic trainers must understand the limits of and restrictions on coverage at their individual institutions.

**Preferred provider organizations**   Preferred provider organizations (PPOs) provide discount health care but also limit where a person can go for treatment of an illness. The coach and/or athletic trainer must be apprised in advance where the ill athlete should be sent. Athletes sent to a facility not on the approved list may be required to pay for care, but if they are sent to a preferred facility, all costs are paid.[2] Added services such as physical therapy may be more easily obtained and at no cost or at a much lower cost than with other insurance policies. PPOs pay on a fee-for-service basis.

**Point of service plan**   The point of service plan is a combination of HMO and PPO plans. It is based on an HMO structure, yet it allows members to go outside the HMO to obtain services. This flexibility is allowed only with certain conditions and under special circumstances.

**Indemnity plan**   The indemnity plan is the most traditional form of billing for health care, in which the provider charges the patient or a third-party payer a fee for services provided. Charges are based on a set fee schedule.

Third-party reimbursement involves reimbursement by the policyholder's insurance company for services performed.

Third-party payers: Private insurance carriers, HMOs, PPOs.

**Capitation**    Capitation is a form of reimbursement used by managed care providers in which members make a standard payment each month regardless of how much service is rendered to the member by the provider.

### Third-Party Reimbursement for Athletic Trainers

Currently, unless an athletic trainer is also a licensed physical therapist, it is difficult if not impossible to obtain third-party reimbursement for health care services provided. Because the majority of athletic trainers are now employed in for-profit clinical or industrial settings, this lack of reimbursement has become a major concern for their future. State licensing or credentialing of the athletic trainer has, to date, not helped with obtaining reimbursement. Insurance companies have not been willing to cover services provided by the athletic trainer. Athletic trainers working in the clinical setting perform many of the same functions as physical therapists in the clinic and are also responsible for obtaining referrals to the clinic through contacts in the local high schools. Securing third-party reimbursement for athletic training services should be a priority, especially for the clinical athletic trainer.[9]

## Accident Insurance

Besides general health insurance, low-cost accident insurance is available to the student. This insurance covers accidents on school grounds while the student is in attendance. The purpose of this insurance is to protect the student against financial loss from medical and hospital bills, to encourage an injured student to receive prompt medical care, to encourage prompt reporting of injuries, and to relieve a school of financial responsibility.

The school's general insurance may be limited; thus accident insurance for a specific activity such as sports may be needed to provide additional protection.[5] This type of coverage is limited and does not require knowledge of fault, and the amount it pays is limited. For serious sport injuries requiring surgery and lengthy rehabilitation, accident insurance is usually not adequate. This inadequacy can put families with limited budgets into a real financial bind. Of particular concern is insurance that does not adequately cover catastrophic injuries.

## INSURANCE TO PROTECT THE COACH

### Personal Liability Insurance

Most individual schools and school districts have general liability insurance to protect against damages that may arise from injuries occurring on school property. Liability insurance covers claims of negligence on the part of individuals. Its major concern is whether supervision was reasonable and whether unreasonable risk of harm was perceived by the sports participant.[8]

Because of the amount of litigation based on alleged negligence, premiums have become almost prohibitive for some schools. Typically, when a victim sues, the lawsuit is a shotgun approach, with the coach, athletic

Because of the amount of litigation for alleged negligence, all professionals involved with the sports program must be fully protected by personal liability insurance.

trainer, physician, school administrator, and school district all named. If a protective piece of equipment is involved, the product manufacturer is also sued.

All coaches should carry professional liability insurance and must clearly understand the limits of coverage. Liability insurance typically covers negligence in a civil case. If a criminal complaint is also filed, liability insurance will not cover the coach.

### Catastrophic Insurance

Although catastrophic injuries in sports participation are relatively uncommon, if they do occur, the consequences to the athlete, family, institution, and society can be staggering. In the past, when available funds had been completely depleted, the family was forced to seek funding elsewhere, usually through a lawsuit. Organizations such as the NCAA and NAIA provide plans that deal with the problem of a lifetime of extensive medical and rehabilitative care because of a permanent disability.[5] Benefits begin when expenses have reached $25,000 and are then extended for a lifetime. At the secondary school level, a program is offered to districts by the National Federation of State High School Associations (NFSHSA). This plan provides medical, rehabilitation, and transportation costs in excess of $10,000 not covered by other insurance benefits.[8] Costs for catastrophic insurance are based on the number of sports and the number of hazardous sports offered by the institution.

To offset the shotgun mentality and to cover what is not covered by a general liability policy, errors and omissions liability insurance has evolved. This insurance is designed to cover school employees, officers, and the district against suits claiming malpractice, wrongful actions, errors and omissions, and acts of negligence.[8] Even when working in a program that has good liability coverage, each person within that program who works directly with students must have his or her own personal liability insurance.

As indicated, insurance that covers the athlete's health and safety can be very complex. Coaches must be concerned that every athlete is adequately covered by a good, reliable insurance company. In some athletic programs the filing of claims becomes the responsibility of the athletic trainer. This task can be highly time consuming, taking the athletic trainer away from his or her major role of directly working with the athlete. Because of the intricacies and time involved with claim filing and follow-up communications with parents, doctors, and vendors, a staff person other than the coach should be assigned this responsibility.

## INSURANCE BILLING

It is essential that insurance claims be filed immediately and correctly.[9] The coach working in an educational setting can facilitate this process by collecting insurance information on every athlete at the beginning of the year. A letter should also be drafted to the parents of the athlete, explaining the limits of the school insurance policy and what the parents must do to file a claim if injury does occur. Schools that have secondary policies should stress to the parents that they must submit all bills to their insurance company before submitting the remainder to the school. In educational institutions, most claims will be filed with a single insurance company, which will pay for medical services provided by individual health care providers.

**COACH'S CORNER**
This checklist contains types of insurance the coach should look into to protect both the athlete and himself or herself.

☐ General health insurance
☐ Accident insurance
☐ Product liability insurance
☐ Catastrophic injury insurance
☐ Personal liability insurance

## SUMMARY

- A great deal of care must be taken in following coaching and athletic training procedures that conform to the legal guidelines governing liability.
- Liability is the state of being legally responsible for the harm one causes another person. The standard of reasonable care assumes that a coach acts according to the reasonable standards of care of any individual with similar educational background or training.
- A coach who fails to use ordinary or reasonable care—care that persons would normally exercise to avoid injury to themselves or to others under similar circumstances—is deemed negligent.
- Although athletes participating in a sports program are considered to assume a normal risk, this assumption in no way exempts those in charge from exercising reasonable care.
- Coaches can significantly decrease risk of litigation by making certain that they have done everything possible to provide a reasonable degree of care to the injured athlete.
- The major types of insurance that coaches should be familiar with are general health insurance, catastrophic insurance, accident insurance, and liability insurance, as well as insurance for errors and omissions.
- Third-party reimbursement is the primary mechanism of payment for medical services in the United States. A number of different health care systems—including health maintenance organizations, preferred provider organizations, point of service plans, indemnity plans, and capitation plans—have been developed to contain costs.
- It is essential that the coach or athletic trainer file insurance claims immediately and correctly.

### Solutions to Critical Thinking Exercises

**3-1** When a coach assumes the duty of caring for an athlete, that coach is also under the obligation to make sure that appropriate care is given. A coach who fails to provide an acceptable standard of care has committed a breach of duty, and the athlete must prove that this breach caused the injury or made the injury worse.

**3-2** The athlete typically has between 1 and 3 years to file suit for negligence. However, a minor may have up to 3 years after the minor reaches the age of 18 to file.

**3-3** Besides general health insurance, low-cost accident insurance often covers accidents on school grounds while the athlete is competing. The purpose of this insurance is to protect the athlete against financial loss from medical and hospital bills, to encourage an injured athlete to receive prompt medical care, to encourage prompt reporting of injuries, and to relieve a school of financial responsibility.

## REVIEW QUESTIONS AND CLASS ACTIVITIES

1. What are the major legal concerns of the coach in terms of liability, negligence, assumption of risk, and torts?
2. What measures can a coach take to minimize the chances of litigation should an athlete be injured?
3. Invite an attorney who is familiar with sport litigation to class to discuss how you can protect yourself from a lawsuit.
4. Discuss how a coach provides reasonable and prudent care in dealing with an injured athlete.
5. Why is it necessary for an athlete to have both general health insurance and accident insurance?
6. Briefly discuss the various methods of third-party reimbursement.
7. Why should a coach carry individual liability insurance?
8. What are the critical considerations for filing insurance claims?

### REFERENCES

1. Appenzeller H: *Safe at first: a guide to help sports administrators reduce their liability,* Chapel Hill, NC, 1999, Carolina Academic Press.
2. De Carlo M: Reimbursement for health care services. In Konin J: *Clinical athletic training,* Thorofare, NJ, 1997, Slack.
3. Gallup E: *Law and the team physician,* Champaign, Ill, 1995, Human Kinetics.
4. Hawkins J, Appenzeller H: Legal aspects of sports medicine. In Mueller F, Ryan A: *Prevention of athletic injuries: the role of the sports medicine team,* Philadelphia, 1991, FA Davis.
5. Health Insurance Association of America: *Fundamentals of health insurance,* Washington, DC, 1997, HIAA.
6. Herbert D: *Legal aspects of sports medicine,* Canton, Ohio, 1990, Professional Reports Corporation.
7. Leverenz L, Helms L: Suing athletic trainers, Parts I and II, *Ath Train* 25(3):212, 1990.
8. Rankin J, Ingersoll C: *Athletic training management: concepts and applications,* St. Louis, 2000, McGraw-Hill.
9. Ray R: *Management strategies in athletic training,* Champaign, Ill, 2000, Human Kinetics.
10. Wong G: *Essentials of amateur sports law,* Westport, Conn, 1994, Praeger.

## ANNOTATED BIBLIOGRAPHY

Appenzeller H: *Youth sports and the law: a guide to legal issues,* Chapel Hill, NC, 2000, Carolina Academic Press.

*Studies various court cases to understand the legal principles involved in sport participation. The objective of the book is to provide better and safer sporting experiences for today's children.*

Gayson E: *Ethics, injury and the law in sports medicine,* New York, 1999, Heinnman-Butterworth.

*Provides an up-to-date review of the status of sports medicine and the law. Addresses the key legal and ethical issues in sports and exercise medicine. For prac-titioners and students preparing for sport and exercise medicine exams.*

Herbert D: *Legal aspects of sports medicine,* Canton, Ohio, 1990, Professional Reports Corporation.

*A discussion of sports medicine, policies, procedures, responsibilities of the sports medicine team, informed consent, negligence, insurance and risk management, medication, drug testing, and other topics.*

Rowell JC: *Understanding medical insurance: a step-by-step guide,* Albany, NY, 1994, Delmar.

*Provides a comprehensive resource for dealing with issues related to insurance.*

## WEBSITES

Legal Information Institute at Cornell: http://www.law.cornell.edu/topics/sports.html

*Part of a series of legal information, this site specifically addresses law in sport, but is rather technical, the relevant area to sports medicine is addressed in the area titled torts.*

Cramer First Aider: http://www.ccsd.k12.wy.us/CCHS_web/sptmed/fstaider.htm

*The Cramer First Aider is a newsletter published by Cramer that provides information about current topics in sports medicine; see the Legal Issues section.*

Sports Lawyers Journal: http://www.law. tulane.edu/journals/slj/abstracts.htm

*Specialized academic and professional publication on legal aspects of sports.*

The Center for Sports Law & Policy Duke University School of Law http://www.law.duke.edu/sportscenter/

Health Insurance Association of America http://www.hiaa.org

*The nation's most prominent trade association representing the private health care system. It is the nation's premier provider of self-study courses on health insurance and managed care.*

# Preventing Injuries through Fitness Training

*When you finish this chapter you will be able to:*

- Identify the concept of periodization and the types of exercise that are performed in each phase.
- Identify the principles of conditioning.
- Explain the importance of the warm-up and cooldown periods.
- Describe the importance of flexibility, strength, and cardiorespiratory endurance for both athletic performance and injury prevention.
- Identify specific techniques and principles for improving flexibility, muscular strength, and cardiorespiratory endurance.

Lack of fitness is one of the primary causes of sports injury.

T o compete successfully at a high level, the athlete must be fit. An athlete who is not fit is more likely to sustain an injury. Coaches recognize that improper conditioning is one of the major causes of sports injuries. Thus coaches should work cooperatively to supervise training and conditioning programs that minimize the possibility of injury and maximize performance.

Fitness does not develop overnight. It takes time and careful preparation to bring an athlete into competition at a level of fitness that will preclude early-season injury. Both the coach and the athlete must possess sound understanding of the principles of training and conditioning relative to flexibility, strength, and cardiorespiratory endurance.

## CONDITIONING SEASONS AND PERIODIZATION

No longer do serious athletes engage only in preseason conditioning and in-season competition. Sports conditioning is a year-round endeavor. The concept of **periodization** is an approach to conditioning that attempts to bring about peak performance while reducing injuries and overtraining in the athlete by developing a training and conditioning program to be followed throughout the various seasons.[10] The idea of periodization takes into account athletes' different training and conditioning needs during different seasons and modifies the program according to individual needs (Table 4-1).

**periodization**
Allows athletes to train year-round with less risk of injury and staleness.

**TABLE 4-1** Periodization Training

| Season | Period/Phase | Type of Training Activity |
|---|---|---|
| Off-season sports | Transition period | Unstructured<br>Recreational |
| | Preparatory period<br>Hypertrophy/endurance phase | Cross training<br>Low intensity<br>High volume<br>Non–sport-specific |
| | Strength phase | Moderate intensity<br>Moderate volume<br>More sport-specific |
| Preseason | Power phase | High intensity<br>Decreased volume<br>Sport-specific |
| In-season | Competition period | High intensity<br>Low volume<br>Skill training<br>Strategic |

## Macrocycle

Periodization organizes a training and conditioning program into cycles. The complete training period, which could be a year in the case of seasonal sports or perhaps 4 years for an Olympic athlete, is referred to as a *macrocycle*. For seasonal sports the macrocycle can be divided into a preseason, an in-season, and an off-season. Throughout the course of this cycle, intensity, volume, and specificity of training are altered so that an athlete can achieve peak levels of fitness for competition. As competition approaches, training sessions change gradually and progressively from high volume, low intensity, non–sport-specific activity to low volume, high intensity, sport-specific training.[10]

### Mesocycle

Within the macrocycle are a series of *mesocycles*, each of which may last for several weeks or even months. A mesocycle is further divided into *preparatory, competition,* and *transition* periods.[7]

**Preparatory Period**  The preparatory period occurs primarily during the off-season when there are no upcoming competitions. In the preparatory period there are three phases; the hypertrophy/endurance phase, the strength phase, and the power phase.

During the hypertrophy/endurance phase, which occurs in the early part of the off-season, training is at a low intensity with a high volume of repetitions, using activities that may or may not be directly related to a specific sport. The goal is to develop a base of endurance, on which more intense training can occur. This phase may last from several weeks to 2 months.

During the strength phase, which also occurs during the off-season, the intensity and volume progress to moderate levels. Weight training activities should become more specific to the sport or event.

The third phase or power phase occurs in the preseason. The athlete trains at a high intensity at or near the level of competition. The volume of training is decreased so that full recovery is allowed between sessions.

**Competition Period**  In certain cases the competition period may last for only a week or less. However, with seasonal sports the competition period may last for several months. In general this period involves high intensity training at a low volume. As training volume decreases, an increased amount of time is spent on skill training or strategy sessions. During the competition period it may be necessary to establish *microcyles,* which are periods lasting from 1 to 7 days. During a weekly microcycle, training should be intense early in the week, progressing to moderate, and finally light the day before a competition. The goal is to make sure that the athlete is at peak levels of fitness and performance on days of competition.[7]

**Transition Period**  The transition period begins after the last competition and comprises the early part of the off-season. The transition period is generally unstructured and the athlete is encouraged to participate in sport activities on a recreational basis. The idea is to allow the athlete to escape both physically and psychologically from the rigor of a highly organized training regimen.

### Cross Training

The concept of cross training is an approach to training and conditioning for a specific sport that involves substitution of alternative activities that have some carryover value to that sport. For example, a swimmer can engage in jogging, running, or aerobic exercise to maintain levels of cardiorespiratory conditioning. Cross training is particularly useful in both the postseason and the off-season to help athletes maintain fitness levels and avoid the boredom that typically occurs from following the same training regimen and using the same techniques for conditioning as during the preseason and competitive season.

## FOUNDATIONS OF CONDITIONING

The SAID principle indicates
that the body will gradually
adapt to the specific demands
imposed on it.

The SAID principle relates to the process of training and conditioning. SAID is an acronym for Specific Adaptation to Imposed Demands. The SAID principle states that when the body is subjected to stresses and overloads of varying intensities, it will gradually adapt over time to overcome whatever demands are placed on it.

Although overload is a critical factor in training and conditioning, the stress must not be great enough to produce damage or injury before the body has had a chance to adjust specifically to the increased demands. Therefore, to reduce the likelihood of injury, coaches should be aware of the principles of training and conditioning. See Focus Box 4-1.

<4-1> **Focus Box**

**Principles of Conditioning**

1. *Warm-up/cooldown.* Give the athletes time to do an appropriate warm-up before engaging in any activity. Do not neglect the cooldown period following a training bout.

2. *Motivation.* Athletes are generally highly motivated to work hard because they want to be successful in their sport. By varying the training program and incorporating different aspects of conditioning, the program can remain enjoyable rather than becoming routine and boring.

3. *Overload.* To see improvement in any physiological component, the system must work harder than it is accustomed to working. Gradually, that system will adapt to the imposed demands.

4. *Consistency.* The athlete must engage in a training and conditioning program on a consistent, regularly scheduled basis if the program is to be effective.

5. *Progression.* Increase the intensity of the conditioning program gradually and within the individual athlete's ability to adapt to increasing workloads.

6. *Intensity.* Stress the intensity of the work rather than the quantity. Coaches and athletic trainers too often confuse working hard with working for long periods. They make the mistake of prolonging the workout rather than increasing tempo or workload. The tired athlete is prone to injury.

7. *Specificity.* Specific goals for the training program must be identified. The program must be designed to address specific components of fitness (i.e., strength, flexibility, cardiorespiratory endurance) relative to the sport in which the athlete is competing.

8. *Individuality.* The needs of individual athletes vary considerably. The successful coach is one who recognizes these individual differences and adjusts or alters the training and conditioning program accordingly to best accommodate the athlete.

9. *Stress.* Expect that athletes will train as close to their physiological limits as possible. Push the athletes but consider other stressful aspects of their lives; allow them time to be away from the conditioning demands of their sport.

10. *Safety.* Make the training environment as safe as possible. Take time to educate athletes about proper techniques, how they should feel during the workout, and when they should push harder or back off.

## Warm-Up

A period of warm-up exercises should take place before a training session begins. The warm-up increases body temperature, stretches ligaments and muscles, and increases flexibility. Related warm-ups, those similar to the activity engaged in, are preferable to unrelated ones because of the rehearsal or practice effect that results.

A proper warm-up before exercise will reduce the tearing of muscle fibers and prevent muscle soreness.

Organizing and Establishing
an Effective Athletic Health
Care System

**Critical Thinking** E x e r c i s e

A track athlete constantly complains of tightness in her lower extremities during workouts. She states that she has a difficult time during her warm-up and cannot seem to "get loose" until her workout is almost complete. She feels that she is always on the verge of "pulling a muscle."

? What should the coach recommend as a specific warm-up routine that should consistently be done before this athlete begins her workout?

Warming up involves general body warming and warming specific body areas for the demands of the sport.

Reduce injuries by increasing:
• Flexibility
• Strength
• Power
• Endurance

Warm-ups have been found to be important in preventing injury and muscle soreness.[24] Muscle injury can result when vigorous exercises are not preceded by a related warm-up. An effective, quick warm-up can also be an effective motivator. If athletes derive satisfaction from a warm-up, they probably will have a stronger desire to participate in the activity. By contrast, a poor warm-up can lead to fatigue and boredom, limiting athletes' attention and ultimately resulting in a poor program. A good warm-up may also improve certain aspects of performance.[25]

The function of the warm-up is to prepare the body physiologically for some upcoming physical work bout. Most coaches view the warm-up period as a precaution against unnecessary musculoskeletal injury and possible muscle soreness. The purpose is to very gradually stimulate the cardiorespiratory system to a moderate degree, thus producing an increased blood flow to working skeletal muscles and resulting in an increase in muscle temperature.

Moderate activity speeds up the metabolic processes that produce an increase in core body temperature. An increase in the temperature of skeletal muscle causes an increased speed of contraction and relaxation, probably because nerve impulse conduction velocity is increased. The elastic properties (the length of stretch) of the muscle are increased, whereas the viscous properties (the rate at which the muscle can change shape) are decreased.

Every workout should be preceded by a warm-up. This activity should include a general warm-up followed by a specific warm-up. The general warm-up elevates the core temperature through the use of static stretching exercises. The specific warm-up involves actions related to the activity to be performed. These actions are sport specific and should gradually increase in intensity. For example, soccer players use the upper extremity considerably less than the lower extremity, so their general warm-up should be directed more toward the lower extremity, perhaps by adding some stretching exercises for the lower extremity. The specific warm-up also relates to the sport: A basketball player should warm up by shooting layups and jump shots and by dribbling, for example, or a tennis player should hit forehand and backhand shots and serves.

The warm-up should last approximately 10 to 15 minutes. Athletes should not wait longer than 15 minutes after the warm-up to get started in the activity, although the effects will generally last up to about 45 minutes. Thus the third-string football player who warms up before the game and then does nothing more than stand around until he gets into the game during the fourth quarter is running a much higher risk of injury. This player should be encouraged to stay warmed up and ready to play throughout the course of a game. In general, sweating is a good indication that the body has been sufficiently warmed up and is ready for more strenuous activity.

The warm-up should begin with 2 or 3 minutes of light jogging to increase metabolic rate and core temperature. The jogging should be followed by flexibility exercises in which the muscles are stretched to take advantage of the increase in muscle elasticity. Finally, the intensity of the warm-up should be increased gradually by performing body movements and skills associated with the specific activity in which the athlete is going to participate.

## Cooldown

After a vigorous workout, a cooldown is essential. This part of the training program helps in returning the blood to the heart for reoxygenation, thus preventing the blood from pooling in the muscles of the arms and the legs. Pooling of the blood in the extremities places additional unnecessary stress and strain on the heart. After vigorous activity, enough blood may not circulate back to the brain, heart, and intestines, and symptoms such as dizziness or faintness may occur without a cooldown period. The cooldown enables the body to cool and return to a resting state. Such a period should last about 5 to 10 minutes.

Although the value of warm-up and workout periods is well accepted, the importance of a cooldown period afterward is often ignored. Persons who stretch during the cooldown period tend to have fewer problems with muscle soreness following strenuous activity.[24]

## WHY IS IT IMPORTANT TO HAVE GOOD FLEXIBILITY?

*Flexibility* may best be defined as the range of motion possible about a given joint or series of joints.[22] Flexibility can be discussed in relation to movement involving only one joint, such as in the knees, or movement involving a whole series of joints, such as the spinal vertebral joints, which must all move together to allow smooth bending, or rotation, of the trunk. Flexibility is specific to a given joint or movement. A person may have good range of motion in the ankles, knees, hips, back, and one shoulder joint. However, if the other shoulder joint lacks normal movement, then this person has a problem that needs to be corrected before he or she can function normally.

For an athlete, good flexibility is considered essential for both successful performance and injury prevention. Lack of flexibility may result in uncoordinated or awkward movements and may predispose a person to muscle strain.

A lack of flexibility in an athlete will likely impair performance. For example, a sprinter with tight, inelastic hamstring muscles may have a problem sprinting at maximum speed because tight hamstrings restrict the ability to flex the hip joint, thus shortening stride length. Most activities in sport require relatively normal amounts of flexibility. However, some athletic activities, such as gymnastics, ballet, diving, karate, and yoga, require increased flexibility for superior performance (Figure 4-1). Increased flexibility may increase an athlete's performance through improved balance and reaction time. Experts in the field of training and conditioning generally agree that good flexibility is essential to successful physical performance.[2]

Most coaches feel that maintaining good flexibility is important in prevention of injury to muscles and tendons, and they will generally

Properly cooling down decreases blood and muscle lactic acid levels more rapidly.

Conditioning should be performed gradually, with work added in small increments.

The "tight" or inflexible athlete performs with a considerable handicap in terms of movement.

**Figure 4-1**

Certain athletic activities
require extreme flexibility for
successful performance.

insist that stretching exercises be included as part of the warm-up before engaging in strenuous activity.

## What Structures in the Body Can Limit Flexibility?

A number of different anatomical structures may limit the ability of a joint to move through a full, unrestricted range of motion. Normal bone structure, fat, and skin or scar tissue may limit the ability to move through a full range of motion.[11]

Muscles and their tendons are most often responsible for limiting range of motion. Performing stretching exercises for the purpose of improving a particular joint's flexibility is an attempt to take advantage of the highly elastic properties of a muscle. Over time it is possible to increase the elasticity, or the length, that a given muscle can be stretched. Athletes who have a good range of motion at a particular joint tend to have highly elastic and flexible muscles.

Connective tissue surrounding the joint, such as ligaments or the joint capsule, may be subject to contractures. Ligaments and joint capsules do have some elasticity; however, if a joint is immobilized for a time, these structures tend to lose some elasticity and actually shorten. This condition is most commonly seen after surgical repair of an unstable joint, but it can also result from long periods of inactivity.

On the other hand, it is also possible for an athlete to have slack ligaments and joint capsules. These individuals are generally referred to as being loose-jointed. An example of this condition is an elbow or knee that extends beyond being straight. Frequently the instability associated with loose-jointedness may present as great a problem in movement as a joint that is too tight.

## Active and Passive Range of Motion

When a muscle actively contracts, it produces a joint movement through a specific range of motion. However, if passive pressure is applied to an extremity, it is capable of moving farther in the range of motion. *Active range of motion* refers to that portion of the total range of motion through which a joint can be moved by an active muscle contraction. The ability to move through the active range of motion is not necessarily a good indicator of the stiffness or looseness of a joint because it applies to the ability to move a joint efficiently, with little resistance to motion. *Passive range of motion* refers to the portion of the total range of motion through which a joint may be moved passively. No muscle contraction is needed to move a joint through a passive range of motion. Passive range of motion begins at the end of and continues beyond active range of motion.

It is essential in sport activities that an extremity be capable of moving through a nonrestricted range of motion.[21] For example, a hurdler who cannot fully extend the knee joint in a normal stride is at a considerable disadvantage because stride length and thus speed are reduced significantly. Passive range of motion is important for injury prevention. Sports contain many situations in which a muscle is forced to stretch beyond its normal active limits. If the muscle does not have enough elasticity to compensate for this additional stretch, the muscle or its tendon will likely be injured.

## Agonist versus Antagonist Muscles

Before discussing the three different stretching techniques, it is essential to define the terms *agonist muscle* and *antagonist muscle*. Most joints in the body are capable of more than one movement. The knee joint, for example, is capable of flexion and extension. Contraction of the quadriceps group of muscles on the front of the thigh causes knee extension, whereas contraction of the hamstring muscles on the back of the thigh produces knee flexion. The muscle that contracts to produce a movement, in this case the quadriceps, is referred to as the agonist muscle. Conversely, the muscle being stretched in response to contraction of the agonist muscle is called the antagonist muscle. In this example of knee extension, the antagonist muscle is the hamstring group.

Some degree of balance in strength must exist between agonist and antagonist muscle groups. This balance is necessary for normal, smooth, coordinated movement and for reducing the likelihood of muscle strain caused by the muscular imbalance. Understanding the relationship between agonist and antagonist muscles facilitates understanding of the three techniques of stretching (see Focus Box 4-2).

## What Are the Different Stretching Techniques?

Maintaining a full, nonrestricted range of motion has long been recognized as an essential component of being fit. Flexibility is important not only for successful physical performance but also in the prevention of injury. The goal of any effective flexibility program should be to improve the range of motion around a given joint by altering the extensibility of the muscles and tendons that produce movement at that joint. Exercises that stretch these muscles and tendons over time will increase the range of movement possible about a given joint.

Stretching techniques for improving flexibility have evolved over the years. The oldest technique for stretching is called **ballistic stretching,** which makes use of repetitive bouncing motions. A second technique, known as **static stretching,** involves stretching a muscle to the point of discomfort and then holding it at that point for an extended time. This technique has been used for many years. Recently another group of stretching techniques known collectively as **proprioceptive neuromuscular facilitation (PNF),** involving alternating contractions and stretches, has also been recommended. Researchers have had considerable discussion about which of these techniques is most effective for improving range of motion.

### Ballistic Stretching

On the track any spring or fall afternoon, runners can be seen warming up by stretching, using bouncing movements to stretch a particular

---

**ballistic stretching**
Older stretching technique that uses repetitive bouncing motions.

---

**static stretching**
Passively stretching an antagonist muscle by placing it in a maximal stretch and holding it there.

---

**proprioceptive neuromuscular facilitation (PNF)**
Stretching techniques that involve combinations of alternating contractions and stretches.

4-2 **Focus Box**

### Guidelines and Precautions for Stretching

The following guidelines and precautions should be incorporated into a sound stretching program:

Warm up using a slow jog or fast walk before stretching vigorously.

To increase flexibility, the muscle must be overloaded or stretched beyond its normal range but not to the point of pain.

Stretch only to the point at which tightness or resistance to stretch or perhaps some discomfort is felt. Stretching should not be painful.

Increases in range of motion will be specific to whatever joint is being stretched.

Exercise caution when stretching muscles that surround painful joints. Pain is an indication that something is wrong; it should not be ignored.

Avoid overstretching the ligaments and capsules that surround joints.

Exercise caution when stretching the low back and neck. Exercises that compress the vertebrae and their disks may cause damage.

Stretching from a seated position rather than a standing position takes stress off the low back and decreases the chances of back injury.

Stretch those muscles that are tight and inflexible.

Strengthen those muscles that are weak and loose.

Always stretch slowly and with control.

Be sure to continue normal breathing during a stretch.

Static and PNF techniques are most often recommended for individuals who want to improve their range of motion.

Ballistic stretching should be done only by those who are already flexible and/or are accustomed to stretching and should be done only after static stretching.

Stretching should be done at least three times per week to see minimal improvement, between five and six times per week to see maximum results.

muscle. This bouncing technique is more appropriately known as ballistic stretching, in which repetitive contractions of the agonist muscle are used to produce quick stretches of the antagonist muscle. The ballistic stretching technique, although apparently effective in improving range of motion, should be used with some caution by sedentary, inactive people because increased range of motion is achieved through a series of jerks or pulls on the resistant muscle tissue. If the forces generated by the jerks are greater than the tissues' extensibility, muscle injury may result. For a conditioned athlete, ballistic stretching will not normally be detrimental and in fact is perhaps the most appropriate stretching technique for most sport activities that require dynamic movements.[21]

Successive forceful contractions of the agonist that result in stretching of the antagonist may cause muscle soreness. For example, forcefully kicking a soccer ball fifty times may result in muscular soreness of the hamstrings (antagonist muscle) as a result of eccentric contraction of the hamstrings to control the dynamic movement of the quadriceps (agonist muscle). Ballistic stretching that is controlled usually does not cause muscle soreness.

### Static Stretching

The static stretching technique is still an extremely effective and popular technique of stretching. This technique involves passively stretching a muscle by placing it in a maximal position of stretch and holding it there for an extended time.[11] Recommendations for the optimal time for holding this stretched position vary, ranging from as short as 3 seconds to as long as 60 seconds. It appears that 20 to 30 seconds may be the best length of time to hold a stretch. The static stretch of each muscle should be repeated three or four times. Much research has been done comparing ballistic and static stretching techniques for the improvement of flexibility. Both static and ballistic stretching are effective in increasing flexibility, and there is no significant difference between the two. However, static stretching offers less danger of exceeding the extensibility limits of the involved joints because the stretch is more controlled. Ballistic stretching may cause muscular soreness (if the athlete is not fit), whereas static stretching generally does not and is commonly used in injury rehabilitation of sore or strained muscles.

Static stretching is certainly a much safer stretching technique, especially for unfit individuals. However, many physical activities involve dynamic movement. Thus, stretching as a warm-up for these types of activities should begin with static stretching followed by ballistic stretching, which more closely resembles the dynamic activity.

### Proprioceptive Neuromuscular Facilitation (PNF) Techniques

PNF techniques were first used by physical therapists for treating patients who had various types of neuromuscular paralysis.[18] Only recently have PNF stretching exercises been used as a stretching technique for increasing flexibility. A number of different PNF techniques are currently being used for stretching, including *slow-reversal-hold-relax, contract-relax,* and *hold-relax* techniques. All involve some combination of alternating contraction and relaxation of both agonist and antagonist muscles (a 10-second pushing phase followed by a 10-second relaxing phase).

Using a hamstring stretching technique as an example (Figure 4-2), the slow-reversal-hold-relax technique is done as follows. With the athlete lying supine with knee extended and the ankle flexed to 90 degrees, the athletic trainer passively flexes the leg at the hip joint to the point at which the athlete feels slight discomfort in the muscle. At this point the athlete begins pushing against the athletic trainer's resistance by contracting the hamstring muscle. After pushing for 10 seconds, the athlete relaxes the hamstring muscles and contracts agonist quadriceps muscle while the athletic trainer applies passive pressure to further stretch the hamstrings. This pressure should move the leg so that the hip joint flexion is increased. The relaxing phase lasts for 10 seconds, at which time the athlete again pushes against the trainer's resistance,

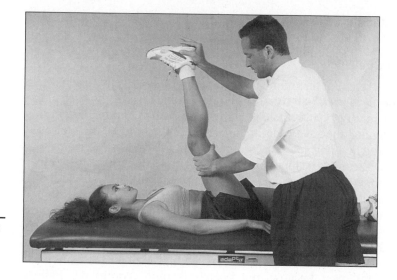

**Figure 4-2**

The slow-reversal-hold-relax
technique can be used to
stretch hamstring muscles.

beginning at this new joint angle. The push-relax sequence is repeated at
least three times.[18]

The contract-relax and hold-relax techniques are variations on the
slow-reversal-hold-relax method. In the contract-relax method, the
hamstrings are isotonically contracted so that the leg actually moves toward the floor during the push phase. The hold-relax method involves
an isometric hamstring contraction against immovable resistance during
the push phase. During the relax phase, both techniques involve relaxation of hamstrings and quadriceps while the hamstrings are passively
stretched. This same basic PNF technique can be used to stretch any
muscle in the body. PNF stretching techniques are perhaps best performed
with a partner, although they may also be done using a wall as resistance.[18]

## Practical Application

Although all three stretching techniques have been demonstrated to effectively improve flexibility, there is still considerable debate as to which
technique produces the greatest increases in range of movement. The
ballistic technique is seldom recommended because of the potential for
causing muscle soreness. However, most sport activities are ballistic in nature (i.e., kicking, running). In highly trained individuals, it is unlikely
that ballistic stretching will result in muscle soreness. Static stretching is
perhaps the most widely used technique. It is a simple technique and
does not require a partner. A fully nonrestricted range of motion can be
attained through static stretching over time.

PNF stretching techniques are capable of producing dramatic increases in range of motion during one stretching session. Studies comparing static and PNF stretching suggest that PNF stretching is capable of
producing greater improvement in flexibility over an extended training
period. The major disadvantage of PNF stretching is that a partner is re-

quired, although stretching with a partner may have some motivational advantages. More and more athletic teams seem to be adopting the PNF technique as the method of choice for improving flexibility.

## Stretching Exercises

Figures 4-3 to 4-14 illustrate stretching exercises that may be used to improve flexibility at specific joints throughout the body. The exercises described may be done statically, or with slight modification they may also be done with a partner using a PNF technique.

Each of these exercises has many possible variations. The exercises selected are those that seem to be the most effective for stretching various muscle groups.

## Assessment of Flexibility

Accurate measurement of the range of joint motion is difficult. Various devices have been designed to accommodate variations in the size of the joints and the complexity of movements in articulations that involve more than one joint. Of these devices, the simplest and most widely used is the goniometer (Figure 4-15). A goniometer is a large protractor with measurements in degrees. By aligning the two arms parallel to the longitudinal axis of the two segments involved in motion about a specific joint, it is possible to obtain relatively accurate measures of range of movement. The goniometer has its place in a rehabilitation setting, in which assessing improvement in joint flexibility is essential for modifying injury rehabilitation programs.

**Figure 4-3**

Arm hang exercise
Muscles stretched: Entire shoulder girdle complex
Instructions: Using a chinning bar, simply hang with shoulders and arms fully extended for 30 seconds. Repeat five times.

**Figure 4-4**

Shoulder towel stretch exercise

Muscles stretched: Internal and external rotators

Instructions: Begin by holding towel above head with hands shoulder width apart. A, Try to pull towel down behind back, first with right hand then with left. B, You should end up in position C. Reverse order to get back to position A. Repeat five times on each side.

A

B

C

**Figure 4-5**

Chest and shoulder stretch exercise

Muscles stretched: Pectoralis and deltoid

Instructions: Stand in a corner, hands on walls, and lean forward. Hold for 30 seconds. Repeat three times.

**Figure 4-6**

Abdominal and anterior chest wall stretch exercise
Muscles stretched: Muscles of respiration in thorax and abdominal muscles
Instructions: Extend upper trunk, support weight on elbows, keeping pelvis on the floor. Hold for 30 seconds. Repeat three times.

A

B

**Figure 4-7**

William's flexion exercise
Muscles stretched: Low back and hip extensors
Instructions: A, Touch chin to right knee and hold, then to left knee and hold. B, Touch chin to both knees and hold. Hold each position for 30 seconds.

## Is There a Relationship between Strength and Flexibility?

It is often said that strength training has negative effects on flexibility. For example, someone who develops large bulk through strength training is often referred to as muscle-bound. The expression "muscle-bound" has negative connotations in terms of the ability of that person to move. People who have highly developed muscles are thought to have lost much of their ability to move freely through a full range of motion.

Occasionally a person develops so much bulk that the physical size of the muscle prevents a normal range of motion. When strength training is not properly done, movement can be impaired. However, weight training, if done properly through a full range of motion, will not impair flexibility. Proper strength training probably improves dynamic flexibility and, if combined with a rigorous stretching program, can greatly enhance powerful and coordinated movements that are essential for success in many athletic activities.[21] In all cases a heavy weight-training program should be accompanied by a strong flexibility program (Figure 4-16).

## WHY ARE MUSCULAR STRENGTH, ENDURANCE, AND POWER IMPORTANT FOR ATHLETES?

The development of muscular strength is an essential component of a training program for every athlete. By definition, **muscular strength** is the ability of a muscle to generate force against some resistance.

**muscular strength**
The maximum force that can be applied by a muscle during a single maximum contraction.

**Figure 4-8**

Low back twister exercise
Muscles stretched: Rotators of lower back and sacrum and hip abductors
Instructions: Lie on back on edge of bed or table. Keep shoulders and arms flat on surface. Cross leg farthest from edge over the top and let it hang off the side of bed, keeping knee straight; hold for 30 seconds. Repeat with other leg. Repeat three times with each leg.
Caution: If keeping the leg straight produces pain, this exercise may be done with the leg bent. Be sure to exercise caution in returning the leg to the starting position.

---

**muscular endurance**
The ability to perform repetitive muscular contractions against some resistance.

---

**power**
The ability to generate force rapidly.

---

**Muscular endurance** is the ability to perform repetitive muscular contractions against some resistance for an extended time. As muscular strength increases, there tends to be a corresponding increase in endurance. For example, an athlete can lift a weight twenty-five times. If muscular strength is increased by 10 percent through weight training, the maximal number of repetitions is increased because it is easier for the athlete to lift the weight.

Most movements in sports are explosive and must include elements of both strength and speed if they are to be effective. If a large amount of force is generated quickly, the movement can be referred to as a **power** movement. Without the ability to generate power, an athlete is limited in his or her performance capabilities.[16] It is difficult to hit a baseball, drive a golf ball, or kick a soccer ball without generating power. For most athletes, the ability to generate power is more critical for successful performance than simply having great strength or muscular endurance.

## Types of Skeletal Muscle Contraction

Skeletal muscle is capable of three different types of contraction: (1) an *isometric contraction,* (2) a *concentric,* or positive, contraction, and (3) an *eccentric,* or negative, contraction. An isometric contraction occurs when the muscle contracts to produce tension, but there is no change in length

**Figure 4-9**

Forward lunge exercise
Muscles stretched: Hip flexors and quadriceps
Instructions: In a kneeling position with one knee on the ground, thrust pelvis forward. Hold for 30 seconds. Repeat three times.

**Figure 4-10**

Lateral trunk stretch exercise
Muscles stretched: Lateral
abdominals and intercostals
Instructions: Standing with
feet spread at shoulder
width, extend right arm
straight up and reach for
the ceiling. Hold for 30
seconds. Repeat three times
on each side.

**Figure 4-11**

Trunk twister exercise
Muscles stretched: Trunk and
hip rotators
Instructions: Place one foot
over opposite knee. Rotate
trunk to bent knee side.

**Figure 4-12**

Hamstring stretch exercise
Muscles stretched: Hip
extensors and knee flexors
Instructions: Lie flat on back.
Raise one leg straight up
with knee extended and
ankle flexed to 90 degrees.
Grasp leg around calf and
pull toward head; hold for 30
seconds. Repeat with
opposite leg. Repeat three
times with each leg.

**Figure 4-13**

Groin stretch exercise
Muscles stretched: Hip
adductors in groin
Instructions: Sit with knees
flexed and soles of feet together. Try to press knees flat
on the floor; if they are flat
to begin with, try to touch
face to floor. Hold for 30 seconds. Repeat three times.

**Figure 4-14**

Achilles heel cord stretch
exercise
Muscles stretched: Foot
plantar flexors. A,
Gastrocnemius; B, Soleus
Instructions: A, Stand facing
wall with toes pointing
straight ahead and with the
knee straight. Lean forward
toward wall, keeping heels
flat on floor. You should feel
stretching high in calf. B,
Stand facing wall with toes
pointing straight ahead and
with the knee flexed. Lean
forward toward wall, keeping
heels flat on floor. You should
feel stretching low in calf.
Hold each position for 30
seconds. Repeat each position
three times for each leg.

A                    B

**Figure 4-15**

Goniometric measurement of
hip joint flexion

of the muscle. Considerable force can be generated against some immovable resistance, even though no movement occurs. In a concentric contraction, the muscle shortens while tension is developed to overcome or move some resistance. In an eccentric contraction, the resistance is greater than the muscular force being produced, and the muscle lengthens while producing tension. For example, when lifting a weight in the hand the biceps muscle in the upper arm is shortening as it contracts, which is a concentric contraction. As the weight is lowered, the biceps muscle is still contracting but now it is lengthening. This movement is an eccentric contraction. Concentric and eccentric contractions must occur to allow most movements.

## What Determines the Amount of Strength?

### Size of the Muscle

Muscular strength is proportional to the size of a muscle as determined by the cross-sectional diameter of the muscle fibers.[14] The greater the cross-sectional diameter or the bigger a particular muscle, the stronger it is, thus, the more force it is capable of generating. The size of a muscle tends to increase in cross-sectional diameter with weight training. This increase in muscle size is referred to as *hypertrophy.* Conversely, a decrease in the size of a muscle is referred to as *atrophy.*

### Number of Muscle Fibers

Strength is a function of the number and diameter of muscle fibers comprising a given muscle. The number of fibers is an inherited characteristic; a person with a large number of muscle fibers to begin with has the potential to hypertrophy to a much greater degree than does someone with relatively few fibers. But anyone can increase his or her strength through exercise.

### Neuromuscular Efficiency

Strength is also directly related to the efficiency of both the nervous and muscular systems (or the neuromuscular system) and the function of the motor unit in producing muscular force. Initial increases in strength during a weight-training program can be attributed primarily to increased neuromuscular efficiency. For a muscle to contract, a nerve impulse must be transmitted from the nervous system to the muscle. Each muscle fiber is innervated by a specific *motor unit.* By overloading a particular muscle, as in weight training, the muscle is forced to work efficiently. Efficiency is achieved by getting more motor units to fire, causing a stronger contraction of the muscle.[1]

### Biomechanical Factors

Strength in a given muscle is determined not only by the physical properties of the muscle but also by biomechanical factors. Bones along with muscles and their tendons form a system of levers and pulleys that collectively generate force to move an external object. The position of

**Figure 4-16**

If strength training is combined with flexibility exercise, a full range of motion may be maintained.

*Critical Thinking* Exercise

A swimmer has been engaged in an off-season weight-training program to increase her muscular strength and endurance. Although she has seen some improvement in her strength, she is concerned that she also seems to be losing flexibility in her shoulders, which she feels is critical to her performance as a swimmer. She has also noticed that her muscles are hypertrophying to some degree and is worried that that may be causing her to lose flexibility. She has just about decided to abandon her weight-training program altogether.

**?** What can the coach recommend that will allow her to continue to improve her muscular strength and endurance while maintaining or perhaps even improving her flexibility?

There are two basic types of muscle fibers:
- Slow-twitch
- Fast-twitch

attachment of a particular muscle tendon on the bone will largely determine how much force this muscle is capable of generating.

### Fast-Twitch versus Slow-Twitch Muscle Fibers

The fibers that make up a muscle are either slow-twitch fibers or fast-twitch fibers.[16] Within a particular muscle, both types of fibers exist, and the ratio in an individual muscle varies with each person. Those muscles that have a primary function of maintaining posture against the pull of gravity require more endurance and have a higher percentage of slow-twitch fibers. Muscles that produce powerful, explosive, and strength movements tend to have a much greater percentage of fast-twitch fibers.

Because this ratio is genetically determined, it may play a large role in determining ability for a given sport activity. For example, sprinters and weight lifters have a large percentage of fast-twitch fibers in relation to slow-twitch ones. One study has shown that sprinters may have as many as 95 percent fast-twitch fibers in certain muscles. Conversely, marathon runners generally have a higher percentage of slow-twitch fibers. The question of whether fiber types can change as a result of training has not been completely resolved.[16] However, both types of fibers can improve their metabolic capabilities through specific strength and endurance training.

### Level of Physical Activity

Loss in muscle strength is definitely related to individual levels of physical activity. Those people who are more active, or perhaps those who continue to strength train, considerably reduce this tendency toward declining muscle strength. In addition, exercise may also have an effect in slowing the decrease in cardiorespiratory endurance and flexibility as well as slowing increases in body fat that tend to occur with aging. Therefore, if total wellness and health is an ultimate goal, strength maintenance is important for all individuals regardless of age or the level of competition.

### Overtraining

Overtraining can have a negative effect on the development of muscular strength. The statement "If you abuse it you will lose it" is very applicable. Overtraining can result in psychological breakdown (staleness) or physiological breakdown, which may involve musculoskeletal injury, fatigue, or sickness. Engaging in proper and efficient resistance training, eating a proper diet, and getting appropriate rest can all minimize the potential negative effects of overtraining.

Gains in muscular strength resulting from resistance training are reversible. Individuals who interrupt or stop resistance training altogether will see rapid decreases in strength gains. "If you don't use it, you'll lose it."

## WHAT PHYSIOLOGICAL CHANGES OCCUR TO CAUSE INCREASED STRENGTH?

Weight training to improve muscular strength unquestionably results in an increased size, or hypertrophy, of a muscle. What causes a muscle to hypertrophy? Over the years, a number of theories have been proposed to explain this increase in muscle size, the majority of which have been discounted.

The primary explanation for this hypertrophy is best attributed to an increase in the size and number of small contractile protein filaments within the muscle, called *myofilaments.* Increases in both size and number of the myofilaments as a result of strength training cause the individual muscle fibers to increase in cross-sectional diameter.[14] This increase is particularly true in men, although women also see some increase in muscle size. More research is needed to further clarify and determine the specific causes of muscle hypertrophy.

## WHAT ARE THE TECHNIQUES OF RESISTANCE TRAINING?

There are a number of different techniques of resistance training for strength improvement, including *isometric exercise, progressive resistance exercise, isokinetic training, circuit training, plyometric exercise,* and *calisthenic exercise.* Regardless of which technique is used, one basic principle of training is extremely important: *For a muscle to improve in strength, it must be forced to work at a higher level than that to which it is accustomed.* In other words, the muscle must be *overloaded.* Without overload the muscle will be able to *maintain* strength as long as training is continued against a level of resistance to which the muscle is accustomed. However, *no additional* strength gains will be realized. This maintenance of existing levels of muscular strength may be more important in weight-training programs that emphasize muscular endurance rather than strength gains. Many individuals can benefit more in terms of overall health by concentrating on improving muscular endurance. However, to most effectively build muscular strength, weight training requires a consistent, increasing effort against progressively increasing resistance. Progressive resistance exercise is based primarily on the principles of overload and progression, although the principle of overload also applies to isometric and plyometric exercise. All three training techniques produce improvement of muscular strength over time. Table 4-2 summarizes the six different techniques for improving muscular strength.

### Isometric Exercise

An **isometric exercise** involves a muscle contraction in which the length of the muscle remains constant while tension develops toward a maximum force against an immovable resistance[3] (Figure 4-17). To develop strength, the muscle should generate a maximum force for 10 seconds at a time, and this contraction should be repeated five to ten times per day.

**isometric exercise**
Contracts the muscle statically without changing its length.

**TABLE 4-2** Techniques for improving muscular strength

| Technique | Action | Equipment/Activity |
|---|---|---|
| Isometric exercise | Force develops while muscle length remains constant | Any immovable resistance |
| Progressive resistance exercise (PRE) | Force develops while the muscle shortens or lengthens | Free weights, Universal, Nautilus, Cybex, Eagle, Body Master |
| Isokinetic training | Force develops while muscle is contracting at a constant velocity | Cybex, Orthotron, Kincom, Biodex |
| Circuit training | Uses a combination of isometric, PRE, or isokinetic exercises organized into a series of stations | May use any of the equipment listed above |
| Plyometric exercise | Uses a rapid eccentric stretch of the muscle to facilitate an explosive concentric contraction | Hops, bounds, and depth jumping |
| Calisthenics | Uses body weight for resistance | No equipment needed (Sit-ups, push-ups, etc.) |

Isometric exercises are capable of increasing muscular strength; unfortunately, strength gains in a particular muscle will occur only in the position in which resistance is applied. At other positions in the range of motion, the strength curve drops off dramatically because of a lack of motor activity at those angles, and there is no corresponding increase in strength.

Another major disadvantage of isometric exercises is that they tend to produce a spike in blood pressure that can result in potentially life-threatening cardiovascular accidents. This sharp increase in blood pressure results from holding the breath and increasing pressure within the chest cavity. Consequently, the heart experiences a significant increase in

**Figure 4-17**

An isometric exercise involves a maximum force against an immovable resistance.

blood pressure. This spike has been referred to as the *Valsalva effect.* To avoid or minimize this effect, breathing should be done during the maximum contraction.

Isometric exercises certainly have a place in a conditioning program. In certain instances, an isometric contraction can greatly enhance a particular movement.[3] A common use for isometric exercises is in injury rehabilitation or reconditioning. Many conditions or ailments resulting either from trauma or overuse must be treated with strengthening exercises. Unfortunately, these problems may get worse with full range-of-motion strengthening exercises. It may be more desirable to make use of isometric exercises until the injury has healed to the point that full-range activities can be performed.

## Progressive Resistance Exercise

Progressive resistance exercise is perhaps the most commonly used and most popular technique for improving muscular strength. Progressive resistance exercise training uses exercises that strengthen muscles through a contraction that overcomes some fixed resistance produced by equipment such as dumbbells, barbells, or various weight machines. Progressive resistance exercise uses isotonic contractions in which force is generated while the muscle is changing in length.[12]

Isotonic contractions may be either *concentric* or *eccentric.* Suppose an athlete is going to perform a biceps curl (see Figure 4-28). To lift the weight from the starting position, the biceps muscle must contract and shorten (**concentric, or positive, contraction**). If the biceps muscle does not remain contracted when the weight is being lowered, gravity causes this weight to simply fall back to the starting position. Thus, to control the weight as it is being lowered, the biceps muscle must continue to contract while gradually lengthening (**eccentric, or negative, contraction**).

Various types of exercise equipment can be used with progressive resistance exercise including free weights (barbells and dumbbells) or weight machines such as Universal, Nautilus, Eagle, Cybex, and Body Master, to name a few (Figure 4-18A). Dumbbells and barbells require the use of iron plates of varying weights that can be easily changed by adding or subtracting equal amounts of weight to both sides of the bar.

Weight machines have a stack of weights that is lifted through a series of levers or pulleys. The stack of weights slides up and down on a pair of bars that restrict the movement to only one plane (Figure 4-18B). Weight can be increased or decreased simply by changing the position of a weight key.

There are advantages and disadvantages to both the free weights and the machines.[17] The weight machines are safer to use than free weights are. For example, athletes who are doing a bench press with free weights must have someone spot (help them lift the weights back onto the support racks if they don't have enough strength to complete the lift); otherwise the weights may be dropped on the chest. The weight machines allow an athlete to easily and safely drop the weight without fear of

**concentric (positive) contraction**
The muscle shortens while contracting against resistance.

**eccentric (negative) contraction**
The muscle lengthens while contracting against resistance.

**Figure 4-18**

A, This Cybex equipment is isotonic. B, Resistance may be easily altered by changing the key in the stack of weights.

injury. It is also a simple process to increase or decrease the weight on the weight machines by moving a single weight key, although changes can generally be made only in increments of 10 or 15 pounds. With free weights, iron plates must be added or removed from each side of the barbell.

Athletes will find a difference in the amount of weight that can be lifted with free weights versus the weight machines. Unlike the weight machines, free weights have no restricted motion and can thus move in many different directions, depending on the forces applied. Also, with free weights, an element of muscular control on the part of the lifter is required to prevent the weight from moving in any direction other than vertical. This control will usually decrease the amount of weight that can be lifted. Regardless of which type of equipment is used, the same principles of **isotonic** training may be applied.[17]

Progressive resistance exercise must incorporate both concentric and eccentric contractions.[12] It is possible to generate greater amounts of force against resistance with an eccentric contraction than with a concentric contraction. Eccentric contractions are more resistant to fatigue than are concentric contractions. The mechanical efficiency of eccentric exercise may be several times higher than that of concentric exercise. Research has clearly demonstrated that the muscle should be overloaded and fa-

**isotonic exercise**

Shortens and lengthens the muscle through a complete range of motion.

**Figure 4-19**

The cam on this Nautilus
machine is designed to
equalize resistance
throughout the full range
of motion.

tigued both concentrically and eccentrically for the greatest strength improvement to occur.

For athletes training specifically for the development of muscular strength, the concentric, or positive, portion of the exercise should require 1 to 2 seconds, whereas the eccentric, or negative, portion of the lift should require 2 to 4 seconds. The ratio of negative to positive should be approximately 2 to 1. Physiologically the muscle will fatigue much more rapidly concentrically than eccentrically.

One suggested disadvantage of any type of isotonic exercise is that the force required to move the resistance is constantly changing throughout the range of movement. Several years ago, Nautilus attempted to address this problem of changing force capabilities by using a cam in its pulley system (Figure 4-19). The cam has been individually designed for each piece of equipment so that the resistance is variable throughout the movement. This change in resistance at different points in the range has been labeled *accommodating resistance,* or **variable resistance.** Whether this design does what it claims to do is debatable. In real-life situations, it does not matter whether the resistance is changing.

> **variable resistance**
> Resistance is varied throughout the range of motion.

### Progressive Resistance Exercise Techniques

Perhaps the most confusing aspect of progressive resistance exercise is the terminology used to describe specific programs. Table 4-3 lists specific terms and their operational definitions, which may provide some clarification.

A considerable amount of research has been done in the area of resistance training to determine optimal techniques in terms of (1) the intensity or the amount of weight to be used, (2) the number of repetitions, (3) the number of sets, (4) the recovery period, and (5) the frequency of training.

There is no such thing as an optimal strength-training program.[5] Achieving total agreement on a program of resistance training that

**TABLE 4-3** Progressive resistance exercise terminology

| Terms | Definitions |
| --- | --- |
| Repetitions | Number of times a specific movement is repeated |
| Repetitions maximum (RM) | Maximum number of repetitions at a given weight |
| Set | A particular number of repetitions |
| Intensity | The amount of weight or resistance lifted |
| Recovery period | The rest interval between sets |
| Frequency | The number of times an exercise is done in a week's period |

includes specific recommendations relative to repetitions, sets, intensity, recovery time, and frequency among researchers and/or other experts in resistance training is impossible. However, the following general recommendations provide an effective resistance training program.

For any given exercise, the amount of weight selected should be sufficient to allow at most six to eight repetitions in each of three sets, with a recovery period of 60 to 90 seconds between sets. Initial selection of a starting weight may require some trial and error to achieve this six to eight repetitions maximum (RM) range. If at least three sets of six repetitions cannot be completed, the weight is too heavy and should be reduced. If it is possible to do more than three sets of eight repetitions, the weight is too light and should be increased. Progression to heavier weights is determined by the ability to perform at least eight RM in each of three sets. When progressing weight, an increase of about 10 percent of the current weight being lifted should still allow at least six RM in each of three sets.[5]

Muscular endurance is defined as the ability to perform repeated muscle contractions against resistance for an extended period. Most weight-training experts believe that muscular strength and muscular endurance are closely related. As one factor improves, the tendency is for the other factor to improve also. When weight training for strength, heavier weights with a lower number of repetitions should be used. Conversely, endurance training uses lighter weights with a greater number of repetitions.[5]

Endurance training should consist of three sets of ten to fifteen repetitions using the same criteria for weight selection, progression, and frequency as recommended for progressive resistance exercise. Thus, training regimens for both muscular strength and endurance are similar in terms of sets and numbers of repetitions. Athletes who possess great strength levels tend to also exhibit greater muscular endurance when asked to perform repeated contractions against resistance.[5]

A particular muscle or muscle group should be exercised consistently every other day. Thus, the frequency of weight training should be at least three times per week but no more than four times per week. Serious weight trainers commonly lift every day; however, they exercise different muscle groups on successive days. For example, Monday, Wednesday, and Friday may be used for upper body muscles, whereas Tuesday, Thursday, and Saturday are used for lower body muscles.

Regardless of what technique is used, to improve strength in a muscle, it must be overloaded in a progressive manner. This criterion is the basis of progressive resistance exercise. The amount of weight used and the number of repetitions performed must be sufficient to make the muscle work at a higher intensity than it is used to. This is the single most critical factor in any strength-training program.

Figures 4-20 to 4-43 describe exercises for strength improvement of shoulder, hip, knee, and ankle joint movements. These exercises are demonstrated using free weights (barbells, dumbbells, weights, and some machine weights). Any of these exercises may be performed on various commercial weight machines such as Cybex or Body Master. Positions may differ slightly when different pieces of equipment are used. However, the joint motions that affect the various muscles are still the same.

**Figure 4-20**

Bench press
Joints affected: Shoulder, elbow
Movement: Pushing away
Position: Supine, feet flat on floor, back flat on bench
Primary muscles: Pectoralis major, tricep

**Figure 4-21**

Incline press
Joints affected: Shoulder, elbow
Movement: Pushing upward and away
Position: Supine at an inclined angle, feet flat on floor, back flat against bench
Primary muscles: Pectoralis major, triceps

*Text continued on page 83.*

**Figure 4-22**

Shoulder rotation
Joint affected: Shoulder
Movement: External rotation
Position: Supine, shoulder at 90-degree angle and elbow flexed at 90-degree angle
Primary muscles: infraspinatus, teres minor

**Figure 4-23**

Military press
Joints affected: Shoulder, elbow
Movement: Pressing the weight overhead
Position: Standing, back straight
Primary muscles: Deltoid, trapezius, tricep

**Figure 4-24**

Lateral pull-downs
Joints affected: Shoulder,
elbow
Movement: Pulling the bar
down behind the neck
Position: Kneeling, back
straight, head up
Primary muscles: Latissimus
dorsi, biceps

**Figure 4-25**

Flys
Joint affected: Shoulder
Movement: Horizontal flexion, bringing arms together over head
Position: Lying on back, feet flat on floor, back flat on bench
Primary muscles: Deltoid, pectoralis major

**Figure 4-26**

Bent-over rows
Joint affected: Shoulder
Movement: Adduction of the scapula
Position: Standing bent over at waist, knee on bench
Primary muscles: Trapezius, rhomboids

**Figure 4-27**

Shoulder medial rotation
Joint affected: Shoulder
Movement: Internal rotation, lifting weight off the floor
Position: Supine, shoulder abducted and elbow flexed
Primary muscles: Subscapularis

**Figure 4-28**

Bicep curls
Joint affected: Elbow
Movement: Elbow flexion, curling the weight up to the shoulder
Position: Standing feet spread at shoulder width, back straight, arms extended
Primary muscles: Biceps

**Figure 4-29**

Tricep extensions
Joint affected: Elbow
Movement: Elbow extension, pressing weight toward ceiling
Position: Standing, elbows pointing directly toward ceiling beside ears
Primary muscles: Triceps

Organizing and Establishing
an Effective Athletic Health
Care System

**Figure 4-30**

Wrist curls
Joint affected: Wrist
Movement: Wrist flexion,
curling weight upward
Position: Seated, forearms on
table, palms up
Primary muscles: Long
flexors of forearm

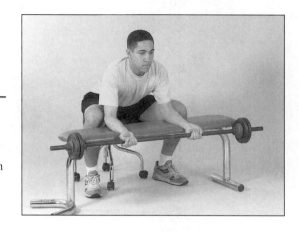

**Figure 4-31**

Wrist extensions
Joint affected: Wrist
Movement: Extension,
curling weight upward
Position: Seated, forearms on
table, palms down
Primary muscles: Long
extensors of forearm

**Figure 4-32**

Leg raises
Joint affected: Hip
Movement: Hip abduction, lifting leg up
Position: Lying on side, weight band strapped around ankle
Primary muscles: Hip abductors

**Figure 4-33**

Leg lifts
Joint affected: Hip
Movement: Hip adduction, lifting bottom leg up
Position: Lying on side, one leg lifted upward, weight band around ankle
Primary muscles: Hip adductors

**Figure 4-34**

Bent-knee leg lifts
Joint affected: Hip
Movement: Hip flexion, lifting knee up
Position: Sitting, knee flexed, weight around ankle
Primary muscles: Iliopsoas

**Figure 4-35**

Reverse leg lifts
Joint affected: Hip
Movement: Hip extension, lifting leg toward ceiling
Position: Prone, knee extended, weight band around ankle
Primary muscles: Gluteus maximus, hamstrings

**Figure 4-36**

Hip medial rotation
Joint affected: Hip
Movement: Internal rotation,
rotating lower leg outward
Position: Sitting, knee flexed,
weight on ankle
Primary muscles: Medial
rotators

**Figure 4-37**

Hip lateral rotation
Joint affected: Hip
Movement: Lateral rotation,
rotating lower leg inward
Position: Sitting, knee flexed,
weight on ankle
Primary muscles: Lateral
rotators

**Figure 4-38**

Quadricep extensions
Joint affected: Knee
Movement: Extension,
straightening knee
Position: Sitting, on knee
machine
Primary muscles: Quadriceps
group

**Figure 4-39**

Hamstring curls
Joint affected: Knee
Movement: Flexion, bending
knee and lifting weight up
Position: Prone, on knee
machine
Primary muscles: Hamstring
group

**Figure 4-40**

Toe raises
Joint affected: Ankle
Movement: Plantar flexion,
pressing up on toes
Position: Standing on both
legs and lifting body weight
Primary muscles:
Gastrocnemius and soleus

**Figure 4-41**

Ankle inversion
Joint affected: Ankle
Movement: Inversion, lifting
the sole of the foot up and in
Position: Sitting, knee flexed,
instep up, weight on foot
Primary muscles: Anterior
tibialis

**Figure 4-42**

Ankle eversion
Joint affected: Ankle
Movement: Eversion, lifting
the sole of the foot up and
out
Position: Sitting, knee flexed,
instep down, weight on foot
Primary muscles: Peroneals

**Figure 4-43**

Ankle dorsiflexion
Joint affected: Ankle
Movement: Dorsiflexion,
lifting the toes upward
Position: Sitting, knee flexed,
heel on edge of table, weight
on foot
Primary muscles: Dorsiflexors
in shin

## Isokinetic Exercise

An **isokinetic exercise** involves a muscle contraction in which the length of the muscle is changing while the contraction is performed at a constant velocity. In theory, maximum resistance is provided throughout the range of motion by the machine. The resistance provided by the machine will move only at some preset speed, regardless of the force applied to it by the individual. Thus, the key to isokinetic exercise is not the resistance but the speed at which resistance can be moved.[8]

Several isokinetic devices are available commercially: Cybex, Biodex, and KinCom are among the more common isokinetic devices (Figure 4-44). In general, these devices rely on hydraulic, pneumatic, and mechanical

**isokinetic exercise**
Resistance is given at a fixed velocity of movement with accommodating resistance.

**Figure 4-44**

Biodex is one of the more widely used types of isokinetic exercise equipment.

pressure systems to produce this constant velocity of motion. The majority of isokinetic devices are capable of resisting both concentric and eccentric contractions at a fixed speed to exercise a muscle.

A major disadvantage of these units is their cost. Many of them come with a computer and printing device and are used primarily as diagnostic and rehabilitative tools in the treatment of various injuries.

Isokinetic devices are designed so that regardless of the amount of force applied against a resistance, the device can only be moved at a certain speed. That speed will be the same whether maximum force or only half the maximum force is applied. Consequently, when training isokinetically, it is absolutely necessary to exert as much force against the resistance as possible (maximum effort) for maximum strength gains to occur. This exertion is another major problem with an isokinetic strength-training program. Anyone who has been involved in a weight-training program knows that on some days it is difficult to find the motivation to work out. Because isokinetic training requires a maximum effort, it is very easy to cheat and not go through the workout at a high level of intensity. In a progressive resistance exercise program, the athlete knows how much weight has to be lifted with how many repetitions. Therefore isokinetic training is often more effective if a partner system is used as a means of motivation toward a maximum effort.

Assuming that a maximum effort is generated on each repetition, a general recommendation for isokinetic training is to use three sets of ten to fifteen repetitions at a selected speed of movement. If the athlete is exerting maximum effort, fatigue will usually occur at some point within each set.

Theoretically, maximum strength gains are best achieved through the isokinetic training method in which the velocity is equal throughout the range of motion if the exercise is done properly with a maximum effort. However, no conclusive research supports this theory.[8]

### Circuit Training

> **circuit training**
> Exercise stations that consist of various combinations of weight training, flexibility, calisthenics, and aerobic exercises.

**Circuit training** uses a series of exercise stations that consist of various combinations of weight training, flexibility, calisthenics, and brief aerobic exercises. Circuits may be designed to accomplish many different training goals. With circuit training, the athlete moves rapidly from one station to the next and performs whatever exercise is to be done at that station within a specified time. A typical circuit consists of eight to twelve stations, and the entire circuit is repeated three times.

Circuit training is definitely an effective technique for improving strength and flexibility. Certainly if the pace or the time interval between stations is rapid and if workload is maintained at a high level of intensity with heart rates at or above target training levels, the cardiorespiratory system benefits from this circuit. However, little research evidence shows that circuit training is very effective in improving cardiorespiratory endurance. It should be and is most often used as a technique for developing and improving muscular strength and endurance. Figure 4-45 provides an example of a simple circuit training setup.

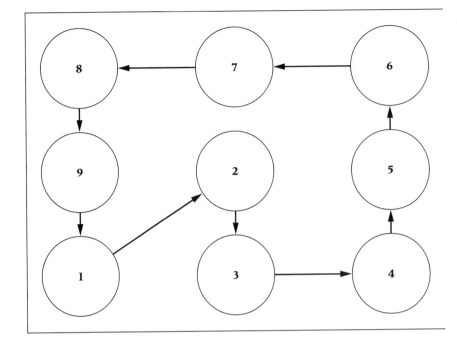

**Figure 4-45**

Sample circuit program. Station 1, squat thrusts, 75% maximum number of repetitions performed in 1 minute; Station 2, general flexion exercise, performed for 1 minute; Station 3, jump rope for 1 minute; Station 4, abdominal curls with weights, 75% maximum number of repetitions; Station 5, two-arm curls, 75% maximum number of repetitions; Station 6, vertical jump; (sargent), 75% maximum number of repetitions performed in 1 minute; Station 7, wrist curls with weight for 1 minute; Station 8, half squat, heels raised, exercise with weight, 75% maximum number of repetitions; Station 9, general flexion exercises.

## Plyometric Exercise

**Plyometric exercise** is a technique of exercise that involves a rapid eccentric (lengthening) stretch of a muscle, followed immediately by a rapid concentric contraction of that muscle for the purpose of producing a forceful explosive movement over a short period.[9] Plyometric exercises involve hops, bounds, and depth jumping for the lower extremity and the use of medicine balls and other types of weighted equipment for the upper extremity. Depth jumping is an example of a plyometric exercise in which an individual jumps to the ground from a specified height and then quickly jumps again as soon as ground contact is made (Figure 4-46).

The greater the stretch put on the muscle from its resting length immediately before the concentric contraction, the greater the resistance the muscle can overcome. Plyometrics emphasize the speed of the stretch phase. The rate of stretch is more critical than the magnitude of the stretch. An advantage to using plyometric exercise is that it can help develop eccentric control in dynamic movements. Plyometrics tend to place a great deal of stress on the musculoskeletal system. The learning and perfection of specific jumping skills and other plyometric exercises must be technically correct and specific to the athlete's age, activity, and physical and skill development.[20]

Recommendations for plyometric exercise are variable, but the athlete should once again adhere to the three sets of six to eight repetitions rule.

> **plyometric exercise**
> Maximizes the myotatic or stretch reflex.

**Figure 4-46**

Depth jumping off a box or platform is a form of plyometric exercise.

Calisthenics, or free exercise,
uses the force of gravity as
resistance.

## Calisthenic Strengthening Exercises

Calisthenics, or free exercise, is one of the more easily available means of developing strength. Isotonic movement exercises can be graded according to intensity by using gravity as an aid, ruling gravity out, moving against gravity, or using the body or body part as a resistance against gravity. Most calisthenics require the athlete to support the body or move the total body against the force of gravity. Push-ups are a good example of a vigorous antigravity free exercise. To be considered maximally effective, the isotonic calisthenic exercise, as in all types of exercise, must be performed in an exacting manner and in full range of motion. In most cases, ten or more repetitions are performed for each exercise and are repeated in sets of two or three.

Some free exercises use an isometric or holding phase instead of using a full range of motion. Examples of these exercises are back extensions and sit-ups. When the exercise produces maximum muscle tension, it is held between 6 and 10 seconds and then repeated one to three times. The exercises illustrated in Figures 4-47 to 4-55 are recommended because they work on specific muscle groups and with a specific purpose. The athlete should work quickly and move from one exercise to the next without delay.

A

B

**Figure 4-47**

Curl-ups. A, Beginning. B, Intermediate.
C, Advanced.
Joints affected: Spinal vertebral joints
Movement: Trunk flexion
Instructions: Lying on back, hands either on chest or behind back, knees flexed to 90-degree angle, feet on floor; curl trunk and head to approximately 45-degree angle.
Primary muscles: Rectus abdominis.

C

*Text continued on page 91.*

A

B

**Figure 4-48**

A, Push-ups. B, Modified push-ups.
Purpose: Strengthening
Muscles: Triceps and pectoralis major
Repetitions: Beginner, 10; intermediate, 20; advanced, 30
Instructions: Keep the upper trunk and legs extended in a straight line; touch floor with chest.
Caution: Avoid hyperextending the back, especially in modified push-ups.

**Figure 4-49**

Tricep extensions
Purpose: Strengthening and range of
motion at shoulder joint
Muscles: Triceps and trapezius
Repetitions: Beginner, 7; intermediate, 12;
advanced, 18
Instructions: Begin with arms extended
and body straight;
lower buttocks until they touch the
ground, then press back up.

**Figure 4-50**

Trunk rotation. A, Beginner. B, Advanced.
Muscles: Internal and external obliques
Repetitions: Beginner, 10 each direction;
intermediate, 15 each direction; advanced,
20 each direction
Instructions: Rotate trunk from side to
side until knees touch the floor, keeping
knees slightly bent.
Caution: This exercise should be done
only by those who already have strong
abdominals.

**Figure 4-51**

Sitting tucks
Purpose: Strengthen abdominals and stretch low back
Muscles: Rectus abdominis and erector muscles in low
back
Repetitions: Beginner, 10; intermediate, 20; advanced, 30
Instructions: Keep legs and upper back off the ground and
pull knees to chest.
Caution: This exercise should be done only by those who
have strong abdominals.

**Figure 4-52**

Bicycle
Purpose: Strengthen hip flexors and stretch lower back
Muscles: Iliopsoas
Repetitions: Beginner, 10 each side; intermediate, 20 each side; advanced, 30 each side
Instructions: Alternately flex and extend legs as if you were pedaling a bicycle.

**Figure 4-53**

Leg lifts. A, Front. B, Back. C, Side (leg up). D, Side (leg down).
Purpose: Strengthen A, hip flexors; B, hip extensors; C, hip abductors; D, hip adductors.
Muscles: A, Iliopsoas; B, gluteus maximus; C, gluteus medius; D, adductor group.
Repetitions: Beginner, 10 each leg; intermediate, 15 each leg; advanced, 20 each leg
Instructions: Raise the exercising leg up as far as possible in each position.

A

B

**Figure 4-54**

A, Chin-ups. B, Modified chin-ups.
Purpose: Strengthening and stretch of shoulder joint
Muscles: Biceps, brachialis, and latissimus dorsi
Repetitions: Beginner, 7; intermediate, 10; advanced, 15
Instructions: Pull up until chin touches top of bar.

**Figure 4-55**

Buttock tucks
Purpose: Strengthen muscles of buttocks
Muscles: Gluteus maximus and hamstrings
Repetitions: Beginner, 10; intermediate, 15; advanced, 20
Instructions: Lying flat on back with knees bent, arch back
and thrust the pelvis upward.

Strength Training Considerations for Female Athletes

Strength is just as important to women as it is to men.[14] The average female is incapable of building significant muscle bulk through weight training. Significant muscle hypertrophy is dependent on the presence of an anabolic steroidal hormone called *testosterone*. Testosterone is considered a male hormone, although all women possess some testosterone in their systems. Women with higher testosterone levels tend to have more masculine characteristics such as increased facial and body hair, a deeper voice, and the potential to develop a little more muscle bulk.

The average woman does not need to worry about developing large bulky muscles with strength building. What does happen is that muscle tone is improved. Muscle tone refers to the firmness, or tension, of the muscle during a resting state. For example, doing sit-ups increases the firmness of the abdominal muscles and makes them more resistant to fatigue.

A woman in weight training will probably see some remarkable gains in strength initially, even though her muscle bulk does not increase. How is this possible? These initial strength gains, which can be attributed to improved neuromuscular system efficiency, tend to plateau, and in the female, minimal improvement in muscular strength will be realized during a continuing strength-training program. These initial neuromuscular strength gains will also be seen in men, although their strength will continue to increase with appropriate training. Women who do possess higher testosterone levels have the potential to further increase their strength because of the development of greater muscle bulk.

Perhaps the most critical difference between men and women regarding physical performance is the ratio of strength to body weight. The reduced *strength/body weight ratio* in women is the result of their higher percentage of body fat.[14] The strength/body weight ratio may be significantly improved through weight training by decreasing the body fat percentage while increasing lean weight. Strength training programs for women should follow the same guidelines as those for men.

> Perhaps the most critical performance difference between men and women is the ratio of strength to weight.

## WHY IS CARDIORESPIRATORY FITNESS IMPORTANT FOR AN ATHLETE?

By definition, **cardiorespiratory endurance** is the ability to perform whole-body large muscle activities for extended periods. The cardiorespiratory system provides a means by which oxygen is supplied to the various tissues of the body. A healthy cardiorespiratory system is critical both for performance and for preventing undue fatigue that may predispose an athlete to injury.[15]

*Aerobic* exercise is great for building cardiorespiratory fitness. An aerobic activity is one in which the intensity of the activity is low enough that the cardiovascular system can supply enough oxygen to continue the activity for long periods. An activity in which the intensity is so great that the demand for oxygen is greater than the body's ability to deliver

> **cardiorespiratory endurance**
> Ability to perform activities for extended periods.

> Cardiorespiratory endurance refers to the body's ability to transport and use oxygen efficiently.

**TABLE 4-4** Comparison of aerobic versus anaerobic activities

| | Mode | Relative Intensity | Intensity | Frequency | Duration | Miscellaneous |
|---|---|---|---|---|---|---|
| Aerobic activities | Continuous, long-duration, sustained activities | Less intense | 60%–90% of MHR | At least three but not more than six times per week | 20–60 min | Less risk to sedentary or older individuals |
| Anaerobic activities | Explosive, short-duration, burst-type activities | More intense | 90%–100% of MHR | Three to four times per week | 10 sec–2 min | Used in sport and team activities |

4–3

***Critical Thinking*** Exercise

A high school shot-putter has been working intensely on weight training to improve his muscular power. In particular he has been concentrating on lifting extremely heavy free weights using a low number of repetitions (three sets of six to eight reps). Although his strength has improved significantly over the last several months, he is not seeing the same degree of improvement in his throws even though his coach says that his technique is very good.

**?** The athlete is frustrated with his performance and wants to know if he can add anything to his training program that might enhance his performance.

oxygen is called an *anaerobic* activity. Short bursts of muscle contraction, as in running or swimming sprints or lifting weights, use predominantly the anaerobic system. However, endurance-type activities that last for a longer time depend a great deal on the aerobic system. In most activities both aerobic and anaerobic systems function simultaneously. Table 4-4 provides a comparison summary between aerobic and anaerobic activities.

The capacity of the cardiorespiratory system to carry oxygen throughout the body depends on the coordinated function of four components: (1) the heart, (2) the blood vessels, (3) the blood, and (4) the lungs. Improvement of cardiorespiratory endurance through exercise occurs because of an increase in the capability of each of these four components in providing necessary oxygen to the working tissues.[4] A basic discussion of the training effects and responses to exercise that occur in the heart should make it easier to understand why the training techniques to be discussed later are effective in improving cardiorespiratory endurance.

How Does Exercise Affect the Function of the Heart?

The heart is the main pumping mechanism and circulates oxygenated blood throughout the body to the various tissues. The heart receives oxygen-poor blood from the venous system and pumps that blood through the pulmonary vessels to the lungs, where carbon dioxide is exchanged for oxygen. The oxygen-rich blood then returns to the heart, from which it exits through the aorta to the arterial system and is circulated throughout the body, supplying oxygen to the tissues (Figure 4-56).[4]

During exercise, muscles use oxygen at a much higher rate, and thus the heart must pump more oxygenated blood to meet this increased demand.

WHAT DETERMINES HOW EFFICIENTLY THE BODY IS USING OXYGEN?

The greatest rate at which oxygen can be taken in and used during exercise is referred to as *maximum aerobic capacity*.[6] Maximum aerobic capacity determines how much oxygen can be used during 1 minute of maximal

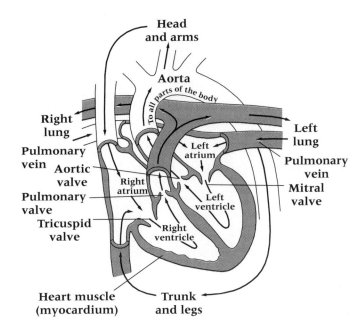

**Figure 4-56**

Anatomy of the heart.

exercise. This rate is most often presented in terms of the volume of oxygen used relative to body weight per unit of time (ml/kg/min). Normal maximum oxygen utilization for most men and women aged 15 to 25 years falls in the range of 38 to 46 ml/kg/min. A world-class male marathon runner may have a maximum aerobic capacity in the 70 to 80 ml/kg/min range whereas a female marathoner may have a 60 to 70 ml/kg/min range.

The performance of any activity requires a certain rate of oxygen use that is about the same for everybody. Generally the greater the rate or intensity of the activity, the greater the oxygen demand. Each person has his or her own maximum rate of oxygen consumption, and the ability to perform an activity is closely related to the amount of oxygen required by that activity.

The maximum rate at which oxygen can be used is to a large extent a genetically determined characteristic. Each person's maximum aerobic capacity falls within a given range. The more active the athlete, the higher the existing maximum aerobic capacity will be within that range. The less active the athlete, the lower the maximum aerobic capacity will be in that range. Thus, athletes engaging in a serious training program can increase aerobic capacity to its highest limit within their range.

The range of maximum aerobic capacity inherited is to a large extent determined by the ratio of fast-twitch to slow-twitch muscle fibers. Athletes with a high percentage of slow-twitch muscle fibers are more resistant to fatigue and are able to use oxygen more efficiently; thus maximum aerobic capacity will be higher.

Organizing and Establishing
an Effective Athletic Health
Care System

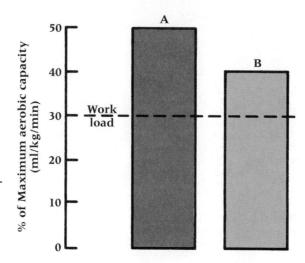

**Figure 4-57**

Athlete A should be able to
work longer than Athlete B
as a result of using a lower
percentage of maximum
aerobic capacity.

*Critical Thinking* Exercise

A female soccer player has a
grade I ankle sprain that is
likely to keep her out of practice for about a week. She has
worked extremely hard on her
fitness levels and is very concerned that not being able to
run for an entire week will
really hurt her cardiorespiratory
fitness.

? What activities should the
coach recommend during her
rehabilitation period that can
help her maintain her existing
level of cardiorespiratory
endurance?

Fatigue is closely related to the percentage of maximum aerobic capacity that a particular activity demands. The greater the percentage of
maximum aerobic capacity that is required during an activity, the less
time the activity can be performed. Fatigue occurs in part when insufficient oxygen is supplied to muscles. For example, Figure 4-57 presents
two athletes, A and B. A has a maximum aerobic capacity of 50
ml/kg/min, whereas B has a maximum aerobic capacity of only 40
ml/kg/min. If A and B are exercising at the same intensity, then A will be
working at a much lower percentage of maximum aerobic capacity than
B is. Consequently, A should be able to sustain his or her activity over a
much longer time. Everyday activities such as walking up stairs or running to catch a bus may be adversely affected if a person's ability to use
oxygen efficiently is impaired. Certainly the ability to perform a sport activity is hindered if an athlete's level of cardiorespiratory endurance is not
what it should be. Thus improvement of cardiorespiratory endurance
must be an essential component of any fitness program.

How Is Maximum Aerobic Capacity Determined?

The most accurate technique for measuring aerobic capacity must be
done in a laboratory. This technique involves exercising a subject on a
treadmill or bicycle ergometer at a specific intensity and then monitoring
heart rate and collecting samples of expired air using somewhat expensive and sophisticated equipment. Obviously for the typical person this
technique is somewhat impractical. Therefore, the technique used most
often is to monitor heart rate as a means of estimating a percentage of
maximum aerobic capacity.[6]

Monitoring heart rate is an indirect method of estimating maximum
aerobic capacity. In general, heart rate and aerobic capacity have a linear relationship, although at very low intensities and at high intensities this linear

y-axis: Percentage of maximum aerobic capacity
x-axis: Heart rate (% maximum)

**Figure 4-58**

Maximum heart rate is
achieved at about the same
time as maximum aerobic
capacity.

**Figure 4-59**

The radial artery provides the
most accurate estimation of
pulse rate.

relationship breaks down (Figure 4-58). The greater the intensity of the exercise, the higher the heart rate. Because of this existing relationship, the
rate of oxygen utilization can be estimated by taking the heart rate.

### Monitoring Heart Rate

Heart rate can be determined by taking a pulse rate at specific sites. The
most accurate site for measuring the pulse rate is the radial artery located
on the thumb side of the wrist joint (Figure 4-59). An accurate heart rate
can be determined by counting the number of beats that occur in 10 seconds and then multiplying that number by six. Heart rate should be monitored within 15 seconds after stopping exercise.

# WHAT TRAINING TECHNIQUES CAN IMPROVE CARDIORESPIRATORY ENDURANCE?

There are a number of different methods through which cardiorespiratory endurance may be improved, including (1) continuous training, (2) interval training, and (3) fartlek training. Regardless of the training technique used for the improvement of cardiorespiratory endurance, one principal goal remains the same: to increase the ability of the cardiorespiratory system to supply a sufficient amount of oxygen to working muscles. Without oxygen, the body is incapable of producing energy for an extended time.

## Continuous Training

Continuous training is a technique that uses exercises performed at the same level of intensity for long periods. Continuous training has four considerations:

- The type of activity
- The frequency of the activity
- The intensity of the activity
- The duration of the activity

### Type of Activity

The type of activity used in continuous training must be aerobic. Aerobic activities are any activities that use large amounts of oxygen, elevate the heart rate, and maintain it at that level for an extended time. Aerobic activities generally involve repetitive, whole body, large-muscle movements performed over an extended time. Examples of aerobic activities include walking, running, swimming, cycling, rowing, cross-country skiing, and so on. The advantage of these aerobic activities as opposed to more intermittent activities, such as racquetball, squash, basketball, or tennis, is that with aerobic activities it is easy to regulate intensity by either speeding up or slowing down the pace. Because it is already known that the given intensity of the workload elicits a given heart rate, these aerobic activities allow athletes to maintain heart rate at a specified *target level*. Intermittent activities involve variable speeds and intensities that cause the heart rate to fluctuate considerably. Although these intermittent activities will improve cardiorespiratory endurance, they are much more difficult to monitor in terms of intensity.

### Frequency of Activity

To see at least minimal improvement in cardiorespiratory endurance, it is necessary for the average person to engage in no less than three exercise sessions per week. A competitive athlete should be prepared to train as often as six times per week. Everyone should take off at least one day per week to give damaged tissues a chance to repair themselves.

Intensity of Activity

The intensity of the exercise is also a critical factor, although recommendations regarding training intensities vary. This is particularly true in the early stages of training, when the body is forced to make a lot of adjustments to increased workload demands.

**Determining exercise intensity by monitoring heart rate** The objective of aerobic exercise is to elevate heart rate to a specified target rate and maintain it at that level during the entire workout. Because heart rate is directly related to the intensity of the exercise and to the rate of oxygen utilization, it becomes a relatively simple process to identify a specific workload (pace) that will make the heart rate plateau at the desired level. By monitoring heart rate, athletes know whether the pace is too fast or too slow to get the heart rate into a target range.

Heart rate can be increased or decreased by speeding up or slowing down pace. As mentioned, heart rate increases proportionately with the intensity of the workload and will plateau after 2 to 3 minutes of activity. Thus the athlete should be actively engaged in the workout for 2 to 3 minutes before measuring his or her pulse.

Several formulas can be used to identify a training *target heart rate*.[23] To calculate a specific target heart rate, maximum heart rate must first be calculated. Exact determination of maximum heart rate involves exercising an individual at a maximal level and monitoring the heart rate using an electrocardiogram. This process is difficult outside a laboratory. An approximate estimate of maximum heart rate for both males and females in the population is about 220 beats per minute. Maximum heart rate is related to age. As age increases, maximum heart rate decreases. A simple estimate of maximum heart rate (HR) is Maximum HR = 220 − Age. For a 20-year-old individual, maximum heart rate is about 200 beats per minute (220 − 20 = 200). Thus if training intensity is to be at 70 percent of maximum heart rate, the target heart rate can be calculated by multiplying 0.7 × (220 − Age).

Another commonly used formula that takes into account current levels of fitness is the Karvonen equation:[19]

*Target HR = Resting HR\* + (0.6 [Maximum HR − Resting HR])*

Resting heart rate generally falls between 60 and 80 beats per minute. A 20-year-old athlete with a resting pulse of 70 beats per minute, according to the Karvonen equation, has a target training heart rate of 148 beats per minute (70 + 0.6 [200 − 70] = 148).

Regardless of the formula used, the American College of Sports Medicine recommends that young healthy individuals train with a target heart rate in the 60 percent to 85 percent range when training continuously. Exercising at a 70 percent level is considered a moderate level

---

\* True resting heart rate should be monitored with the subject lying down.

---

**training effect**
Stroke volume increases
while heart rate is reduced
at a given exercise load.

---

**TABLE 4-5** Rating of
perceived exertion

| Scale | Verbal Rating |
|-------|---------------|
| 6 | |
| 7 | Very, very light |
| 8 | |
| 9 | Very light |
| 10 | |
| 11 | Fairly light |
| 12 | |
| 13 | Somewhat hard |
| 14 | |
| 15 | Hard |
| 16 | |
| 17 | Very hard |
| 18 | |
| 19 | Very, very hard |
| 20 | |

---

**interval training**
Alternating periods of work
with active recovery.

---

because activity can be continued for a long time with little discomfort and still produce a **training effect.** A highly trained athlete will not find it difficult to sustain a heart rate at the 85 percent level.

**Determining exercise intensity through rating of perceived exertion** *Rating of perceived exertion* (RPE) can be used in addition to heart rate monitoring to indicate exercise intensity.[13] During exercise, individuals are asked to rate subjectively on a numerical scale from 6 to 20 exactly how they feel relative to their level of exertion (Table 4-5). More intense exercise that requires a higher level of oxygen consumption and energy expenditure is directly related to higher subjective ratings of perceived exertion. Over time, individuals can be taught to exercise at a specific RPE that relates directly to more objective measures of exercise intensity.

### Duration of Activity

For minimal improvement to occur, the American College of Sports Medicine recommends 20 to 60 minutes of workout/activity with the heart rate elevated to training levels. Generally, the greater the duration of the workout, the greater the improvement in cardiorespiratory endurance. The competitive athlete should train for at least 45 minutes per session.

## ADVANCED TRAINING METHODS

### Interval Training

Unlike continuous training, **interval training** involves activities that are more intermittent. Interval training consists of alternating periods of relatively intense work and active recovery. It allows for performance of much more work at a more intense workload over a longer period than does working continuously. In continuous training, the athlete strives to work at an intensity of about 60 to 85 percent of maximum heart rate. Obviously, sustaining activity at the higher intensity over a 20-minute period is extremely difficult. The advantage of interval training is that it allows work at the 80 percent or higher level for a short period followed by an active period of recovery during which the athlete may be working at only 30 to 45 percent of maximum heart rate. Thus the intensity of the workout and its duration can be greater than with continuous training.

Most sports are anaerobic, involving short bursts of intense activity followed by a sort of active recovery period (for example, football, basketball, soccer, or tennis). Training with the interval technique allows the athlete to be more sport specific during the workout. With interval training, the overload principle is applied by making the training period much more intense. There are several important considerations in interval training. The *training period* is the amount of time that continuous activity is actually being performed, and the *recovery period* is the time between training periods. A *set* is a group of combined training and recovery periods, and a *repetition* is the number of training/recovery periods per set.

*Training time* or *distance* refers to the rate or distance of the training period. The training/recovery ratio indicates a time ratio for training versus recovery.

An example of interval training is a soccer player running sprints. An interval workout would involve running ten 120-yard sprints in under 20 seconds each, with a 1-minute walking recovery period between each sprint. During this training session, the soccer player's heart rate will probably increase to 85 to 90 percent of maximum level during the sprint and will probably fall to the 35 to 45 percent level during the recovery period.

## Fartlek Training

*Fartlek,* a training technique that is a type of cross-country running, originated in Sweden. Fartlek literally means "speed play." It is similar to interval training in that the athlete must run for a specified period; however, specific pace and speed are not identified. The course for a fartlek workout should be a varied terrain with some level running, some uphill and downhill running, and some running through obstacles such as trees or rocks. The object is to put surges into a running workout, varying the length of the surges according to individual purposes. One big advantage of fartlek training is that because the pace and terrain are always changing, the training session is less regimented and allows for an effective alternative in the training routine. Most people who jog or walk around the community are really engaging in a fartlek-type workout.

Again, if fartlek training is going to improve cardiorespiratory endurance, it must elevate the heart rate to at least minimal training levels (60%–85%). Fartlek may best be used as an off-season conditioning activity or as a change-of-pace activity to counteract the boredom of a training program that uses the same activity day after day.

## COACH'S CORNER

The following is a checklist of factors the coach should focus on in a training and conditioning program to make sure the athlete is fit and to prevent injuries.

☐ Incorporate the concept of periodization into the year-round training and conditioning plan

☐ Make sure the athlete does a proper warm-up before training and a cooldown afterwards

☐ Incorporate flexibility training

☐ Use ballistic, static, or PNF stretching techniques

☐ Select specific and appropriate stretching exercises to improve flexibility

☐ Incorporate training techniques to improve muscular strength, endurance, or power

☐ Use isometric, progressive resistance exercise, isokinetic, plyometric, or calisthenic techniques or some combination of these to achieve the goal of strength development

☐ Select specific strengthening exercises to be included in a workout

☐ Incorporate training techniques to improve cardiorespiratory fitness

☐ Use continuous training to improve aerobic capacity

☐ Use interval training or fartlek training to improve anaerobic function

## SUMMARY

- Proper physical conditioning for sports participation should prepare the athlete for a high-level performance while helping to prevent injuries inherent to that sport.

- Year-round conditioning is essential in most sports to assist in preventing injuries. Periodization is an approach to conditioning that attempts to bring about peak performance while reducing injuries and overtraining in the athlete by developing a training and conditioning program to be followed throughout the various seasons.

- Physical conditioning must follow the SAID principle—an acronym for specific adaptation to imposed demands. It must work toward making the body as lean as possible, commensurate with the athlete's sport.

- A proper warm-up should precede conditioning, and a proper cooldown should follow. It takes at least 15 to 30 minutes of gradual warm-up to bring the body to a state of readiness for vigorous sports training and participation. Warming up consists of general, unrelated activities followed by specific, related activities.

- Optimum flexibility is necessary for success in most sports. Too much flexibility can allow joint trauma to occur, whereas too little flexibility can result in muscle tears or strains. The safest and most effective means of increasing flexibility are static stretching and the PNF techniques.

- Strength is that capacity to exert a force or the ability to perform work against a resistance. There are numerous means to develop strength, including isometric exercise, progressive resistance exercise, isokinetic exercise, circuit training, plyometric exercise, and calisthenics.

- Cardiorespiratory endurance is the ability to perform whole-body, large-muscle activities repeatedly for long periods. Maximum aerobic capacity is the greatest determinant of the level of cardiorespiratory endurance. Improvement of cardiorespiratory endurance may be accomplished through continuous, interval, or fartlek training.

---

*Solutions to Critical Thinking* Exercises

---

**4-1** The warm-up should begin with a 5- to 7-minute slow jog during which the athlete should break into a light sweat. At that point, she should engage in stretching (using either static or PNF techniques), concentrating on quadriceps, hamstrings, groin, and hip abductor muscles. She should repeat each specific stretch four times, holding the stretch for 15 to 20 seconds. Once her workout begins, she should gradually and moderately increase the intensity of the activity. The coach should also stress the importance of stretching during the cooldown that follows the workout.

**4-2** Weight training will not have a negative effect on flexibility as long as the lifting technique is done properly. Lifting the weight through a complete and full range of motion will improve strength and simultaneously maintain range of motion. This female swimmer is not likely to bulk up to the point at which range of motion will be affected by muscle size. The coach should also recommend that she continue to incorporate active stretching into her training regimen.

**4-3** The shot put, like many other dynamic movements in sport, requires not only great strength, but also the ability to generate that strength very rapidly. To develop muscular power, the athlete must engage in dynamic, explosive training techniques that will help him develop his ability. Power-lifting techniques such as squats and power cleans should be helpful. In addition, plyometric exercises using weights for added resistance will help him learn to improve his speed of muscular contraction against some resistive force.

**4-4** Alternative activities such as swimming or riding a stationary exercise bike should be incorporated into this athlete's rehabilitation program immediately. If the pressure on the ankle when riding an exercise bike is initially too painful, she should use a bike that incorporates upper extremity exercise. The coach should recommend that the soccer player engage in a minimum of 30 minutes of continuous training and some higher intensity interval training to maintain both aerobic and anaerobic fitness.

## REVIEW QUESTIONS AND CLASS ACTIVITIES

1. Why is year-round conditioning so important for injury prevention?
2. In terms of injury prevention, list as many advantages as you can for conditioning.
3. How does the SAID principle relate to sports conditioning and injury prevention?
4. What is the value of proper warm-ups and cooldowns to sports injury prevention?
5. Critically observe how a variety of sports use warm-up and cooldown procedures.
6. Compare ways to increase flexibility and how those ways may decrease or increase the athlete's susceptibility to injury.
7. How may increasing strength decrease susceptibility to injury?
8. Compare different techniques of increasing strength. How may each way be an advantage or a disadvantage to the athlete in terms of injury prevention?
9. Discuss the relationship between maximum aerobic capacity and heart rate.
10. Differentiate between aerobic and anaerobic training methods.
11. How is continuous training different from interval training?

## REFERENCES

1. Akima H, Takahashi H, Kuno SY: Early phase adaptations of muscle use and strength to isokinetic training, *Med Sci Sports Exerc* 31(4):588, 1999.
2. Anderson B: *Stretching,* ed 20, Bolinas, Calif, 2000, Shelter Publishers.
3. Baker D, Wilson G, Carlyon B: Generality vs. specificity: a comparison of dynamic and isometric measures of strength and speed-strength, *Eur J Appl Physiol* 68:350, 1994.
4. Bassett DR, Howley ET: Limiting factors for maximum oxygen uptake and determinants of endurance performance, *Med Sci Sports Exerc* 32(1):70, 2000.
5. Berger R: *Conditioning for men,* Boston, 1973, Allyn & Bacon.
6. Bergh U, Ekblom B, Astrand PO: Maximal oxygen uptake "classical" versus "contemporary" viewpoints, *Med Sci Sports Exerc* 32(1):85, 2000.
7. Bompa TO: *Periodization training for sports,* Champaign, Ill, 1999, Human Kinetics.
8. Brown LE: *Isokinetics in human performance,* Champaign, Ill, 2000, Human Kinetics.
9. Chu DA: Plyometrics in sports injury rehabilitation and training, *Ath Ther Today* 4(3):7, 1999.
10. Conroy M: The use of periodization in the high school setting, *Streng Cond J* 21(1):52, 1999.
11. Cross KM, Worrell TW: Effects of a static stretching program on the incidence of lower extremity musculotendinous strains, *J Ath Train* 34(1):11, 1999.
12. De Lorme TL, Watkins AL: *Progressive resistance exercise,* New York, 1951, Appleton-Century-Crofts.
13. Glass S, Whaley M, Wegner M: A comparison between ratings of perceived exertion among standard protocols and steady state running, *Int J Sports Med* 12:77, 1991.
14. Gravelle BL, Blessing DL: Physiological adaptation in women concurrently training for strength and endurance, *J Streng Cond Res* 14(1):5, 2000.
15. Hawley J, Myburgh K, Noakes T: Maximal oxygen consumption: a contemporary perspective. In Fahey T, editor: *Encyclopedia of sports medicine and exercise physiology,* New York, 1995, Garland.
16. Hickson R, Hidaka C, Foster C: Skeletal muscle fiber type, resistance training and strength-related performance, *Med Sci Sports Exerc* 26:593, 1994.
17. Hilbert S, Plisk SS: Free weights versus machines, *Streng Cond J* 21(6):66, 1999.
18. Holcomb WR: Improved stretching with proprioceptive neuromuscular facilitation, *Streng Cond J* 22(1):59, 2000.
19. Karvonen MJ, Kentala E, Mustala O: The effects of training on heart rate: a longitudinal study, *Ann Med Exp Biol* 35:305, 1957.
20. Radcliffe JC, Farentinos RC: *High-powered plyometrics,* Champaign, Ill, 1999, Human Kinetics.
21. Schilling BK, Stone MH: Stretching: acute effects on strength and power performance, *Streng Cond J* 22(1):44, 2000.
22. Surburg P: Flexibility/range of motion. In Winnick JP, editor: *The Brockport physical fitness training guide,* Champaign, Ill, 1999, Human Kinetics.
23. Swain D, Abernathy K, Smith C: Target heart rates for the development of cardiorespiratory fitness, *Med Sci Sports Exerc* 26:112, 1994.
24. Thomas M: The functional warm-up, *Streng Cond J* 22(2):51, 2000.
25. Zentz C: Warm up to perform up, *Ath Ther Today* 5(2):59, 2000.

## ANNOTATED BIBLIOGRAPHY

Alter J: *The science of stretching*, Boston, 1988, Houghton Mifflin.

*This text explains the principles and techniques of stretching and details the anatomy and physiology of muscle and connective tissue. It includes guidelines for developing a flexibility program and illustrated stretching exercises and warm-up drills.*

Anderson B: *Stretching*, Bolinas, Calif, 2000, Shelter.

*An extremely comprehensive best-selling text on stretching exercises for the entire body.*

Baechle T, Groves B: *Essentials of strength training and conditioning*, Champaign, Ill, 2000, Human Kinetics.

*Explains the various concepts of exercise, identifies correct lifting techniques, corrects common weight-training errors, and lists personal goals for weight training.*

Brooks G, Fahey T, White T: *Exercise physiology: human bioenergetics and its applications*, ed 3, Mountain View, Calif, 2000, Mayfield.

*An up-to-date advanced text in exercise physiology that contains a comprehensive listing of the most current journal articles relative to exercise physiology.*

Chu D: *Jumping into plyometrics*, Champaign, Ill, 1998, Human Kinetics.

*Detailing plyometric exercises for a variety of sports, this guide explains how plyometrics work and how to incorporate plyometrics into a comprehensive strength and power-training program.*

Moran G, McGlynn G: *Dynamics of strength training*, St. Louis, 2000, McGraw-Hill.

*Provides a comprehensive resource using an individualized approach to strength training, including conditioning and cardiorespiratory fitness. Emphasizes the physiological basis of muscle strength and endurance. Illustrates the most efficient and effective training techniques.*

## WEBSITES

Health and Fitness Worldguide Forum: http://www.worldguide.com/Fitness/hf.html

*Includes coverage of anatomy, strength, cardiovascular exercise, eating well, and sports medicine.*

Stretching and Flexibility: Everything you never wanted to know: http://www.cs.huji.ac.il/papers/rma/stretching_toc.html

*Prepared by Brad Appleton, detailed information on stretching and stretching techniques is presented, including normal ranges of motion, flexibility, how to stretch, the physiology of stretching, and the types of stretching including PNF.*

Tips on Fitness: http://www.geocities.com/HotSprings/2894

*Provides information on exercise, flexibility, and nutritional guidelines in an easy-to-read and straightforward format.*

Mesomorphosis Interactive: Cardiovascular exercise principles and guidelines: http://mesomorphosis.com/tackett.cardiol.htm

*Topics discussed include warm-up, stretching, cooldown, frequency of exercise, and duration of exercise; there are also links to related pages that may be informative.*

Fitness World: http://www.fitnessworld.com

*Presents information about fitness in general and includes access to Fitness Management magazine.*

Kaiser Permanente Health Reference: http://www.scl.ncal.kaiperm.org/healthinfo/index.html

*Click on Cardiovascular Exercise and find several topics including how to start, target heart rate, and injuries.*

Chapter

# 5

# Nutritional Considerations

*When you finish this chapter you will be able to:*

- Identify the six classes of nutrients and describe their major functions.
- Explain the importance of good nutrition in enhancing performance and preventing injuries.
- Describe the advantages or disadvantages of supplementing various nutrients in the athlete's diet.
- Explain the advantages and disadvantages of a preevent meal.
- Explain the distinction between body weight and body composition.
- Explain the principle of caloric balance and how to assess it.
- Describe methods for losing and gaining weight.
- List the signs of bulimia and anorexia nervosa.

T he relation of nutrition, diet, and weight control to overall health and fitness is an important aspect of any training and conditioning program for an athlete. Athletes who practice sound nutritional habits reduce the likelihood of injury by maintaining a higher standard of healthful living. Eating a well-balanced diet can positively contribute to the development of strength, flexibility and cardiorespiratory endurance. Unfortunately, misconceptions, fads, and in many cases, superstitions regarding nutrition affect dietary habits, particularly in the athletic population.

Many athletes associate successful performance with the consumption of special foods or supplements. An athlete who is performing well may be reluctant to change dietary habits regardless of whether the diet is physiologically beneficial to overall health. The psychological aspect of allowing the athlete to eat whatever he or she is most comfortable with can greatly affect performance. The problem is that these eating habits tend to become accepted as beneficial and may become traditional when in fact they may be physiologically detrimental to athletic performance. Thus, many nutrition "experts" may disseminate nutritional information based on traditional rather than experimental information. The coach must possess a strong knowledge base in nutrition so that he or she may serve as an informational resource for the athlete.

## THE NUTRIENTS

People usually think of losing weight when they hear the word *diet*. Actually, diet refers to a person's usual food selections. What people choose

Six classes of nutrients:
- CHO
- Fats
- Proteins
- Vitamins
- Minerals
- Water

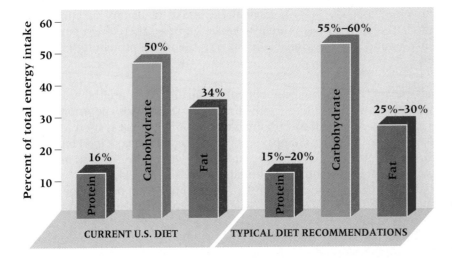

**FIGURE 5-1**

Comparison of calories from
carbohydrates, fats, and
proteins

to eat is their diet. Although people have different food likes and dislikes, everyone must eat to survive. Nutrition is the science of certain food substances, *nutrients,* and what they do in the body.[23] Nutrients perform three major roles:[21]

1. Grow, repair, and maintain all body cells
2. Regulate body processes
3. Supply energy for cells

The various nutrients are categorized into six major classes: *carbohydrates, fats* (often called *lipids*), *proteins, water, vitamins,* and *minerals.* Most foods are actually mixtures of these nutrients. Some nutrients can be made by the body, but an *essential nutrient* must be supplied by the diet. Not all substances in food are considered nutrients. There is no such thing as the perfect food; that is, no single natural food contains all of the nutrients needed for health. A summary of current percentages and recommended percentages of calories from carbohydrates, fats, and proteins is shown in Figure 5-1.

> Nutrient-dense foods supply adequate amounts of vitamins and minerals in relation to caloric value.

## Carbohydrates (CHO)

Athletes have increased energy needs. *Carbohydrates* are the body's most efficient source of energy and should be relied on to fill that need.[10] Carbohydrates should account for at least 55 percent or more of total caloric intake and some recommendations go as high as 60 to 70 percent. Carbohydrates are classified as simple (sugars) or complex (starch and most forms of fiber). During digestion, complex carbohydrates are broken down into *glucose.* The glucose that is not needed for immediate energy is stored as glycogen in the liver and muscle cells. Glucose can be released from glycogen later if needed. The body, however, can store only a limited amount of glucose as glycogen. Any extra amount of glucose is

> Carbohydrates are sugars, starches, or fiber.

Organizing and Establishing
an Effective Athletic Health
Care System

5-1

**Critical Thinking** Exercise

A female softball player has
been told by her coach that she
is slightly overweight and
needs to lose a few pounds.
The athlete has been watching
television and reading about
how important it is to limit the
dietary intake of fat for losing
weight. She has decided to go
on a diet that is essentially fat
free and is convinced that this
diet will help her lose weight.

? What should the coach tell
her about avoiding excessive
intake of fat as a means of
losing weight?

Fats may be saturated or
unsaturated.

Dietary recommendations:
• CHO 55 percent
• Fats 30 percent
• Proteins 15 percent

Proteins are made up of
amino acids.

converted to body fat. An inadequate intake of dietary carbohydrate
causes the body to use protein to make glucose. Therefore a supply of
glucose must be kept available to prevent the use of protein for energy.

### Fats

*Fats* are another essential component of the diet. They are the most con-
centrated source of energy, providing more than twice the calories per
gram when compared to carbohydrates or proteins. Fat is used as a primary source of energy. Some dietary fat is needed to make food more fla-
vorful and for sources of the fat-soluble vitamins. Also, a minimal
amount of fat is essential for normal growth and development.[23]

In the United States, dietary fat represents a high percentage of the
total caloric intake (see Figure 5-1). For many Americans, a substantial
amount of the fat is from saturated fatty acids. This intake is believed to
be too high and may contribute to the prevalence of obesity, certain cancers, and coronary artery disease. The recommended intake should be
limited to less than 25 percent of total calories with saturated fat reduced
to less than 10 percent of total calories.

### Proteins

*Proteins* make up the major structural components of the body. They are
needed for growth, maintenance, and repair of all body tissues. In addition, proteins are needed to make enzymes, many hormones, and antibodies that help fight infection. In general, the body tends not to use
much protein for energy; instead it relies on fats and carbohydrates. Protein intake should be around 12 to 15 percent of total calories.

The basic units that make up proteins are called *amino acids.* Most of
the body's proteins are made up of about twenty different amino acids.
The majority of the amino acids can be produced as needed in the body.
The others cannot be made to any significant degree and therefore must
be supplied by the diet. These are referred to as the *essential* amino acids.
A diet that contains large amounts of protein will not support growth, repair, and maintenance of tissues if the essential amino acids are not available in the proper proportions.[22] Most of the proteins from animal foods
contain all the essential amino acids that humans require. Examples are
the proteins found in meat, fish, poultry, eggs, milk, and other dairy
products.

### Vitamins

Although they are required in very small amounts when compared to
carbohydrates, fats, proteins, and water, *vitamins* perform essential roles
primarily as regulators of body processes. Over the years, researchers
have identified thirteen vitamins and determined their specific roles in
the body.

People mistakenly think that vitamins provide energy. In fact, the
body cannot break them down to release energy. Table 5-1 provides information about vitamins, including rich food sources, deficiency symptoms, and toxicity potential from high doses.

**TABLE 5-1** Vitamins

| Vitamin | Major Function | Most Reliable Sources | Deficiency | Excess (Toxicity) |
|---|---|---|---|---|
| A | Maintains skin and other cells that line the inside of the body; bone and tooth development; growth; vision in dim light | Liver, milk, egg yolk, deep green and yellow fruits and vegetables | Night blindness, dry skin, growth failure | Headaches, nausea, loss of hair, dry skin, diarrhea |
| D | Normal bone growth and development | Exposure to sunlight; fortified dairy products; eggs and fish liver oils | Rickets in children—defective bone formation leading to deformed bones | Appetite loss, weight loss, failure to grow |
| E | Prevents destruction of polyunsaturated fats caused by exposure to oxidizing agents; protects cell membranes from destruction | Vegetable oils, some in fruits and vegetables, whole grains | Breakage of red blood cells leading to anemia | Nausea and diarrhea; interferes with vitamin K if vitamin D is also deficient. Not as toxic as other fat-soluble vitamins |
| K | Production of blood-clotting substances | Green leafy vegetables; normal bacteria that live in intestines produce K that is absorbed | Increased bleeding time | |
| B$_1$ (thiamin) | Needed for release of energy from carbohydrates, fats, and proteins | Cereal products, pork, peas, and dried beans | Lack of energy, nerve problems | |
| B$_2$ (riboflavin) | Energy from carbohydrates, fats, and proteins | Milk, liver, fruits and vegetables, enriched breads and cereals | Dry skin, cracked lips | |
| B$_3$ (niacin) | Energy from carbohydrates, fats, and proteins | Liver, meat, poultry, peanut butter, legumes, enriched breads and cereals | Skin problems, diarrhea, mental depression, and eventually death (rarely occurs in U.S.) | Skin flushing, intestinal upset, nervousness, intestinal ulcers |
| B$_6$ | Metabolism of protein; production of hemoglobin | White meats, whole grains, liver, egg yolk, bananas | Poor growth, anemia | |
| B$_{12}$ | Production of genetic material; maintains central nervous system | Foods of animal origin | Neurological problems, anemia | Severe loss of coordination from nerve damage |
| Folate (folic acid) | Production of genetic material | Wheat germ, liver, yeast, mushrooms, green leafy vegetables, fruits | Anemia | |
| C (ascorbic acid) | Formation and maintenance of connective tissue; tooth and bone formation; immune function | Fruits and vegetables | Scurvy (rare), swollen joints, bleeding gums, fatigue, bruising | Kidney stones, diarrhea |
| Pantothenic acid | Energy from carbohydrates, fats, and proteins | Widely found in foods | Not observed in humans under normal conditions | |
| Biotin | Use of fats | Widely found in foods | Rare under normal conditions | |

107

Organizing and Establishing
an Effective Athletic Health
Care System

5–2

*Critical Thinking* Exercise

A volleyball player complains
that she constantly feels tired
and lethargic even though she
thinks that she is eating well
and getting a sufficient amount
of sleep. A teammate has
suggested that she begin taking
vitamin supplements, which,
the teammate claims, will give
her more energy and make her
more resistant to fatigue. The
athlete comes to the coach to
ask advice about what kind of
vitamins she needs to take.

**?** What facts should the coach
explain to the athlete about
vitamin supplementation, and
what recommendations should
be made?

The fat-soluble vitamins:
• Vitamin A
• Vitamin D
• Vitamin E
• Vitamin K

The water-soluble vitamins:
• Vitamin C
• Thiamin
• Riboflavin
• Niacin
• Folate
• Biotin
• Pantothenic acid
• Vitamin $B_6$
• Vitamin $B_{12}$

The antioxidants:
• Vitamin C
• Vitamin E
• Beta carotene

Vitamins are classified into two groups: The *fat-soluble vitamins* are dissolved in fats and stored in the body; the *water-soluble vitamins* are dissolved in watery solutions and are not stored. The fat-soluble vitamins that dissolve in fat rather than water are vitamins A, E, D, and K. Extra amounts of the fat-soluble vitamins are not easy to eliminate from the body in urine, which is mostly water. Instead they are stored in the liver or body fat until needed, making them potentially toxic.[21]

The water-soluble vitamins are vitamin C, known as *ascorbic acid,* and the B-complex vitamins, including thiamin ($B_1$), riboflavin ($B_2$), niacin ($B_3$), $B_6$, folate, $B_{12}$, biotin, and pantothenic acid. Vitamin C is used for building bones and teeth, maintaining the tissues that hold muscles and other tissues together (connective tissues), and strengthening the immune system. Unlike fat-soluble vitamins, the water-soluble ones cannot be stored to any significant extent in the body and should be supplied in the diet each day.

### Antioxidant Nutrients

Certain nutrients, called antioxidants, may prevent premature aging, certain cancers, heart disease, and other health problems.[14] An antioxidant protects vital cell components from the destructive effects of certain agents, including oxygen. Vitamins C and E and beta carotene are antioxidants. Beta carotene is a plant pigment found in dark green, deep yellow, or orange fruits and vegetables. The body can convert beta carotene to vitamin A.[14] In the early 1980s, researchers reported that smokers who ate large quantities of beta carotene–rich fruits and vegetables were less likely to develop lung cancer than were other smokers. Since that time, more evidence is accumulating about the benefits of a diet rich in the antioxidant nutrients.

Some experts believe athletes should increase their intake of antioxidants, even if it means taking supplements. Others are more cautious. Excess beta carotene pigments circulate throughout the body and may turn the skin yellow. However, the pigment is not believed to be toxic like its nutrient cousin, vitamin A. On the other hand, increasing intake of vitamins C and E is not without some risk. Excesses of vitamin C are not well absorbed; the excess is irritating to the intestines and creates diarrhea. Although less toxic than vitamins A or D, too much vitamin E causes health problems.

### Minerals

More than twenty *mineral* elements need to be supplied by the diet.[10] Some of these minerals are listed in Table 5-2. Other mineral elements are found in the body. The role of minerals is unclear. Minerals are needed for a variety of jobs such as forming strong bones and teeth, generating energy, activating enzymes, and maintaining water balance. Most minerals are stored in the body, especially in the bones and liver. Although each of these minerals is important in its own way, two minerals, calcium and iron, require special attention.

**TABLE 5-2** Major minerals

| Mineral | Major Role | Most Reliable Sources | Deficiency | Excess |
|---|---|---|---|---|
| Calcium | Bone and tooth formation; blood clotting; muscle contraction; nerve function | Dairy products | May lead to osteoporosis | Calcium deposits in soft tissues |
| Phosphorus | Skeletal development; tooth formation | Meats, dairy products, and other protein-rich foods | Rarely seen | |
| Sodium | Maintenance of fluid balance | Salt (sodium chloride) added to foods and sodium-containing preservatives | | May contribute to the development of hypertension |
| Iron | Formation of hemoglobin; energy from carbohydrates, fats, and proteins | Liver and red meats, enriched breads and cereals | Iron-deficiency anemia | Can cause death in children from supplement overdose |
| Copper | Formation of hemoglobin | Liver, nuts, shellfish, cherries, mushrooms, whole grain breads and cereals Seafood and meats | Anemia | Nausea and vomiting |
| Zinc | Normal growth and development | | Skin problems, delayed development, growth problems | Interferes with copper use; may decrease HDL levels |
| Iodine | Production of the hormone thyroxin | Iodized salt, seafood | Mental and growth retardation; lack of energy | |
| Fluorine | Strengthens bones and teeth | Fluoridated water | Teeth are less resistant to decay | Damage to tooth enamel |

## Water

Water is the most essential nutrient.[23] A person can live for weeks, months, even years without the other nutrients, but will perish after a few days without water. About 60 percent of the adult's body weight is water. Many materials used in the body are water soluble, that is, dissolved in water. Although water does not supply any calories, an adequate supply of water is needed for energy production. Water also takes part in digestion and maintaining the proper environment inside and outside of cells. When the body burns fuels for energy, it produces a great deal of heat energy. Sweating is how the body uses water to keep itself from overheating.

The average adult requires a minimum of 2.5 liters of water or about ten glasses of water a day.[23] Because water is so vital, the healthy body carefully manages its internal water levels. When body water weight drops by 1 to 2 percent, you begin to feel thirsty. Drinking water causes the internal water levels to return to normal. If thirst signals are ignored and body water continues to decrease, *dehydration* results. People who are dehydrated cannot generate enough energy and feel weak. Other symptoms include nausea, vomiting, and fainting.

Dehydration is more likely to occur when you are outdoors, and sweating heavily while engaging in some strenuous activity. To prevent dehydration make sure to replace the lost water by drinking plenty of fluids. Don't rely on thirst as a signal that it's time to have a drink. By the time thirst develops the body is already slightly dehydrated. Many people ignore their thirst, or if they do heed it, they don't drink enough. Most people replace only about 50 percent of the water they lose through sweating.[19] It is recommended that athletes stop and take a drink of water each time they pass a water fountain to minimize the chances of dehydration. An athlete should consume fluids before, during, and after practice or competition.

Replacing fluid after heavy sweating is far more important than replacing electrolytes.

## Electrolyte Requirements

Electrolytes, including sodium, chloride, potassium, magnesium, and calcium, are electrically charged ions in solution. They maintain the balance of water outside the cell. Electrolyte replenishment may be needed when a person is not fit, suffers from extreme water loss, participates in a marathon, or has just completed an exercise period and is expected to perform at near-maximum effort within the next few hours. In most cases, electrolytes can be sufficiently replaced with a balanced diet. Free access to water (ad libitum) before, during, and after activity should be the rule. Electrolyte losses are primarily responsible for muscle cramping and intolerance to heat. Sweating results not only in a body water loss but in some electrolyte loss as well.[19]

Electrolytes: sodium, chloride, potassium, magnesium, and calcium

## Using Sports Drinks

During physical activity it is essential to replace fluids lost through sweating. It has been shown that replacing lost fluids with a sports drink is

**Recommendations for fluid replacement***

- Athletes should begin all exercise sessions well hydrated.
- To ensure proper hydration the athlete should consume 17 to 20 ounces of water or a sports drink 2 to 3 hours before exercise and then 7 to 10 ounces 20 minutes before exercise.
- Fluid replacement beverages should be easily accessible during activity and should be consumed at a minimal rate of 7 to 10 ounces every 10 to 20 minutes.
- During activity the athlete should consume the maximal amount of fluid that can be tolerated.
- A cool, flavored beverage at 50 to 59° F is recommended.
- Addition of proper amounts of carbohydrates and electrolytes to a fluid replacement solution is recommended for exercise events that last longer than 1 hour.
- A 6 percent carbohydrate solution appears to be optimal.
- For exercise lasting less than 1 hour the addition of carbohydrates and electrolytes does not seem to enhance physical performance.

*Based on recommendations from ACSM[1] and NATA.[3]*

more effective than using water alone.[19] Research has shown that because of the flavor of the sports drinks an athlete is likely to drink more than plain water. In addition, sports drinks replace both fluids and electrolytes that are lost in sweat and also provide energy to the working muscles.

Water is a good thirst quencher but it is not a good rehydrator because water "turns off" your thirst before you're completely rehydrated. Water also "turns on" the kidneys prematurely so you lose fluid in the form of urine much more quickly than when drinking a sports drink. The small amount of sodium in sports drinks allows the body to hold onto the fluid consumed rather than losing it through urine.[3]

Not all sports drinks are the same. How a sports drink is formulated dictates how well it works in providing rapid rehydration and energy. The optimal level of carbohydrate is 14 grams per 8 ounces of water for quickest absorption and energy. Thus sports drinks should be used without diluting. Research has shown that full-strength sports drinks are absorbed just as fast as water. Most contain no carbonation or artificial preservatives, making them satisfying during exercise and causing no stomach bloating. Also most sports drinks contain a minimal number of calories. It has been shown that sports drinks are effective in improving performance during both endurance activities and short-term high-intensity activities such as soccer, basketball, and tennis that last from 30 minutes to an hour.[3] Focus Box 5-1 provides recommendations for fluid replacement.

## THE PRODUCTION OF ENERGY FROM FOODSTUFFS

Energy is produced when cells break down CHO, fats, or proteins to release energy stored in these compounds. As can be seen in Figure 5-2, carbohydrates provide the major proportion of energy for short-term, high-intensity muscular contractions. As the duration and the intensity of the activity increases, breathing also increases, supplying more oxygen for the cells and maximizing energy production. When the activity is prolonged, such as in an endurance sport, the percentage of fat and carbohydrate used for fuel is similar. Under usual conditions, proteins supply less than about 5 percent of energy. However, athletes engaged in endurance activities receive as much as 10 to 15 percent of their energy needs from protein.[13]

## WHAT IS A NUTRITIOUS DIET?

### The Food Pyramid

The Basic Four Food Groups Plan, first introduced in the mid-1950s, has recently been redesigned into a food pyramid concept that is believed to do a better job of educating Americans about the relationship of food choices to health. Figure 5-3 illustrates the food groupings, the minimum number of servings that should be eaten daily, and examples of foods from each group. Carbohydrate-rich foods (the breads and cereals group) form the foundation of the diet, which reflects the recommendations in the Dietary Guidelines for Americans that suggest a need for people to consume a greater percentage of total calories from this group. The other food groups are shown according to their relative importance in a healthy diet. One major change from the Basic Four plan is that the fruits and vegetables are separated into two distinct groups, each with a specified number of servings. Note that fats and sugars form the small apex of the pyramid. This placement indicates that foods rich in fat and sugar should provide the smallest proportion of total calories; no minimum number of servings is suggested because many Americans consume far too much fat and sugar.[21]

### Nutrient Dense Foods versus Junk Foods

Foods that contain considerable amounts of vitamins, minerals, and proteins in relation to their caloric content are referred to as being *nutrient dense*. Candy, chips, doughnuts, cakes, and cookies are often referred to as junk foods. These foods are not nutrient dense because they provide too many calories from fats and sugars in relation to vitamins and minerals. If an athlete's overall diet is nutritious, and he or she can afford the extra calories, it's okay to eat occasional fatty or sugary foods. However, many people who live on diets that are rich in these kinds of foods displace more nutritious food items in their diets. This behavior is not a healthy one to practice in the long run.[10]

## NUTRITION AND PHYSICAL ACTIVITY

Vitamin requirements do not increase during exercise.

Athletes often believe that exercise increases requirements for nutrients such as proteins, vitamins, and minerals and that it is possible and desirable to saturate the body with these nutrients.[22] There is no scientific

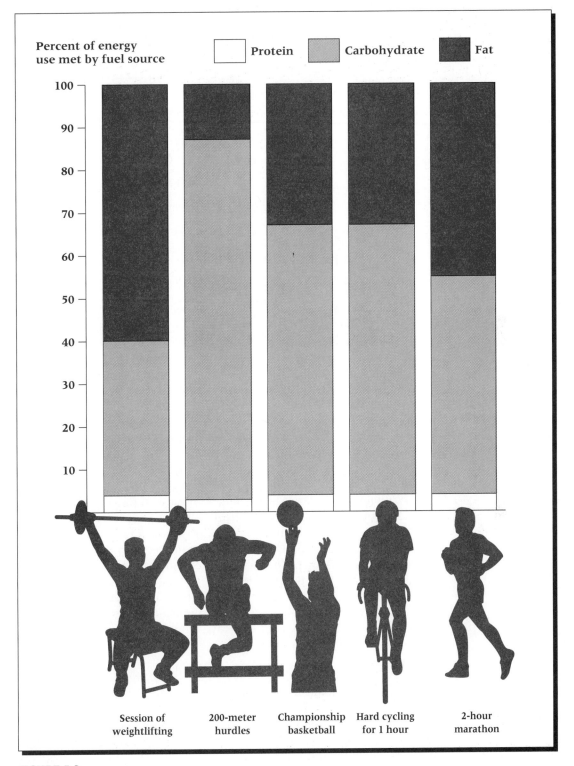

**FIGURE 5-2**

The relative portions of CHO, fat, and protein fuels used during physical activity

Organizing and Establishing
an Effective Athletic Health
Care System

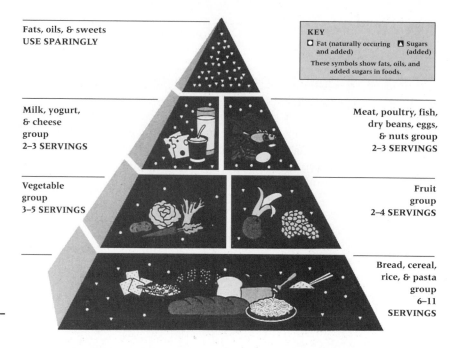

**Fats, oils, & sweets
USE SPARINGLY**

KEY
☐ Fat (naturally occuring ◼ Sugars
and added)          (added)

These symbols show fats, oils, and
added sugars in foods.

**Milk, yogurt,
& cheese
group
2–3 SERVINGS**

**Meat, poultry, fish,
dry beans, eggs,
& nuts group
2–3 SERVINGS**

**Vegetable
group
3–5 SERVINGS**

**Fruit
group
2–4 SERVINGS**

**Bread, cereal,
rice, & pasta
group
6–11
SERVINGS**

**FIGURE 5-3**

USDA food guide pyramid

U.S. RDA helps consumers
compare nutritional values of
foods.

basis for ingesting levels of these nutrients above U.S. Recommended Dietary Allowances (RDA) levels. Exercise increases the need for energy, not for proteins, vitamins, and minerals.[13] Thus it is necessary to explore some of the more common myths that surround the subject of nutrition's role in physical performance.

## Vitamin Supplementation

Many athletes believe that taking large amounts of vitamin supplements can lead to superior health and performance. A megadose of a nutrient supplement is essentially an overdose; the amount ingested far exceeds the RDA levels. The rationale used for such excessive intakes is that if a pill that contains the RDA for each vitamin and mineral makes an athlete healthy, then taking a pill that has ten times the RDA should make that athlete ten times healthier. There is no truth to this kind of logic. For an athlete eating a balanced diet, vitamin supplementation is probably not necessary. Supplementing with excessive amounts of fat-soluble vitamins can produce toxic effects.

## Mineral Supplementation

Obtaining adequate levels of certain minerals can be a problem for some athletes. Calcium and iron intakes may be low for athletes whose diets do not include dairy products, red meats, or enriched breads and cereals. However, athletes must first determine whether they need extra minerals to prevent wasting their money and overdosing. The following sections explore some of the minerals that can be low in the diet and some suggestions for improving the quality of the diet so that supplements may not be necessary.

### Calcium Deficiency

Calcium is the most abundant mineral in the body. It is essential for bones and teeth and for muscle contraction and conduction of nerve impulses. If calcium intake is too low to meet needs, the body can remove calcium from the bones. Over time, the bones become weakened and appear porous on x-ray films. These bones are brittle and often break spontaneously. This condition is called **osteoporosis** and is estimated to be eight times more common among women than men. Osteoporosis becomes a serious problem for women after menopause.[11]

Exercise causes calcium to be retained in bones, so physical activity is beneficial. However, younger females who exercise to extremes so that their normal hormonal balance is upset are prone to develop premature osteoporosis. For females who have a family history of osteoporosis, calcium supplementation, preferably as calcium carbonate or citrate rather than phosphate, may be advisable.[18]

Milk products are the most reliable sources of calcium. Many athletes dislike milk or complain that it upsets their stomach. Those athletes may lack an enzyme called *lactase* that is needed to digest milk sugar, lactose. This condition is referred to as lactose intolerance, or **lactase deficiency.** The undigested lactose enters the large intestine, where the bacteria that normally reside there use it for energy. The bacteria produce large quantities of intestinal gas, which causes discomfort and cramps. Many lactose-intolerant people also suffer from diarrhea. Fortunately, scientists have produced the missing enzyme, lactase. Lactase is available without prescription in forms that can be added to foods before eating or taken along with meals.

### Iron Deficiency

Iron deficiency is also a common problem, especially for young females. Lack of iron can result in iron-deficiency **anemia.**[16] Iron is needed to properly form hemoglobin. In anemia, the oxygen-carrying ability of the red blood cells is reduced so that muscles cannot obtain enough oxygen to generate energy. An anemic person feels tired and weak. Obviously, athletes cannot compete at their peak level while suffering from an iron deficiency.

### Protein Supplementation

Athletes often believe that more protein is needed to build bigger muscles. It is true that a relatively small amount of protein is needed for developing muscles in a training program. Many athletes, particularly those who are weight training heavily or body builders, routinely take commercially produced protein supplements. To build muscle, athletes should consume 1 to 1.5 grams of extra protein per kilogram (0.5 to 0.7 grams per pound) of body weight every day.[22] This range goes from slightly

---

**osteoporosis**
A decrease in bone density.

**lactase deficiency**
Difficulty digesting dairy products.

**anemia**
Lack of iron.

above to about double the protein RDA (0.8 grams per kilogram of desirable body weight). Anyone eating a variety of foods, but especially protein-rich foods can easily meet the higher amounts. Thus protein supplements are not needed for athletes because their diets typically exceed even the most generous protein recommendations. An active adult usually requires 0.6 grams per pound or 66 percent more than the RDA.

## Sugar and Performance

Ingesting large quantities of glucose in the form of honey, candy bars, or pure sugar immediately before physical activity has a significant impact on performance. As carbohydrates are digested, large quantities of glucose enter the blood. This increase in blood sugar (glucose) levels stimulates the release of the hormone insulin. Insulin allows the cells to use the circulating glucose so that blood glucose levels soon return to normal. It was hypothesized that this decline in blood sugar levels was detrimental to performance and endurance. However, recent evidence indicates the effect of eating large quantities of carbohydrates is beneficial rather than negative.[19]

Nevertheless, some athletes are sensitive to high carbohydrate feedings and experience problems with increased levels of insulin. Also, some athletes cannot tolerate large amounts of the simple sugar fructose. For these individuals, too much fructose leads to intestinal upset and diarrhea. Athletes should test themselves with various high-carbohydrate foods to see if they are affected, but they should not try this test before a competitive event.[23]

## Caffeine and Performance

Caffeine is a central nervous system stimulant. Most people who consume caffeine in coffee, tea, or carbonated beverages are aware of its effect of increasing alertness and decreasing fatigue. Chocolate contains compounds that are related to caffeine and have the same stimulating effects. However, large amounts of caffeine cause nervousness, irritability, increased heart rate, and headaches. Also, headaches are a withdrawal symptom experienced when a person tries to stop consuming caffeinated products.

Although small amounts of caffeine do not appear to harm physical performance, cases of nausea and lightheadedness have been reported. Caffeine may enhance the use of fat during endurance exercise, thus delaying the depletion of glycogen stores, which would help endurance performance. Caffeine also appears to help make calcium more available to the muscle during contraction, which helps the muscle work more efficiently. However, Olympic officials rightfully consider caffeine to be a drug. It should not be present in an Olympic competitor's blood in levels greater than that resulting from drinking five or six cups of coffee.

## Alcohol and Performance

Alcohol provides energy for the body; each gram of pure alcohol (ethanol) supplies 7 calories. However, sources of alcohol provide very little other nutritional value in regard to vitamins, minerals, and proteins. The depressant effects of alcohol on the central nervous system include decreased physical coordination, slowed reaction times, and decreased mental alertness. Also, this drug increases the production of urine, resulting in body water losses (diuretic effect). Therefore use of alcoholic beverages by the athlete cannot be recommended before, during, or after physical activity.

## Organic, Natural, and Health Foods

Many athletes are concerned about the quality of the foods they eat—not just the nutritional value of the food but also its safety. Organic foods are foods grown without the use of synthetic fertilizers and pesticides.[21] People who advocate the use of organic farming methods claim that these foods are nutritionally superior and safer than the same products grown using chemicals such as pesticides and synthetic fertilizers.

Technically, the description of organic food is meaningless. All foods (except water) are organic, that is, contain the element carbon. Organically produced foods are often quite expensive when compared to the same foods produced by conventional means. There is no advantage to consuming organic food products. They are not more nutritious than those foods produced by conventional methods. Nevertheless, for some, the psychological benefit of believing that they are doing something "good" for their bodies justifies the extra cost.

Natural foods have been subjected to very little processing and contain no additives such as preservatives or artificial flavors. Processing can protect nutritional value. Preservatives save food that would otherwise spoil and have to be destroyed. Furthermore, many foods in their natural form are quite poisonous. The green layer often found under the skin of potatoes is poisonous if eaten in large amounts. There are poisonous mushrooms, and molds in peanuts can cause liver cancer.

Both organic and natural foods could be described as health foods. However, there is no benefit derived from eating a diet consisting of health foods, even for the athlete.

## Herbs

The use of herbs as natural alternatives to drugs and medicines has clearly become a trend among American consumers.[8] Most herbs, as edible plants, are safe to take as foods, and they are claimed to have few side effects as natural medicines, although occasionally a mild allergy-type reaction may occur.

Nutritionally, herbs can offer the body nutrients that are reported to nourish the brain and glands, and aid hormone production. Unlike vitamins, which work best when taken with food, it is not necessary to take herbs with other foods.[8]

Herbs in their whole form are not drugs. As medicines, herbs are essentially body balancers that work with the body functions, to help the body heal and regulate itself. Herbal formulas can be general for overall strength and nutrient support, or specific to a particular ailment or condition.

**TABLE 5-3** Most widely used herbs and purposes for use

| Herb | Uses |
|------|------|
| *dong quai* | to treat menstrual symptoms |
| *echinacea* | to promote wound healing and strengthen immune system |
| *garlic* | as an antibiotic, antibacterial, antifungal agent, to prevent and relieve coronary-artery disease by reducing total blood cholesterol and triglyceride levels and raising HDL levels |
| *ginkgo biloba* | to improve blood circulation, especially in the brain |
| *ginseng* | to reduce impotence, weakness, lethargy, and fatigue |
| *kava* | to reduce anxiety, relax muscle tension, produce analgesic effects, act as a local anesthetic, provide antibacterial benefit |
| *ma huang (ephedrine)* | derived from the ephedra plant, has been used in China for medicinal purposes including increased energy, appetite suppression, increased fat burning, and preservation of muscle tissue from breakdown; a central nervous system stimulant drug used in many diet pills; in 1995, FDA revealed adverse reactions to ephedrine including heart attacks, strokes, paranoid psychosis, vomiting, fever, palpitations, convulsions, and comas |
| *saw palmetto* | to treat inflamed prostate; also used as a diuretic and as a sexual enhancement agent |
| *St. John's wort* | used as an antidepressant; also used to treat nervous disorders, depression, neuralgia, kidney problems, wounds, and burns |
| *valerian* | to treat insomnia, anxiety, stress |
| *yohimbe* | to increase libido and blood flow to sexual organs in the male |

Hundreds of herbs are widely available today at all quality levels. They are readily available at health-food stores. However, unlike both food and medicine, there are no federal or governmental controls to regulate the sale and ensure the quality of the products being sold. Thus extreme caution must be exercised by the consumer of herbal products.

Table 5-3 lists the most popular and widely used herbal products sold in health-food stores. Some additional potent and complex herbs, such as capsicum, lobelia, sassafras, mandrake, tansy, canada snake root, wormwood, woodruff, poke root, and rue may be useful in small amounts and as catalysts, but should not be used alone.

### Vegetarianism

Many athletes are health conscious and try to do things that are good for their bodies. *Vegetarianism* has emerged as an alternative to the usual American diet. All vegetarians use plant foods to form the foundation of their diet; animal foods are either totally excluded or included in a variety of eating patterns. Athletes who choose to become vegetarians do so for economic, philosophical, religious, cultural, or health reasons. Vegetarianism is no longer considered to be a fad if it is practiced intelligently. However, the vegetarian diet may create deficiencies if nutrient needs are not carefully considered. Athletes who follow this eating pattern need to plan their diet carefully so that their calorie needs are met.

## Preevent Nutrition

The importance and content of the preevent meal have been heatedly debated among coaches, athletic trainers, and athletes. The trend has been to ignore logical thinking about what should be eaten before competition in favor of upholding the tradition of "rewarding" the athlete for hard work by serving foods that may hamper performance. For example, the traditional steak-and-eggs meal before football games is great for coaches and trainers; however, the athlete gains nothing from this meal. The important point is that too often people are concerned primarily with the preevent meal and fail to realize that those nutrients consumed over several days before competition are much more important than what is eaten 3 hours before an event. The purpose of the preevent meal should be to provide the competitor with sufficient nutrient energy and fluids for competition while taking into consideration the digestibility of the food and, most importantly, the eating preferences of the individual athlete. Figure 5-4 gives examples of preevent meals.

**FIGURE 5-4**

Sample preevent meals

**MEAL 1**
³/₄ c Orange juice
¹/₂ c Cereal with 1 tsp sugar
1 slice whole wheat toast with:
   1 tsp Margarine
   1 tsp Honey or jelly     **or**
8 oz Skim or lowfat milk
Water
(Approximately 450–500 kcal)

³/₄ c Orange juice
1–2 Pancakes with:
   1 tsp Margarine
   2 tbsp Syrup
8 oz Skim or lowfat milk
Water
(Approximately 450–500 kcal)

**MEAL 2**
1 c Vegetable soup
1 Turkey sandwich with:
   2 Slices bread
   2 oz Turkey (white or dark)
   1 oz Cheese slice     **or**
   2 tsp Mayonnaise
8 oz Skim or lowfat milk
Water
(Approximately 550–600 kcal)

1 c Spaghetti with tomato sauce and cheese
¹/₂ c Sliced pears (canned) on 1/4 c cottage cheese
1–2 Slices (Italian) bread with 1–2 tsp margarine (avoid garlic)
¹/₂ c Sherbet
1–2 Sugar cookies
4 oz Skim or lowfat milk
Water
(Approximately 700 kcal)

The athlete should be encouraged to be conscious of his or her diet. However, no experimental evidence indicates that performance may be enhanced by altering a diet that is basically sound. A nutritious diet may be achieved in several ways, and the diet that is optimal for one athlete may not be the best for another. In many instances, the individual is the best judge of what he or she should or should not eat in the preevent meal or before exercising. A person's best guide is to eat whatever he or she is most comfortable with.

### Liquid Food Supplements

Liquid food supplements (Gatorpro, Exceed) have been recommended as extremely effective preevent meals and are being used by high school, college, university, and professional teams with some indications of success. These supplements supply from 225 to 400 calories per average serving. Athletes who have used these supplements report elimination of the usual pregame symptoms of dry mouth, abdominal cramps, leg cramps, nervous defecation, and nausea.

Under ordinary conditions it usually takes approximately 4 hours for a full meal to pass through the stomach and the small intestine. Pregame emotional tension often delays the emptying of the stomach; therefore the undigested food mass remains in the stomach and upper bowel for a prolonged time, even up to or through the actual period of competition, and frequently causes nausea, vomiting, and cramps. This unabsorbed food mass is of no value to the athlete. According to team physicians who have experimented with the liquid food supplements, one of their major advantages is that they clear both the stomach and the upper bowel before game time, thus making available the caloric energy that would otherwise still be in an unassimilated state. There is merit in the use of such food supplements for pregame meals.

## GLYCOGEN SUPERCOMPENSATION (LOADING)

For endurance events, maximizing the amount of glycogen that can be stored, especially in muscles, may make the difference between finishing first or at the "end of the pack." Glycogen supplies in muscle and liver can be increased by reducing the training program a few days before competing and by significantly increasing carbohydrate intake during the week before the event. Reducing training for at least 48 hours before the competition allows the body to eliminate any metabolic waste products that may hinder performance. The high-carbohydrate diet restores glycogen levels in muscle and the liver. This practice is called **glycogen supercompensation.** (In the past this practice has been called glycogen loading.) The basis for this practice is that the quantity of glycogen stored in muscle directly affects the endurance of that muscle.

Glycogen supercompensation is accomplished over a 6-day period divided into three phases. In phase 1 (days 1 to 2), training should be very hard and dietary intake of carbohydrates fairly normal, accounting for about 60 percent of total calorie intake. During phase 2 (days 3 to 5),

**glycogen
supercompensation**
High-carbohydrate diet.

training is cut back and the individual eats at least 70 percent or more of the diet in carbohydrates. Studies have indicated that glycogen stores may be increased from 50 to 100 percent, theoretically enhancing endurance during a long-term event. Phase 3 (day 6) is the day of the event, during which a normal diet must be consumed.

The effect of glycogen supercompensation in improving performance during endurance activities has not yet been clearly demonstrated. Glycogen supercompensation should not be done more than two to three times during the course of a year. Glycogen loading is only of value in long-duration events that produce glycogen depletion, such as a marathon.

## Fat Loading

Recently some endurance athletes have tried fat loading in place of carbohydrate loading. Their intent was to have a better source of energy at their disposal. The deleterious effects of this procedure outweigh any benefits that may be derived. Fat loading can lead to cardiac protein and potassium depletion, causing arrhythmias and increased levels of serum cholesterol as a result of the ingestion of butter, cheese, cream, and marbled beef.

## WEIGHT CONTROL AND BODY COMPOSITION

The need for gain or loss of weight in an athlete often poses a problem because the individual's ingrained eating habits are difficult to change. The coach's inability to adequately supervise the athlete's meal program in terms of balance and quantity further complicates the problem. An intelligent and conscientious approach to weight control requires some knowledge of what is involved on the part of both the coach and the athlete. Such understanding allows athletes to better discipline themselves as to the quantity and kinds of foods they should eat.

## Body Composition

**Body composition** refers to both the fat and nonfat components of the body. That portion of total body weight that is composed of fat tissue is referred to as the percent body fat. That portion of the total body weight that is composed of nonfat or lean tissue, which includes muscles, tendons, bones, connective tissue, and so on, is referred to as lean body weight. Body composition measurements are the most accurate way to determine precisely how much weight an athlete may gain or lose.[7]

> **body composition**
> Percent body fat plus lean body weight.

The average college-age female has between 20 and 25 percent of her total body weight made up of fat. The average college-age male has between 12 and 15 percent body fat. Male endurance athletes may get their fat percentage as low as 8 to 12 percent, and female endurance athletes may reach 10 to 18 percent. The recommendation is that body fat percentage not go below 5 percent in males and 12 percent in females, because below these percentages the internal organs tend to lose their protective padding of essential fat, potentially subjecting them to injury.[12]

## Assessing Body Composition

Measuring the thickness of skin folds is based on the fact that about 50 percent of the fat in the body is contained in the subcutaneous fat layers and is closely related to total fat. The remainder of the fat in the body is found around organs and vessels and serves a shock-absorptive function. The skin-fold technique involves measurement of the thickness of the subcutaneous fat layer with a skin-fold caliper.[7]

## Assessing Caloric Balance

Changes in body weight are almost entirely the result of changes in caloric balance.

Positive caloric balance = weight gain
Negative caloric balance = weight loss

*Caloric balance = Number of Calories Consumed – Number of Calories Expended*

Calories may be expended by three different processes: (1) basal metabolism; (2) work (work may be defined as any activity that requires more energy than sleeping); and (3) excretion. If more calories are consumed than expended, the positive caloric balance results in weight gain. Conversely, weight loss results from a negative caloric balance in which more calories are expended than are consumed.

Caloric balance is determined by the number of calories consumed regardless of whether the calories are contained in fat, carbohydrate, or protein. There are differences in the caloric content of these three foodstuffs:

Carbohydrate = 4 calories per gram

Protein = 4 calories per gram

Fat = 9 calories per gram

Alcohol = 7 calories per gram

(Alcohol should not be considered as a foodstuff, but cannot be classified under the other headings. Alcohol contains 7 calories per gram.)

Estimations of caloric intake for college athletes range between 2,000 and 5,000 calories per day. Estimations of caloric expenditure range between 2,200 and 4,400 calories on the average. Energy demands are considerably higher in endurance athletes, who may require as many as 7,000 calories.

## Methods of Weight Loss

There are several ways to lose weight: (1) dieting, (2) increasing the amount of physical exercise, or (3) a combination of diet and exercise.

Weight loss through dieting alone is difficult, and in most cases, dieting is an ineffective means of weight control. Long-term weight control through dieting alone is successful only 20 percent of the time.[15] Through dieting, 35 to 45 percent of the weight decrease results from a loss of lean tissue. The minimum caloric intake for a female should not go below 1,000 to 1,200 calories per day, and for a male, not below 1,200 to 1,400 calories per day.[17]

Weight loss through exercise involves an 80 to 90 percent loss of fat tissue with almost no loss of lean tissue. Weight loss through exercise

( 5-2 )    *Focus Box*

**Guidelines for Weight Loss**

The American College of Sports Medicine has made the following statements and recommendations regarding weight loss:[15]

- Prolonged fasting and diet programs that severely restrict caloric intake
  are scientifically undesirable and can be medically dangerous.
- Fasting and diet programs that severely restrict caloric intake result in
  the loss of large amounts of water, electrolytes, minerals, glycogen
  stores, and other fat-free tissue (including proteins within fat-free tissues), with minimal amounts of fat loss.
- Mild calorie restriction (500 to 1,000 calories less than the usual daily intake) results in a smaller loss of water, electrolytes, minerals, and other
  fat-free tissue and is less likely to cause malnutrition.
- Dynamic exercise of large muscles helps to maintain fat-free tissue, including muscle mass and bone density, and results in losses of body
  weight. Weight loss resulting from an increase in energy expenditure is
  primarily in the form of fat weight.
- A nutritionally sound diet resulting in mild calorie restriction coupled
  with an endurance exercise program, along with behavioral modification of existing eating habits, is recommended for weight reduction. The
  rate of sustained weight loss should not exceed 1 kilogram (2 pounds)
  per week.
- To maintain proper weight control and optimal body fat levels, a lifetime
  commitment to proper eating habits and regular physical activity is
  required.

alone is almost as difficult as losing weight through dieting. However, exercise will not only result in weight reduction but may also enhance cardiorespiratory endurance, improve strength, and increase flexibility.[4] For
this reason, exercise has some distinct advantages over dieting in any
weight-loss program.

The most efficient method of decreasing body fat is through some
combination of diet and exercise.[9] A moderate caloric restriction combined with a moderate increase in caloric expenditure will result in a negative caloric balance. This method is relatively fast and easy compared
with either of the other methods because habits are moderately changed.

In any weight-loss program, the goal should be to lose $1^1/_2$ to 2
pounds per week. Weight loss of more than 4 to 5 pounds during a
week's time may be attributed to dehydration as opposed to a loss of body
fat. The American College of Sports Medicine has established specific
guidelines for losing weight, which are listed in Focus Box 5-2.[15]

## Methods of Weight Gain

The aim of a weight-gaining program should be to increase lean body
mass, that is, increase muscle as opposed to body fat. Muscle mass should
be increased only by muscle work combined with an appropriate increase

in dietary intake. It cannot be increased by the intake of any special food or vitamin.[5]

The recommended rate of weight gain is approximately 1 to 2 pounds per week. Each pound of lean body mass gained represents a positive caloric balance, which is an intake in excess of an expenditure of approximately 2,500 calories. One pound of fat represents the equivalent of 3,500 calories; lean body tissue contains less fat, more protein, and more water and represents approximately 2,500 calories. To gain 1 pound of muscle, an excess of approximately 2,500 calories is needed; to lose one pound of fat, approximately 3,500 calories must be expended in activities in excess of intake.[5] Adding 500 to 1,000 calories daily to the usual diet will provide the energy needs of gaining 1 to 2 pounds per week and fuel the increased energy expenditure of the weight-training program. Weight training must be part of the program. Otherwise, the excess intake of energy will be converted to fat.

## EATING DISORDERS

There is an epidemic in this society, especially in sports. This problem is the inordinate concern with being overweight. Out of this obsession has emerged the eating disorders bulimia and anorexia nervosa. (Female athletic triad is discussed in Chapter 23.) Both these disorders are increasingly seen in athletes.[20] Focus Box 5-3 provides tips for identifying athletes with eating disorders.

### Bulimia

The bulimic person is commonly female, ranging in age from adolescence to middle age. One out of every 200 American girls ages 12 to 18 years (1 to 2 percent of the population) will develop patterns of bulimia and/or anorexia nervosa.[2] The bulimic individual typically gorges herself with thousands of calories after a period of starvation and then purges herself through induced

5–3

*Critical Thinking* Exercise

An ice hockey attackman is at an excellent level of fitness and has superb skating ability and stick work. He is convinced that the only thing keeping him from moving to the next level is his body weight. In recent years he has engaged more in weight-training activities to improve his endurance and, to a lesser extent, to increase strength.

? What recommendations should the coach make for him to be successful in his weight-gaining efforts?

---

5-3    *Focus Box*

**Recognizing the Athlete with an Eating Disorder**

Signs to look for are when athletes display:

- Social isolation and withdrawal from friends and family
- A lack of confidence in athletic abilities
- Ritualistic eating behavior (e.g., organizing food on plate)
- An obsession with counting calories
- An obsession with constantly exercising, especially just before a meal
- An obsession with weighing self
- A constant overestimation of body size
- Patterns of leaving the table directly after eating to go into the restroom
- Problems related to eating disorders (e.g., malnutrition, menstrual irregularities, or chronic fatigue)
- Family history of eating disorders

vomiting and further fasting or through the use of laxatives or diuretics. This secretive binge-eating and purging cycle may go on for years.

Typically the bulimic athlete is white and belongs to a middle- or upper-middle-class family. She is perfectionistic, obedient, overcompliant, highly motivated, very successful academically, well-liked by her peers, and a good athlete.[6] She most commonly participates in gymnastics, track, and dance. Male wrestlers and gymnasts may also develop bulimia. The formal definition of bulimia is as follows: recurrent episodes of rapid, uncontrollable ingestion of large amounts of food in a short time, usually followed by purging, either by forced vomiting and/or abuse of laxatives or diuretics.

Binge-purge patterns of eating can cause stomach rupture, disrupt heart rhythm, and cause liver damage. Stomach acids brought up by vomiting cause tooth decay and chronically inflame the mucous lining of the mouth and throat.[20]

### Anorexia Nervosa

Thirty to fifty percent of all individuals diagnosed as having anorexia nervosa also develop some symptoms of bulimia. Anorexia nervosa is characterized by a distorted body image and a major concern about weight gain. As with bulimia, anorexia nervosa affects mostly females. It usually begins in adolescence and can be mild without major consequences or can become life threatening. As many as 15 to 21 percent of those individuals diagnosed as anorexic will ultimately die from this disorder. Despite being extremely thin, the athlete sees herself as too fat. These individuals deny hunger and are hyperactive, engaging in abnormal amounts of exercise such as aerobics or distance running.[2] In general, the anorexic individual is highly secretive and the coach and athletic trainer must be sensitive to eating problems. Early intervention is essential. Any athlete with signs of bulimia or anorexia nervosa must be confronted in a kind, sympathetic manner by the coach. When detected, individuals with eating disorders must be referred for psychological or psychiatric treatment. Unfortunately, simply referring an anorexic person to a health education clinic for help is not usually effective. The key to treatment of anorexia seems to be getting the patient to realize that a problem exists and that he or she could benefit from outside professional help. The individual must voluntarily accept such help if treatment is to be successful.[17]

*5–4*

***Critical Thinking*** Exercise

A tennis coach observes that one of her players has lost a significant amount of weight. Also, the athlete's level of play has begun to decrease. The coach becomes seriously concerned when another player tells the coach that she thinks her roommate was purposely throwing up after a team meal on a recent road trip.

**?** How should the coach handle this situation?

### COACH'S CORNER

This checklist contains factors the coach should consider to ensure the athlete is consuming a nutritious diet.

☐ Generally, does the athlete consume a reasonably well-balanced diet?
☐ Is it necessary for the athlete to take a daily vitamin supplement?
☐ Does the athlete need to take a mineral supplement because of some dietary deficiency?
☐ Is the athlete consuming a sufficient amount of water to stay hydrated?
☐ Are athletes using sports drinks to replace lost fluids and electrolytes?

☐ Is the athlete consuming excess caffeine, sugar, or protein in an effort to enhance performance?
☐ Does the athlete take herbs or consume other types of health foods?
☐ What does the athlete eat for the preevent meal?
☐ Does the athlete appear to be able to balance his or her intake of food with energy expenditure to maintain weight and body composition at an appropriate level?
☐ Is there anything the athlete is doing to make you suspect that the athlete may have an eating disorder?

## SUMMARY

- The classes of nutrients are carbohydrates, fats, proteins, vitamins, minerals, and water.
- Carbohydrates, fats, and proteins provide the energy required for muscular work and also play a role in the function and maintenance of body tissues.
- Protein supplementation is not necessary.
- Vitamins are substances found in foods, which have no caloric value but are necessary to regulate body processes.
- Antioxidants are nutrients that protect the body against various destructive agents.
- Minerals are also involved in regulation of bodily functions and are used to form important body structures.
- Water is the most essential nutrient and should be used with sports drinks in fluid replacement.
- A nutritious diet consists of eating a variety of foods in the amounts recommended on the food pyramid. An athlete whose diet meets those recommendations may not need nutrient supplements.
- Some people need extra iron and calcium.
- The preevent meal should be (1) higher in carbohydrates, (2) easily digested, (3) eaten 2 to 4 hours before an event, and (4) acceptable to the athlete.
- Glycogen supercompensation involves maximizing the stores of carbohydrate in muscle and liver before a competitive event.
- Body composition analysis indicates the percentage of total body weight composed of fat tissue versus the percentage composed of lean tissue.
- Changes in body weight are caused almost entirely by a change in caloric balance, which is a function of the number of calories taken in and the number of calories expended.
- Weight can be lost by increasing caloric expenditure through exercise, by decreasing caloric intake through reducing food intake, or most effectively, by using a combination of moderate caloric restriction and a moderate increase in physical exercise during the course of each day.

- Bulimia is an eating disorder that involves periodic binging and subsequent purging.

- Anorexia nervosa is a form of mental illness in which a person reduces food intake and increases energy expenditure to the extent that the loss of body fat threatens health and life.

---

*Solutions to Critical Thinking* Exercises

---

**5-1** In terms of weight control, the important consideration is the total number of calories that this athlete consumes relative to the total number of calories she expends. It makes no difference whether the calories consumed are CHO, fat, or protein. Because fat contains more than twice the number of calories as either CHO or protein, this athlete can eat significantly more food and still have about the same calorie intake if the diet is high in CHO. The coach should also stress the necessity of consuming at least some fat in the diet, which is necessary for the production of certain enzymes and hormones.

**5-2** If this athlete is truly consuming anything close to a well-balanced diet, vitamin supplementation is generally not necessary. However if taking a one-a-day vitamin supplement makes her feel better, no harm is done. The fact that she feels tired could be related to a number of medical conditions (e.g., mononucleosis). An iron deficiency anemia may be detected through a laboratory blood test. The coach should refer the athlete to a physician for blood work.

**5-3** This athlete must understand the importance of adding lean tissue muscle mass rather than increasing his percent body fat. It is true that caloric intake must be increased so that he is in a positive caloric balance of about 500 calories per day. Additional calorie intake should consist primarily of CHO. Additional supplementation with protein is not necessary. It is absolutely essential that this athlete incorporate a weight-training program using heavy weights that will overload the muscle, forcing it to hypertrophy over time.

**5-4** Treating eating disorders is difficult even for health care professionals specifically trained to counsel these individuals. The coach should approach the athlete as a support person and not with accusation, showing concern about her weight loss and expressing a desire to help her secure appropriate counseling. Remember that the athlete must first be willing to admit that she has an eating disorder before treatment and counseling will be effective. Eliciting the support of close friends and family can help with treatment.

## REVIEW QUESTIONS AND CLASS ACTIVITIES

1. What is the value of good nutrition in terms of an athlete's performance and injury prevention?
2. Ask coaches of different sports about the type of diet they recommend for their athletes and their rationale for doing so.
3. Have a nutritionist talk to the class about food myths and fallacies.
4. Have each member of the class prepare a week's food diary; then compare it with other class members' diaries.
5. What are the daily dietary requirements according to the food pyramid? Should the requirements of the typical athlete's diet differ from those on the food pyramid? If so, in what ways?
6. Have the class debate the value of vitamin and mineral supplements.

7. Describe the advantages and disadvantages of supplementing iron and calcium.
8. Is there some advantage to preevent nutrition?
9. Are there advantages and/or disadvantages in the vegetarian diet for the athlete?
10. Discuss the importance of having an athlete monitor body composition.
11. Explain the most effective technique for losing weight.
12. Contrast the signs and symptoms of bulimia and anorexia nervosa. If a coach is aware of an athlete who may have an eating disorder, what should he or she do?

## REFERENCES

1. American College of Sports Medicine: Position stand on exercise and fluid replacement, *Med Sci Sports Exerc* 28:1, 1996.
2. Brownell K, Fairburn C: *Eating disorders and obesity: a comprehensive handbook,* New York, 1999, Guilford Press.
3. Casa D, Armstrong L, Hillman S: National Athletic Trainers Association position statement: fluid replacement for athletes, *Journal of Athlete Training* 35(2):212, 2000.
4. Clarkson P et al: Methods and strategies for weight loss in athletics, *Sports Sci Exchange* 9(1):1–5, 1998.
5. Clarkson PM: Nutritional supplements for weight gain, *Sports Sci Exchang* 11(1):1, 1998.
6. Claude-Pierre P: *The secret language of eating disorders,* New York, 1999, Vintage Books.
7. DeLorenzo A et al: Comparison of different techniques to measure body composition in moderately active adolescents, *Br J Sports Med* 32(3):215, 1998.
8. Foster S: *101 medicinal herbs,* Loveland, Colo, 1998, Interweave Press.
9. Grilo CM: The role of physical activity in weight loss and weight loss management, *Med Exerc Nutr Health* 4(2):60, 1995.
10. Larson-Duyff R: *The American Dietetic Association's complete food and nutrition guide,* New York, 1998, John Wiley and Sons.
11. Lewis RD, Modlesky CM: Nutrition, physical activity, and bone health in women, *Int J Sport Nutr* 8(3):250, 1998.
12. Marks BL, Rippe JM: The importance of fat free mass maintenance in weight loss programmes, *Sports Med* 22(5):273, 1996.
13. McArdle W, Katch F, Katch V: *Sports and exercise nutrition,* Baltimore, 1999, Lippincott, Williams and Wilkins.
14. Papas A, Quillen J: *Antioxidant status: diet, nutrition, and health,* Boca Raton, Fla, 1998, CRC Press.
15. Parr RB: Weight loss: what works and what doesn't, *Am Coll Sports Med Health Fitness J* 2(2):12, 1998.
16. Peterson D: Athletes and iron deficiency: is it true anemia or "sport anemia"? *Physician Sportsmed* 26(2):24, 1998.
17. Rhea DJ, Jambor EA, Wiginton K: Preventing eating disorders in female athletes, *Journal of Physical Education, Recreation and Dance* 67(4): 66–68, 1996.
18. Sanborn CF et al: Disordered eating and the female athlete triad, *Clin Sports Med* 19(2):199, 2000.
19. Shi X, Gisolfi CV: Fluid and carbohydrate replacement during intermittent exercise, *Sports Med* 25(3):157, 1998.
20. Sundgot-Borgen J: Eating disorders in athletes. In Sundgot-Borgen J, editor: *Nutrition in sport,* Oxford, 2000, Blackwell.
21. Wardlaw GM, Insel PM: *Perspectives in nutrition,* ed. 4, Boston, 1998, WCB/McGraw-Hill.
22. Williams C, Nicholas C-W: Nutrition needs for team sport, *Sci Sports Exchange* 11(3):1, 1998.

23. Williams M: *Nutrition for health, fitness, and sport,* St Louis, 1998, WCB/McGraw-Hill.

## ANNOTATED BIBLIOGRAPHY

Clark N: *Nancy Clark's sports nutrition guidebook,* Champaign, Ill, 1996, Human Kinetics.

*Complete guide to eating for the vigorous person. Provides the basics of sports nutrition and includes over 100 fast recipes for meals that enhance physical performance.*

Sheldan M: *Wellness encyclopedia for food and nutrition,* New York, 2000, Rebus.

*Covers every type of whole, fresh food found in supermarkets, specialty shops, and health-food stores. Also presents the latest information on what makes up a healthy diet and on the connection between diet and disease protection.*

Weil A: *Eating well for optimum health: the essential guide to food, diet, and nutrition,* New York, 2000, Knopf.

*Offers a thorough rundown of nutritional basics and a primer of micronutrients such as vitamins, minerals, and fiber.*

Williams M: *Nutrition for fitness and sport,* Boston, 1998, WCB/McGraw-Hill.

*Provides the reader with thorough coverage of the role nutrition plays in enhancing health, fitness, and sport performance. Current research and practical activities are incorporated throughout.*

## WEBSITES

Food and Nutrition Information Center: http://www.nalusda.gov/fnic

*Part of the information centers at the National Agricultural Library, this site provides access to information on healthy eating habits, food composition, and many additional resources.*

Yahoo Health and Nutrition Information: http://www.yahoo.com/Health/ Nutrition

*Includes diet analysis information, nutritional facts, and links to many informative sites.*

Eating Disorders: http://www. something_fishy.com/ed.htm

*Eating disorder information can be found here, including information about anorexia, bulimia, and overeating as well as information about how to access support groups.*

Athletes and Eating Disorders: http:// www. uq. net.au/~zzedainc/ n3frames.html

*Part of the Eating Disorders Resources Website; recent statistics of an NCAA study are provided including a section on the coach's responsibility; also includes information about warning signs and the female athlete triad.*

The American Dietetic Association: http://www.eatright.org

*This site includes access to the journal published by the American Dietetic Association and provides informative nutritional tips and a section entitled "gateway to nutrition".*

Gatorade Sports Science Institute http://www.gssiweb.com/

*This Website provides information for coaches, athletic trainers, physicians, nutritionists, and others in the field of sports medicine, sports nutrition, and exercise science.*

Healthy Biz 2000 http://www. healthybiz2000.com/trainer.html

*Information about sports nutrition and nutritional supplements for fitness and weight loss.*

# PART

2

# TECHNIQUES FOR PREVENTING AND MINIMIZING SPORT-RELATED INJURIES

# Protective Sports Equipment

*When you finish this chapter you will be able to:*

- Discuss legal concerns related to the use of protective equipment.
- Identify the different types of protective equipment available for various parts of the body.
- Describe the proper technique for fitting a football helmet and shoulder pads.
- Discuss what consideration should be given to shoe selection.
- Discuss the efficacy of knee and ankle braces in reducing injuries.

Because of the nature of sports activity, injuries often occur. One of the main responsibilities of the coach is to try to minimize the likelihood of injury. A number of factors either singly or collectively can contribute to the incidence of injury. Certainly the selection, fitting, and maintenance of protective equipment are critical in injury prevention. Thus it is essential that the coach have some knowledge about the types of protective equipment available for a particular sport and how that equipment should best be fitted and maintained to reduce the possibility of athletic injury.

This protection is particularly important in direct contact and collision sports such as football, hockey, and lacrosse, but it can also be important in indirect contact sports such as basketball and soccer. When protective sports equipment is selected and purchased, a major commitment is made to safeguard athletes' health and welfare.[13]

## SAFETY STANDARDS FOR SPORTS EQUIPMENT AND FACILITIES

There is serious concern about the standards for protective sports equipment, particularly material durability standards—concerns that include who should set these standards, mass production of equipment, equipment testing methods, and requirements for wearing protective equipment.

Standards are also needed for protective equipment maintenance, both to keep it in good repair and to determine when to throw it away. Too often, old, worn-out, and ill-fitting equipment is passed down

Old, worn-out, ill-fitting equipment should never be passed down to younger, less-experienced players; it compounds their risk of injury.

*Focus Box*

**Equipment Regulatory Agencies**

American National Standards Institute
1819 L Street NW
Washington, DC 20036
(202) 293-8020
http://www.ansi.org

Amercian Society for Testing Materials
100 Barr Harbor Drive
West Conshohocken, PA 19428-2959
(610) 832-9585
http://www.astm.org

Athletic Equipment Manufacturers Association
Dorothy Cutting
Cornell University Athletic Department
P.O. Box 729
Ithaca, NY 14851
(607) 255-4115
http://www.wisc.edu/ath/aema/

National Athletic Trainers Association
2952 Stemmons Freeway
Dallas, TX 75247-6196
(214) 637-6282
http://www.nata.org

National Collegiate Athletic Association
700 W. Washington Street
P.O. Box 6222
Indianapolis, IN 46206-6222
http://www.ncaa.org

National Association of Intercollegiate Athletics
6120 S. Yale Avenue
Suite 1450
Tulsa, OK 74136
(918) 494-8828
http://www.naia.org

National Federation of State High School
Athletic Associations
P.O. Box 690
Indianapolis, IN 46200
(317) 972-6900
http://www.nfhs.org

National Operating Committee on Standards
for Athletic Equipment
P.O. Box 12290
Overland, KS 66282-2290
http://www.nocsae.org

Sporting Goods Manufacturers Association
200 Castlewood Drive
North Palm Beach, FL 33418
(561) 842-4100
http://sgma@ix.netcom.com

U.S. Consumer Product Safety Commission
4330 East-West Highway
Bethesda, MD 20814-4408
(301) 504-0990
http://www.cpsc.gov

from the varsity players to the younger and often less-experienced players, compounding their risk of injury. Coaches must learn to be less concerned with the color, look, and style of a piece of equipment and more concerned with its ability to prevent injury. Many national organizations are addressing these issues. Engineering, chemistry, biomechanics, anatomy, physiology, physics, computer science, and other related disciplines are applied to solve problems inherent in safety standardization of sports equipment and facilities. Focus Box 6-1 lists regulatory agencies.

## LEGAL CONCERNS IN USING PROTECTIVE EQUIPMENT

As with other aspects of sports participation there is increasing litigation related to the use of protective equipment. Both manufacturers and those who purchase sports equipment must foresee all possible uses and misuses of the equipment and must warn the user of any potential risks inherent in using or misusing that equipment.

6–1

*Critical Thinking* Exercise

A student coach must acquire a basic understanding of protective sports equipment.

? What competencies in protective sports equipment must coaches have?

If an injury occurs as the result of an athlete using a piece of equipment and if that piece of equipment is determined to be defective or inadequate for its intended purpose the manufacturer is considered liable. If a piece of protective equipment is modified in any way either by the athlete or by the coach (e.g., removing some pads from inside a football helmet) the liability on the part of the manufacturer is voided, and thus the individual who modified the equipment becomes liable.

If the coach in some way modifies a piece of equipment and an athlete wearing that equipment is injured, it is likely that any lawsuit would involve both the coach individually and the employing institution. This becomes a case of tort (described in Chapter 3) in which the injured athlete must show that the coach was negligent in his or her decision to alter a piece of equipment and that the negligence resulted in injury. The coach would then be legally liable for that action.

## USING OFF-THE-SHELF VS. CUSTOM PROTECTIVE EQUIPMENT

6–2

*Critical Thinking* Exercise

C- and B-level high school football players are issued their equipment. These athletes and their parents know very little about the equipment's potential for preventing injury.

? What is the responsibility of the coach in educating the team and their parents about equipment safety limits?

"Off-the-shelf" equipment is premade and packaged by the manufacturer and when taken out of the package may be used immediately without modification. Examples of off-the-shelf equipment are neoprene sleeves, sorbethane shoe inserts, and protective ankle braces. Customized equipment is constructed according to the individual characteristics of the athlete. Using off-the-shelf items may cause problems with sizing and exact fit. In contrast, a custom-made piece of equipment can be specifically sized and made to fit the protective and support needs of the individual.

## HEAD PROTECTION

Direct-collision sports such as football and hockey require special protective equipment, especially for the head. Football involves more body contact than does hockey, but hockey players generally move faster and therefore create greater impact forces. Besides direct head contact stemming from hitting the boards, hockey has the added injury elements of swinging sticks and fast-moving pucks. Other sports using fast-moving projectiles are baseball, with its pitched ball and swinging bat, and track and field, with the javelin, discus, and heavy shot, which can also produce serious head injuries.[13]

### Football Helmets

Football helmets must withstand repeated blows that are of high mass and low velocity.

The National Operating Committee on Standards for Athletic Equipment (NOCSAE) has developed standards for football helmet certification.[9] An approved helmet must protect against concussive forces that may injure the brain.[9]

Schools must provide the athlete with quality equipment, especially the football helmet. All helmets must have a NOCSAE certification. The fact that a helmet is certified does not mean that it is completely fail-safe. Athletes and their parents must be apprised of the dangers that are inherent in any sport, particularly football. To make this point especially clear, NOCSAE has adopted the following recommended warning to be placed on all football helmets:

> *Warning: Do not strike an opponent with any part of this helmet or face mask. This is a violation of football rules and may cause you to suffer severe brain or neck injury: including paralysis or death. Severe brain or neck injury may also occur accidentally while playing football.* NO HELMET CAN PREVENT ALL SUCH INJURIES. USE THIS HELMET AT YOUR OWN RISK.

Each player's helmet must have a visible exterior warning label ensuring that players have been made aware of the risks involved in the game of American football. The label must be attached to each helmet by both the manufacturer and the reconditioner.[9]

Each player must read this warning, after which it is read aloud by the coach or equipment manager. The athlete then signs a statement agreeing that he or she understands this warning (Figure 6-1).

When fitting helmets, always wet the player's hair to simulate playing conditions; this will make the initial fitting easier. Closely follow the manufacturer's directions for a proper fit (see Focus Box 6-2).

The football helmet must be routinely checked for proper fit, especially in the first few days that it is worn (Figure 6-2). If air bladder helmets are used by a team that travels to a different altitude and air pressure, the helmet fit must be routinely rechecked.

Chin straps are also important in maintaining the proper head and helmet relationship. Two basic types of chin straps are in use today—a

**Figure 6-1**

The air and fluid-filled football helmet

---

( 6-2 ) **Focus Box**

**Proper Football Helmet Fit**

To properly fit a football helmet:

- The helmet should fit snugly around all parts of the player's head (front, sides, and crown), and there should be no gaps between the pads and the head or face.
- It should cover the base of the skull. The pads placed at the back of the neck should be snug but not to the extent of discomfort.
- It should not come down over the eyes. It should sit (front edge) ¾ inch (1.91 cm) above the player's eyebrows.
- The ear holes should match.
- It should not shift when manual pressure is applied.
- It should not recoil on impact.
- The chin strap should be an equal distance from the center of the helmet.
- Straps must keep the helmet from moving up and down or side to side.
- The cheek pads should fit snugly against the sides of the face.
- The face mask should be attached securely to the helmet, allowing a complete field of vision.

( 6-3 )

**Critical Thinking** Exercise

The coach is responsible for explaining the potential risks involved in wearing a football helmet to the football players.

? What are the most critical points to stress?

**Figure 6-2**

Fitting a football helmet: A, Pull down on face mask; helmet must not move. B, Turn helmet to position on the athlete's head. C, Push down on helmet; there must be no movement. D, Try to rock helmet back and forth; there must be no movement. E, Check for a snug jaw pad fit. F, Proper adjustment of the chin strap is necessary to ensure proper helmet fit.

Even high-quality helmets are of no use if not properly fitted or maintained.

Ice hockey helmets must withstand the high-velocity impact of a stick or puck and the low-velocity forces of falling or hitting a board.

two-snap and a four-snap strap. Many coaches prefer the four-snap chin strap because it keeps the helmet from tilting forward and backward.

Jaw pads are also essential to keep the helmet from rocking laterally. They should rest snugly against the player's cheekbones. Even if a helmet's ability to withstand the forces of the game is certified, it is of no avail if the helmet is not properly fitted or maintained.

## Ice Hockey Helmets

As with football helmets, there has been a concerted effort to upgrade and standardize ice hockey helmets.[13] In contrast to football, blows to the head in ice hockey are usually singular rather than multiple. An ice hockey helmet must withstand both high-velocity impacts (e.g., being hit with a stick or a puck, which produces a force that has low mass and high velocity) and the high mass–low velocity forces produced by running into the boards or falling on the ice. In each instance, the hockey helmet, like the football helmet, must be able to spread the impact over a large surface area through a firm exterior shell and at the same time be able to decelerate forces that act on the head through a proper energy-absorbing liner. All hockey players must wear protective helmets that carry the stamp of approval from the Canadian Standards Association (CSA).

## Baseball/Softball Batting Helmets

Like ice hockey helmets, the baseball/softball helmet must withstand high-velocity impacts. Unlike football and ice hockey, baseball and softball have not produced a great deal of data on batting helmets.[13] It has been suggested, however, that baseball/softball helmets do not adequately dissipate the energy of the ball during impact (Figure 6-3). A possible answer is to add external padding or to improve the helmet's suspension. The use of a helmet with an ear flap can afford some additional protection to the batter. Each on-deck batter and runner is required to wear a baseball/softball head protector that carries a NOCSAE stamp similar to that on football helmets.

## FACE PROTECTION

Devices that provide face protection fall into four categories: full face guards, mouth guards, ear guards, and eye protection devices.

### Face Guards

Face guards are used in a variety of sports to protect the face from carried or flying objects during a collision with another player (Figure 6-4). Since the adoption of face guards and mouth guards for use in football, mouth injuries have been reduced more than 50 percent (Figure 6-5), but the incidence of neck injuries has increased significantly. The catcher in baseball, hockey players, lacrosse players, and football players should all be adequately protected against facial injuries, particularly lacerations and fractures (Figure 6-6).

A variety of face masks and bars is available to the player, depending on the position played and the protection needed. In football no face protection should have fewer than two bars. Proper mounting of the face

**Figure 6-3**

There is some question about how well baseball batting helmets protect against high-velocity impacts.

In sports, the face may be protected by:
- Face guards
- Mouth guards
- Ear guards
- Eye protection devices

**Figure 6-4**

Sports such as fencing require complete face protection.

**Figure 6-5**

Face guards used in football

A

B

**Figure 6-6**

A, Baseball catcher's mask.
B, Lacrosse helmet and
faceguard

A properly fitted mouth
guard protects the teeth,
absorbs blows to the chin,
and can help prevent
concussion.

mask and bars is imperative for maximum safety. All mountings should be made in such a way that the bar attachments are flush with the helmet. A 3-inch (7.62 cm) space should exist between the top of the face guard and the lower edge of the helmet. No helmet should be drilled more than one time on each side, and this drilling must be done by a factory-authorized reconditioner. Attachment of a bar or face mask not specifically designed for the helmet can invalidate the manufacturer's warranty.

Ice hockey face masks have been shown to reduce the incidence of facial injuries. In high school face masks are required for all players, not just the goalkeeper. Helmets should be equipped with commercial plastic-coated wire-mesh guards that must meet standards set by the Hockey Equipment Certification Council (HECC) and the American Society for Testing Materials (ASTM). The openings in the guard must be small enough to prevent a hockey stick from penetrating. Plastic guards such as polycarbonate face shields have been approved by the HECC/ASTM and by the CSA Committee on Hockey Protective Equipment. In addition to face protectors, goalkeepers should wear commercial throat protectors.

### Laryngotracheal (Throat) Protection

A laryngotracheal injury, though relatively uncommon, can be fatal. Baseball catchers, lacrosse goalies, and ice hockey goalies are most at risk. Throat protection should be mandatory in these sports.[13]

### Mouth Guards

The majority of dental traumas can be prevented if the athlete wears a customized intraoral mouth guard, as compared with an extraoral type (Figure 6-7). In addition to protecting the teeth, the intraoral mouth guard absorbs the shock of chin blows and helps reduce the chance of cerebral concussion. Mouth guards serve also to minimize lacerations to the lips and cheeks and fractures to the lower jaw.[2]

The mouth guard should provide a tight fit, comfort, unrestricted breathing, and unimpeded speech during competition.[1] The athlete's air passages should not be obstructed in any way by the mouthpiece. It is best when the mouthpiece is retained on the upper jaw and projects backward only as far as the last molar, thus permitting speech.

**Figure 6-7**

Moldable and customized
mouth protectors

Cutting down mouth guards to cover only the front four teeth should never be condoned. It invalidates the manufacturer's warranty against dental injuries, and a cut-down mouth guard can easily become dislodged and lead to an obstructed airway, which poses a serious life-threatening situation for the athlete. Maximum protection is afforded when the mouth guard is composed of a flexible, resilient material and is form fitted to the teeth and upper jaw.[2]

Three types of mouth guards generally used in sports include the ready-made stock variety, a commercial mouth guard formed after submersion in boiling water, and the custom-fabricated type, which is formed over a mold made from an impression of the athlete's maxillary arch.

Many high schools and colleges now require that mouth guards be worn at all times during competition and must be visible to the officials.

## Ear Guards

With the exception of boxing and wrestling, most contact sports do not make a special practice of protecting the ears. Both boxing and wrestling can cause irritation of the ears to the point that permanent deformity can result. To avoid this problem special ear guards should be routinely worn. Recently a very effective ear protector has been developed for the water polo player (Figure 6-8).

A

B

**Figure 6-8**

Ear protection: A, Wrestler's ear guard. B, Water polo player's ear protection

Techniques for Preventing
and Minimizing
Sport-Related Injuries

## Glasses

For the athlete who must wear corrective lenses, glasses can be both a blessing and a nuisance. They may slip on sweat, get bent when hit, fog from perspiration, detract from peripheral vision, and be difficult to wear with protective headgear. Even with all these disadvantages, properly fitted and designed glasses can provide adequate protection and withstand the rigors of the sport. If the athlete has glass lenses, they must be case-hardened to prevent them from splintering on impact. When a case-hardened lens breaks, it crumbles, eliminating the sharp edges that may penetrate the eye. The cost of this process is relatively low. The only disadvantages involved are that the glasses are heavier than average and they may be scratched more easily than regular glasses.[8]

Another possible sports advantage of glass-lensed glasses is a process through which the lenses can become color tinted when exposed to ultraviolet rays from the sun and then return to a clear state when removed from the sun's rays. These lenses are known as photochromic lenses. Plastic lenses for glasses are popular with athletes. They are much lighter in weight than glass lenses and they can be made scratch resistant with a special coating.

## Contact Lenses

The athlete who is able to wear contact lenses without discomfort can avoid many of the inconveniences of glasses.[8] The greatest advantage to contact lenses is that they "become a part of the eye" and move with it.

Contact lenses come mainly in two types: the corneal type, a hard plastic lens that covers just the iris of the eye, and the scleral type, a soft plastic lens that is a little larger. Peripheral vision, astigmatism, and corneal waviness are improved through the use of contact lenses. Unlike regular glasses, contact lenses do not normally cloud during temperature changes. They also can be tinted to reduce glare. For example, yellow lenses can be used against ice glare and blue ones against glare from snow. Generally, athletes prefer the soft, hydrophilic lenses to the hard type. The soft lenses require a shorter adjustment time than the hard lenses do, they can be more easily replaced, and they are more adaptable to the sports environment.

## Eye and Glasses Guards

Eye protection must be worn by all athletes who play sports that use fast-moving projectiles.

It is essential that athletes take special precautions to protect their eyes, especially in sports that use fast-moving projectiles and implements (Figure 6-9). Besides the more obvious sports of ice hockey, lacrosse, and baseball, the racquet sports also cause serious eye injury. Athletes not wearing glasses should wear closed eye guards to protect the orbital cavity. Athletes who normally wear glasses with plastic or case-hardened lenses are to some degree already protected against eye injury from an implement or projectile; however, greater safety is afforded if the athlete wears a polycarbonate frame that surrounds and fits over the athlete's

**Figure 6-9**

glasses. The protection that the guard offers is excellent, but it does hinder vision in some planes.[8]

Polycarbonate eye shields can be attached to football face masks, hockey helmets, and baseball/softball helmets.

Athletes playing sports that involve small, fast projectiles should wear closed eye guards.

## TRUNK AND THORAX PROTECTION

Trunk and thorax protection is essential in many contact and collision sports. Areas that are most exposed to impact forces must be covered with some material that offers protection against soft-tissue compression (Figures 6-10 and 6-11).

### Football Shoulder Pads

There are two general types of pads, flat and cantilevered. The player who uses the shoulder a great deal in blocking and tackling requires the bulkier cantilevered type, whereas the quarterback and ball receiver use the flat type (Figure 6-12). Over the years the shoulder pad's front and rear panels have been extended along with the cantilever. The following are rules for fitting the football shoulder pad:[13]

- The width of the shoulder is measured to determine the proper size of pad.
- The inside shoulder pad should cover the tip of the shoulder in a direct line with the lateral aspect of the shoulder.
- The epaulets and cups should cover the deltoid muscle and allow movements required by the athlete's specific position.
- The neck opening must allow the athlete to raise the arm over the head without placing undue pressure on the neck yet must not allow the pad to slide back and forth.
- If a split-clavicle shoulder pad is used, the channel for the top of the shoulder must be in the proper position.

**Figure 6-10**

Full-body protection: Baseball chest protector for catchers

**Figure 6-11**

Football shoulder pads protect both the shoulder and thorax. A, B, C, Football shoulder pads. D, Lacrosse shoulder pad

■ Straps underneath the arm must hold the pads firmly in place, but not so they constrict soft tissue. A collar and drop-down pads may be added to provide additional protection.

Some coaches use a combination of football and ice hockey shoulder pads to prevent injuries high on the upper arm and shoulder. A pair of supplemental shoulder pads is placed under the regular football pads. The deltoid cap of the hockey pad is connected to the main body of the hockey pad by an adjustable lace (Figure 6-13). The distal end of the deltoid cap is held in place by a Velcro strap. The chest pad is adjustable to ensure proper fit for any size athlete. The football shoulder pads are placed over the hockey pads. The coach should inspect the pads for a proper fit. Larger football pads may be needed.

## Sports Bras

Manufacturers have made significant efforts to develop athletic support bras for women who participate in all types of physical activity. In the past, the primary concern was for breast protection against external forces that could cause bruising. Most sports bras are now designed to minimize excessive vertical and horizontal movements of the breasts that occur with running and jumping.[11] Several styles of sports bras are now available.

1. A *compressive bra* is perhaps the most common and is recommended for women with medium size breasts. Compressive bras function like wide elastic bandages, binding the breasts to the chest wall (Figure 6-14A).

Epaulet

Shoulder
cup

Breastplate

Extended
deltoid
pad

Belt
strap

Pectoral
pad

**Figure 6-12**

Football shoulder pads
should be made to protect
the player against direct force
to the entire shoulder
complex.

2. *Support bras* are a bit more heavy duty and provide good upward support with elastic material. They tend to have wide bands under the breasts with wide shoulder straps in the back. They are designed for women with larger breasts (Figure 6-14B).

3. For women with smaller breasts it is not as critical to provide compression or support and thus a less elastic lightweight bra is sufficient (Figure 6-14C).

**Figure 6-13**

Customized foam is placed on the underside of the shoulder pad to provide additional protection.

**Figure 6-14**

Female athletes should wear sports bras made of elastic material. A, Compressive bra. B, Supportive bra. C, Lightweight bra.

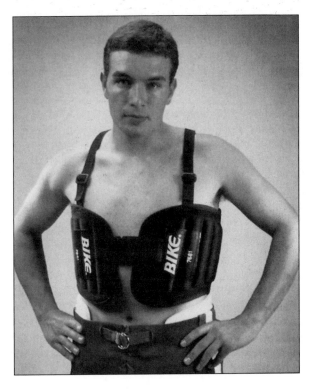

**Figure 6-15**

Protective rib belt

In contact sports additional padding may be placed inside the cup if needed. Women competing in ice hockey, for example, wear protective plastic chest pieces that attach to their shoulder pads to protect the breast tissue from contusions.

### Thorax Protection

Several manufacturers provide off-the-shelf pads for thorax protection. Many of the thorax protectors and rib belts can be modified, replacing stock pads with customized thermomoldable plastic protective devices[13] (Figure 6-15). Recently many lightweight pads have been developed to protect the athlete against external forces. A jacket for the protection of a rib injury incorporates a pad composed of air-inflated, interconnected cylinders that protect against severe external forces. This same principle has been used in the development of other protective pads.

**Figure 6-16**

Girdle-style hip and coccygeal pad

### Hips and Buttocks

Pads in the region of the hips and buttocks are often needed by athletes in collision and high-velocity sports such as hockey and football. Other athletes needing protection in this region are amateur boxers, snow skiers, equestrians, jockeys, and water skiers. Two popular commercial pads are the girdle and belt types (Figure 6-16).

**Figure 6-17**

A cup, held in place by an
athletic supporter, used for
protecting the genitals
against high-velocity
projectiles

All athletic socks should be
clean and dry and without
holes. Socks of the wrong
size can irritate the skin.

### Groin and Genitalia

Sports involving high-velocity projectiles (e.g., hockey, lacrosse, and baseball) require cup protection for male participants. The cup comes as a stock item that fits into place in a jockstrap or athletic supporter (Figure 6-17).

## LOWER EXTREMITY PROTECTIVE EQUIPMENT

### Footwear

It is essential that the coach and equipment personnel make every effort to select and fit their athletes with proper shoes and socks (Figure 6-18).

#### Socks

Poorly fitted socks can create a variety of problems for the foot. For example, socks that are too short apply excessive pressure to the fourth and fifth toes. Socks that are too long can cause skin irritation because of wrinkles. All socks should be clean, dry, and without holes to avoid irritations. Manufacturers provide double-knit tubular socks without heels that decrease friction considerably within the shoe. The heelless tubular sock is especially good for the basketball player. The sock's material also should be noted. Cotton socks can be too bulky; a combination of materials such as cotton and some lightweight synthetic material is less bulky and dries faster.

#### Shoe Selection

The athletic and fitness shoe manufacturing industry has become extremely sophisticated and offers a number of options when it comes to purchasing shoes for different activities.[16] Figure 6-18 shows the major parts of a shoe. The following guidelines can help in selecting the most appropriate shoe:

- *Toe Box.* There should be plenty of room for the toes in the fitness shoe. Most experts recommend a ½- to ¾-inch distance between the longest toe and the front of the shoe. A few fitness shoes are made in

**Figure 6-18**

Parts of a well-designed
sports shoe

varying widths. If an athlete has a very wide or narrow foot, most shoe salespersons can recommend a specific shoe for that foot. The best way to make sure there is adequate room in the toe box is to have the foot measured and then try on the shoe.

- *Sole.* The sole should possess two qualities. First, it must provide a shock absorptive function; second, it must be durable. Most shoes have three layers on the sole: a thick spongy layer, which absorbs the force of the foot strike under the heel; a midsole, which cushions the midfoot and toes; and a hard rubber layer, which comes in contact with the ground. The average runner's feet strike the ground between 1,500 and 1,700 times per mile. Thus it is essential that the force of the heel strike be absorbed by the spongy layer to prevent overuse injuries from occurring in the ankles and knees. "Heel wedges" are sometimes inserted either on the inside or outside surface of the sole underneath the heel counter to accommodate and correct for various structural deformities of the foot that may alter normal biomechanics of the running gait. A flared heel may be appropriate for running shoes but is not recommended in aerobic or court shoes. The sole must provide good traction and must be made of a tough material that is resistant to wear. Most of the better-known brands of shoes have well-designed, long-lasting soles.

- *Heel counters.*   The heel counter is the portion of the shoe that prevents the foot from rolling from side to side at heel strike. The heel counter should be firm but well fitted to minimize movement of the heel up and down or side to side. A good heel counter may prevent ankle sprains and painful blisters.

- *Shoe uppers.*   The upper part of the shoe is made of some combination of nylon and leather. The uppers should be lightweight, quick drying, and well ventilated. The uppers should have some type of extra support in the saddle area, and there should be some extra padding in the area of the Achilles tendon just above the heel counter.

- *Arch support.*   The arch support should be made of some durable yet soft supportive material and should smoothly join with the insole. The support should not have any rough seams or ridges inside the shoe, which may cause blisters.

- *Price.*   Unfortunately, in many instances price is the primary consideration in buying athletic shoes. When buying athletic shoes, remember that in many activities shoes are important for performance and prevention of injury. Thus it is worth a little extra investment to buy a quality pair of shoes.

**Shoe fitting**   Fitting sports footgear is always difficult, mainly because the individual's left foot varies in size and shape from the right foot. Therefore measuring both feet is imperative. To fit the sports shoe properly, the athlete should approximate the conditions under which he or she will perform, such as wearing athletic socks, jumping up and down,

**TABLE 6-1** Shoe comparisons

| | Tennis | Aerobic | Running |
|---|---|---|---|
| Flexibility | Firm sole, more rigid than running shoe | Sole between running and tennis shoe | Flexible ball of foot |
| Uppers | Leather or leather with nylon | Leather or leather with nylon | Nylon or nylon mesh |
| Heel flare | None | Very little | Flared for stability |
| Cushioning | Less than a running shoe | Between running and tennis shoe | Heel and sole well padded |
| Soles | Polyurethane | Rubber or polyurethane | Carbon-based material for greater durability |
| Tread | Flattened | Flat or pivot dot | Deep grooves for grip |

and running. It is also desirable to fit the athlete's shoes at the end of the day to accommodate the gradual increase in size that occurs from the time of awakening. The athlete must carefully consider this choice because he or she will be spending countless hours in those shoes (Table 6-1).

During performance conditions the new shoe should feel snug but not too tight.[6] The sports shoe should be long enough that all toes can be fully extended without being cramped. Its width should permit full movement of the toes, including flexion, extension, and some spreading. A good point to remember is that the wide part of the shoe should match the wide part of the foot to allow the shoe to crease evenly when the athlete is on the balls of the feet. The shoe should bend (or "break") at its widest part; when the break of the shoe and the ball joint coincide, the fit is correct. However, if the break of the shoe is in back or in front of the normal bend of the foot (metatarsophalangeal joint), the shoe and the foot will be opposing one another, causing abnormal skin and structural stresses to occur. Two measurements must be considered when fitting shoes: (1) the distance from the heel to the bend in the foot and (2) the distance from the heel to the end of the longest toe. An individual's feet may be equal in length from the heels to the balls of the feet but different between heels and toes. Shoes, therefore, should be selected for the longer of the two measurements. Other factors to consider when buying the sports shoe are the stiffness of the sole and the width of the shank, or narrowest part of the sole. A shoe with a too rigid, nonyielding sole places a great deal of extra strain on the foot tendons. A shoe with too narrow a shank also causes extra strain because it fails to adequately support the athlete's inner, longitudinal arches. Two other shoe features to consider are innersoles to reduce friction and built-in arch supports.[6]

A properly fitted shoe will bend where the foot bends.

6–4

*Critical Thinking* Exercise

A high school basketball player is given advice on purchasing a pair of basketball shoes.

? What fitting factors must be taken into consideration when purchasing basketball shoes?

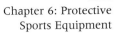

**Figure 6-19**

Variations in cleated shoes—
the longer the cleat, the
higher the incidence of
injury.

**The specialty soled shoe**  The cleated or specialty soled sports shoe presents some additional problems in selection. For example, American football shoes use the multi-short-and-cleated polyurethane sole and often use a five-in-front-and-two-in-back cleat arrangement that is common with the soccer-type sole. Both football and soccer shoes have cleats no longer than ½ inch (1.27 cm) (Figure 6-19). Special-soled shoes are also worn when playing on a synthetic surface. If cleated shoes are used, no matter what the sport, the cleats must be properly positioned under the two major weight-bearing joints and must not be felt through the soles of the shoes.

### Using Orthotics

An orthotic is a device for correcting biomechanical problems that exist in the foot that can potentially cause an injury.[15] The orthotic is a plastic, thermoplastic, rubber, sorbethane, or leather support that is placed in the shoe as a replacement for the existing insole.[10] Ready-made orthotics can be purchased in sporting goods or shoe stores. Some athletes need orthotics that are custom made by a physician, podiatrist, athletic trainer, or physical therapist. These are more expensive but can be well worth the expense if the athlete's feet cause pain and discomfort, especially when exercising (Figure 6-20).

### Heel Cups

Heel cups should be used for a variety of conditions including plantar fasciitis, a heel spur, Achilles tendonitis, and heel bursitis (Figure 6-21). Heel cups may be either hard plastic or spongy rubber. The heel cup helps to compress the fat pad under the heel, providing more heel cushioning during weight-bearing activities.

### Commercial Ankle Supports

Currently, semirigid ankle braces such as the Air Stirrup are being used successfully to restrain ankle motion. Compared with ankle taping, these devices do not loosen significantly during exercise (Figure 6-22).[4] Commercial ankle stabilizers, used either alone or in combination with ankle taping, are becoming increasingly popular in sports.[7]

**Figure 6-20**

Commercially manufactured
orthotic devices

### Shin and Lower Leg Protection

The shin is commonly neglected in contact and collision sports. Commercially marketed hard-shelled, molded shin guards are used in field hockey and soccer (Figure 6-23).

### Thigh and Upper Leg Protection

Thigh and upper leg protection is necessary in collision sports such as football, soccer, and hockey. Generally, pads slip into ready-made pock-

**Figure 6-21**

Heel cups and pads, including
lifts of orthotic felt

**Figure 6-22**

Commercial ankle supports
for an injured ankle

ets in the uniform (Figure 6-24). In some instances customized pads should be constructed and held in place with tape or an elastic wrap. Neoprene sleeves can be used for support following strain to the quadriceps, hamstrings, or groin muscles (Figure 6-25).[3]

## Knee Braces

Because of the high incidence of injury to the knee joint, manufacturers have designed a host of different knee braces for a variety of purposes. *Protective knee braces* are used prophylactically to prevent injuries to the medial collateral ligament in contact sports such as football (Figure 6-26A).[12] Although these protective braces have been widely used in the past, the American Orthopedic Society for Sports Medicine has expressed concern about their efficacy in reducing injuries to the collateral ligaments. Several studies have actually shown an increase in the incidence of injuries to the medial collateral ligament in athletes wearing these braces.[12]

*Rehabilitative braces* are widely used following surgical repair or reconstruction of the knee joint to allow for controlled progressive immobilization (Figure 6-26B). These braces have hinges that can be easily adjusted to allow range of motion to be progressively increased over time.

*Functional knee braces* may be worn both during and following the rehabilitative period to provide support during functional activities (Figure 6-26C).[14] Functional braces can be purchased ready made or can be custom made. Some physicians strongly recommend that their patients consistently wear these braces during physical activity whereas others do not feel that they are necessary.[5]

**Figure 6-23**

Soccer shin guards

Techniques for Preventing
and Minimizing
Sport-Related Injuries

**Figure 6-24**

Protective thigh pads

*Neoprene braces with medial and lateral supports* may be used by individuals who have sustained injury to the collateral ligaments and feel that they need extra support medially and laterally (Figure 6-26D).

A variety of *neoprene sleeves* may also be used to provide some support for patellofemoral conditions (Figure 6-26E).[3]

## ELBOW, WRIST, AND HAND PROTECTION

As with the lower extremity, the upper extremity requires protection from injury and prevention of further injury after trauma. Although the elbow joint is less commonly injured than the ankle, knee, or shoulder, it is still vulnerable to instability, contusion, and muscle strain. A variety of off-the-shelf protective neoprene sleeves and pads and hinged adjustable rehabilitative braces can offer protection to the elbow (Figure 6-27).

**Figure 6-25**

Neoprene thigh sleeve for
muscle strains

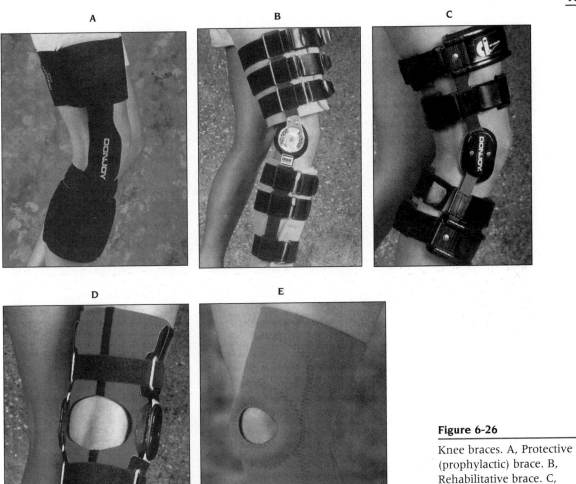

**Figure 6-26**

Knee braces. A, Protective (prophylactic) brace. B, Rehabilitative brace. C, Functional brace. D, Neoprene brace with medial and lateral supports. E, Neoprene patellar brace

In sports medicine, injuries to the wrist, hand, and fingers are often trivialized and considered insignificant. But injuries to the distal aspect of the upper extremity can be functionally disabling, especially in those sports that involve throwing and catching. In both contact and noncontact sport activities the wrist, hand, and particularly the fingers are susceptible to fracture, dislocation, ligament sprains, and muscle strains. Protective gloves are essential in preventing injuries in sports like lacrosse and ice hockey (Figure 6-28). It is also common to use both off-the-shelf and custom-molded splints both for support and to immobilize an injury (Figure 6-29).

A

B

C

**Figure 6-27**

Elbow braces and supports. A, Rehabilitation elbow brace. B, Neoprene elbow sleeve. C, Elbow pad

**Figure 6-28**

Hand protection is essential in lacrosse and ice hockey.

A

C

**Figure 6-29**

Wrist supports. A, Off-the-shelf neoprene wrist support. B and C, Custom molded wrist and thumb splints

## COACH'S CORNER

The following checklist contains factors the coach must consider when selecting, purchasing, and fitting athletic equipment to help minimize liability.

☐ Buy sports equipment from reputable manufacturers.

☐ Buy the safest equipment that resources will permit.

☐ Make sure that all equipment is assembled correctly.

☐ Ensure that the person who assembles equipment is competent to do so and follows the manufacturer's instructions to the letter.

☐ Maintain all equipment properly, according to the manufacturer's guidelines.

☐ Use equipment only for the purpose for which it was designed.

☐ Warn athletes who use the equipment about all possible risks that using the equipment could entail.

☐ Use great caution in the construction or customizing of any piece of equipment.

☐ Use no defective equipment.

☐ Routinely inspect all equipment for defects, and render all defective equipment unusable.

## SUMMARY

• The proper selection and fitting of sports equipment are essential in the prevention of many sports injuries.

• Because of the current number of lawsuits, both durability of material and fit and wear requirements must meet sports equipment standards.

• Manufacturers must foresee all the possible uses and misuses of their equipment and warn the user of any potential risks.

• Head protection in many collision and contact sports is of particular concern: The helmet must be used as intended and not as a weapon; proper fit is also a requirement.

- A warning label on the outside of the helmet must indicate that it is not fail-safe, and the helmet must be used as intended.

- Face protection is of major importance in sports that have fast-moving projectiles, that use implements that come in close proximity to other athletes, and that are characterized by body collisions.

- The customized mouth guard, fitted to individual requirements, provides the best protection for the teeth and also helps protect against concussions.

- Eyes must be protected against projectiles and sports implements.

- The safest eye guard for the athlete not wearing glasses is the closed type that completely protects the orbital cavity.

- Many sports require protection of various parts of the athlete's body. American football players, ice hockey players, and baseball/softball catchers are examples of players who require body protection.

- Socks must be clean, without holes, and made of appropriate materials.

- Shoes must be suited to the sport and must be fitted to the larger foot, the wide part of the foot must match the wide part of the shoe, if the shoe has cleats, they must be positioned at the metatarsophalangeal joints.

- The hand, wrist, and elbow are also vulnerable to sports trauma and require special protective devices.

---

## Solutions to Critical Thinking Exercises

**6-1** The student coach must acquire the following protective equipment competencies:
- Identify good-quality and poor-quality commercial protective equipment.
- Properly fit commercial protective equipment.
- Construct protective and supportive devices.

**6-2** The coach initiates the following steps:
1. A team meeting is called in which the risks entailed in the use and fitting of the equipment are fully explained.
2. A defective piece of equipment must be immediately reported and repaired.
3. A letter is sent out to each parent or guardian explaining equipment limitations. This letter is signed and returned to the athletic trainer.
4. A meeting of parents, team members, and coaches is called to further explain equipment limitations.

**6-3** The coach should explain that the helmet cannot prevent serious neck injuries. Striking an opponent with any part of the helmet or face mask can place abnormal stress on cervical structures. Most severe neck injuries occur from striking an opponent with the top of the helmet; this action is known as axial loading.

**6-4** The coach advises the following:
- Purchase shoes to fit the large foot.
- Fit shoes wearing athletic socks.
- Purchase shoes at the end of the day.
- Each foot is measured from the heel to the end of the largest toe.

- Shoes feel snug but comfortable when jumping up and down and performing cutting motions.
- Shoe length and width allow full toe function.
- Wide part of foot matches the wide part of the shoe.
- Shoe bends at widest part of shoe.

## REVIEW QUESTIONS AND CLASS ACTIVITIES

1. What are the legal responsibilities of the equipment manager and coach in terms of protective equipment?
2. Invite an attorney to class to discuss product liability and its impact on the coach and equipment manager.
3. What are the various sports with high-risk factors that require protective equipment?
4. How can the coach select and use safety equipment to decrease the possibility of sports injuries and litigation?
5. Why is continual inspection and/or replacement of used equipment important?
6. What are the standards for fitting football helmets? Are there standards for any other helmets?
7. Invite your school equipment manager to class to demonstrate all the protective equipment and how to fit it to the athlete.
8. Why are mouth guards important, and what are the advantages of custom-made mouth guards over the stock type?
9. What are the advantages and disadvantages of glasses and contact lenses in athletic competition?
10. How do you fit shoulder pads for different-sized players and their positions?
11. Why is breast protection necessary? Which types of sport bras are available and what should the athlete look for when purchasing one?
12. How do you properly fit shoes? What type of shoes should you use for various sports and different floor and field surfaces?
13. What types of knee braces are on the market today? Do they provide adequate support and protection from injury?

### REFERENCES

1. Amis T et al: Influence of intra-oral maxillary sports mouthguards on the airflow dynamics of oral breathing, *Med Sci Sports Exerc* 32(2):284, 2000.
2. Banky J: Mouthguards and dental injury: an update, *Sports Coach* 22(3):30, 1999.
3. Birmingham TB, Inglis JT, Kramer JF: Effect of a neoprene sleeve on knee joint kinesthesis: influence of different testing procedures, *Med Sci Sports Exerc* 32(2):304, 2000.
4. Bot SDM, van Mechelen W: The effect of ankle bracing on athletic performance, *Sports Med* 27(3): 171, 1999.
5. Brownstein B: Migration and design characteristics of functional knee braces, *J Sport Rehab* 7(1):33, 1998.
6. Cuddy S: The right running shoe: the first step in avoiding running injuries, *Sports Med Update* 13(3): 8, 1998.
7. Fiolkowski P: Considerations in the use of ankle braces, *Ath Ther Today* 3(4):38, 1998.
8. International Federation of Medicine: Position statement: eye injuries and eye protection in sports, *Ath Ther Today* 4(5):6, 1999.
9. Mazzola G: At your service: reconditioning your football helmets, *Coach Ath Dir* 68(4):40, 1998.

Techniques for Preventing
and Minimizing
Sport-Related Injuries

10. Nigg BM, Nurse MA, Stefanyshyn DJ: Shoe inserts and orthotics for sport and physical activities, *Med Sci Sports Exerc* 31(7 suppl):S421, 1999.

11. Page KA, Steele JR: Breast motion and sports brassiere design: implications for future research, *Sports Med* 27(4):205, 1999.

12. Sauers EL, Harter RA: Efficacy of prophylactic knee braces: current research perspectives, *Ath Ther Today* 3(4):14, 1998.

13. Street S, Runkle D: *Athletic protec-tive equipment: care, selection, and fitting*, Boston, 1999, McGraw-Hill.

14. Styf J: The effects of functional knee bracing on muscle function and performance, *Sports Med* 28(2):77, 1999.

15. Swanik CB: Orthotics in sports medicine, *Ath Ther Today* 5(1):5, 2000.

16. Wischnia B, Carrozza P: Spring 2000 shoe buyer's guide, *Runner's World* 35(3):37, 2000.

## ANNOTATED BIBLIOGRAPHY

Street S, Runkle D: *Athletic protective equipment: care, selection, and fitting*, Boston, 1999, McGraw-Hill.

*This reference book provides an overview of available athletic equipment and its usage. The text is a resource for athletic trainers, coaches, and physical education teachers.*

## WEBSITES

Riddell: http://riddell.com/index.htm

*Riddell is an equipment manufacturing company, and this site gives information about the safety of the products they sell and the necessary standards for safety equipment.*

Healthyway Sporting Protective Eyewear: http://www1.sympatico.ca/healthyway/HEALTHYWAY/feature_vis3c.html

*Emphasizes the importance of protective eyewear for young athletes and provides links to related informative sites.*

National Institute for Sports Science and Safety (NISSS): http://www.nisss.org

*Research, design, and testing of sports equipment and sports protective equipment.*

The Training Room: http://www.thetrainingroom.net

*Sports orthopedic braces, orthotics, protective sports equipment, and athletic injury treatment.*

Athletic Protective Equipment: http://rapid-wear.com

Douglas Protective Equipment: http://www.douglascustompads.com

*Manufacturer and distributor of football, hockey, and baseball protective padding. Custom fitting players at all levels for over 12 years.*

# Emergency Situations and Injury Assessment

*When you finish this chapter you will be able to:*

- Establish a plan for handling emergency situations at your institution.
- Explain the importance of knowing cardiopulmonary resuscitation (CPR) and how to manage an obstructed airway.
- Describe techniques for control of hemorrhage.
- Assess the types of shock and their management.
- Describe the various phases of injury assessment.
- Explain the importance of controlling swelling during initial injury management.
- Describe techniques for moving and transporting the injured athlete.

M ost sports injuries do not result in life-or-death emergency situations, but when such situations do arise, prompt care is essential. Time becomes the critical factor, and assistance to the injured athlete must be based on knowledge of what to do and how to do it—how to perform effective first aid immediately. There is no room for uncertainty, indecision, or error. A mistake in the initial management of injury can prolong the time required for rehabilitation and can potentially create a life-threatening situation for the athlete.

In situations in which an athletic trainer is not available to provide care, the responsibility falls on the shoulders of the coach. Therefore it is critical that the coach be well prepared to handle whatever emergency situation may arise.

## THE EMERGENCY PLAN

*Time becomes critical in an emergency situation.*

The prime concern of emergency aid is to maintain cardiovascular function and, indirectly, central nervous system function, because failure of any of these systems may lead to death. The key to emergency aid in the sports setting is the initial evaluation of the injured athlete. Time is of the essence, so this evaluation must be done rapidly and accurately so that proper aid can be rendered without delay. In some instances these first steps not only will be lifesaving but also may determine the degree and extent of permanent disability.

As discussed in Chapter 1, the sports medicine team—the coach, the athletic trainer, and the team physician—must at all times act reasonably and prudently. This behavior is especially important during emergencies. **All sports programs must have a prearranged emergency plan that can be implemented immediately when necessary.** The following issues must be addressed when developing the emergency system:

1. Phones should be readily accessible. Cellular phones are best because they provide the coach with immediate access to either the emergency medical system or the athletic trainer, who may be with another team. If cellular phones are not available, the location of the telephone should be well known by coaches, athletes, managers, and athletic trainers. These phone locations should be clearly marked. (Use 911 if available.)

2. A specific person should be assigned to make an emergency phone call. The emergency medical system can usually be accessed by dialing 911. This number gets you a dispatcher who has access to the rescue squad and the police and fire departments. The person making the emergency phone call must provide the following information:
   a. Type of emergency situation
   b. Type of suspected injury
   c. Present condition of the athlete
   d. Current assistance being given (e.g., CPR)
   e. Location of telephone being used
   f. Exact location of emergency (give names of streets and cross streets) and how to enter facility

3. Keys to gates or padlocks must be easily accessible. Both coaches and athletic trainers should have the appropriate key.

4. There should be separate emergency plans for each sport's fields, courts, or gymnasiums.

5. All coaches, athletic trainers, athletic directors, school nurses, and maintenance personnel should be apprised of the emergency plan at a meeting held annually before the beginning of the school year. Each individual must know his or her responsibilities should an emergency occur.

6. A responsible adult should always be assigned to accompany the injured athlete to the hospital.

Individuals providing emergency care to the injured athlete must cooperate and act professionally. Too often, the rescue squad personnel, a physician, an athletic trainer, or a coach disagree over exactly how the injured athlete should be handled and transported. The coach or athletic trainer is usually the first individual to deal with the emergency situation. The athletic trainer has generally had more training and experience in moving and transporting an injured athlete than the physician has. **If an athletic trainer or physician is not available, the coach should not**

All sports programs must have an emergency plan.

**hesitate to dial 911 to let the rescue squad handle an emergency situation.** If the rescue squad is called and responds, the emergency medical technicians (EMTs) should have the final say on how the athlete is to be transported while the coach and athletic trainer assume an assistive role.

To alleviate potential conflicts, it is a good idea for either the coach or the athletic trainer to establish procedures and guidelines and to arrange practice sessions at least once a year with all parties concerned for handling the injured athlete. The rescue squad may not be experienced in dealing with someone who is wearing a helmet or other protective equipment. The coach should make sure before an incident occurs that the EMTs understand how athletes wearing various types of athletic equipment should be managed. When dealing with the injured athlete, all egos should be put aside. Certainly the most important consideration is what is the best for the athlete.

### Parent Notification

If the injured athlete is a minor, it is essential that actual consent to treat the athlete be obtained from the parent. **Actual consent may be given in writing either before or during an emergency.** Actual consent is notification that the parent has been informed about what the coach, athletic trainer, or other medical personnel thinks is wrong and what that person intends to do, and parental permission is granted to give treatment for a specific incident. If the athlete's parents cannot be contacted, then the predetermined wishes of the parent given at the beginning of a season or school year can be acted upon. If there is no informed consent, then implied consent on the part of the athlete to save his or her life takes precedence.

## PRINCIPLES OF ASSESSMENT

The coach cannot deliver appropriate medical care to the injured athlete until some systematic assessment of the situation has been made. This assessment (Figure 7-1) helps to determine the nature of the injury and provides direction in the decision-making process concerning the emergency care that must be rendered. The *primary survey* refers to assessment of potentially life-threatening problems including airway, breathing, circulation (ABC), severe bleeding, or shock. It takes precedence over all other aspects of victim assessment and should be used to correct life-threatening situations.[9] Once the condition of the victim is stabilized, the *secondary survey* is used to take a closer look at the injury sustained by the athlete. The secondary survey gathers specific information about the injury from the athlete, systematically assesses vital signs and symptoms, and allows for a more detailed evaluation of the injury. The secondary survey is done to uncover problems that do not pose an immediate threat to life but that may do so if they remain uncorrected.[9] Certainly the coach should be most concerned about the primary survey.

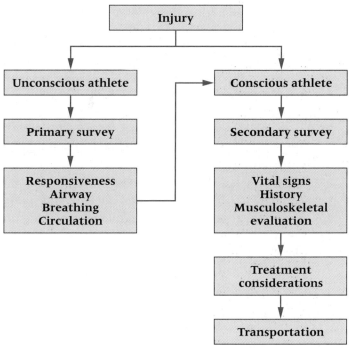

**Figure 7-1**

Flow chart showing
appropriate emergency
procedures for the injured
athlete

An injured athlete who is conscious and stable does not require a primary survey. However, the unconscious athlete must be monitored for life-threatening problems throughout the assessment process.

## The Unconscious Athlete

The state of unconsciousness provides one of the greatest dilemmas in sports. **With an unconscious athlete, a coach acting alone without an athletic trainer should always call the rescue squad before attempting to move the athlete regardless of whether the situation is life threatening.** Unconsciousness may be defined as a state of insensibility in which there is a lack of conscious awareness. This condition can be brought about by a blow to either the head or the solar plexus, or it may result from general shock. It is often difficult to determine the exact cause of unconsciousness.

The unconscious athlete must always be considered to have a life-threatening injury, which requires an immediate primary survey. Here are guidelines that should be followed when dealing with the unconscious athlete:

1. The coach should immediately note the body position and determine the level of consciousness and responsiveness.
2. Airway, breathing, and circulation (ABC) should routinely be established immediately.

3. Injury to the neck and spine is always a possibility in the unconscious athlete.

4. If the athlete is wearing a helmet, it should never be removed until neck and spine injury have been unequivocally ruled out. However, the face mask must be cut away and removed to allow for CPR.

5. If the athlete is supine and not breathing, establish ABC immediately.

6. If the athlete is supine and breathing, do nothing until consciousness returns.

7. If the athlete is prone and not breathing, logroll him or her carefully to supine position and establish ABC immediately.

8. If the athlete is prone and breathing, do nothing until consciousness returns, and wait for the rescue squad.

9. Monitor and maintain life support for the unconscious athlete until emergency medical personnel arrive.

## PRIMARY SURVEY

### Treatment of Life-Threatening Injuries

Life-threatening injuries take precedence over all other injuries sustained by the athlete. Situations that are considered life threatening include those that require CPR (i.e., obstruction of the airway, no breathing, no circulation), profuse bleeding, and shock. **Whenever there is a life-threatening situation, the coach should always call the rescue squad.**

### Overview of Emergency CPR

*All coaches should be currently certified in CPR so that if an athletic trainer is not available, the coach can perform the techniques correctly.* It is essential that a careful evaluation of the injured athlete be made to determine whether CPR should be conducted. The following is an overview of adult CPR and is not intended to be used by persons who are not certified in CPR. It should also be noted that, because of the serious nature of CPR, updates should routinely be studied through courses offered by the American Red Cross, the American Heart Association, or the National Safety Council.

#### Establish Unresponsiveness

First, establish unresponsiveness of the athlete by tapping or gently shaking his or her shoulder and shouting, "Are you okay?" Note that shaking should be avoided if the athlete has a possible neck injury. If the athlete is unresponsive, the emergency medical system (EMS) should be activated immediately by dialing 911. Carefully position the athlete in the supine position. If the athlete is in a position other than supine, he or she must be carefully rolled over as a unit, avoiding any twisting of the body, because CPR can be administered only with the athlete lying flat on the

**7–1**

**_Critical Thinking_** Exercise

A football defensive back is making a tackle and on contact drops his head to tackle the ball carrier. He hits the ground and does not move. When the coach gets to him, the athlete is lying prone, is unconscious, but is breathing.

? How should the coach manage this situation?

back with knees straight or slightly flexed. In cases of suspected cervical spine injury, care must be taken to minimize cervical movement during logrolling. Then proceed with the ABCs of CPR.[6]

### Equipment Considerations

Protective equipment worn by an athlete may complicate life-saving CPR procedures. A great deal of controversy exists even among athletic trainers as to whether equipment should be removed or left in place. The presence of a football, ice hockey, or lacrosse helmet with a face mask and various types of shoulder pads associated with each sport obviously makes CPR more difficult if not impossible.

Removing the face mask should be the first step.[8] The face mask does not hinder the evaluation of the airway but it may hinder treatment. A number of techniques using various instruments have been recommended to remove the face mask, including electric screwdrivers, which work well as long as the screws are not rusted; or wire cutters, bolt cutters, trainers' scissors, or scalpels, none of which work very well. Three devices, the Anvil Pruner, the Trainer's Angel, and the FM Extractor have been effective in quickly cutting the plastic clips (Figure 7-2).[4] The coach should be proficient in removing the face mask within 30 seconds.

In 1992, the Occupational Safety and Health Administration (OSHA) mandated the use of barrier devices to protect the coach from transmission

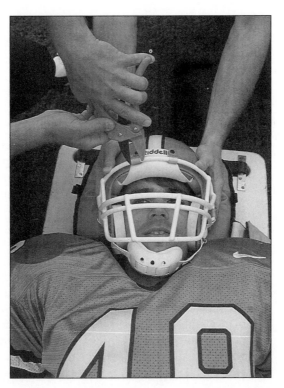

**Figure 7-2**

A Trainer's Angel is effective in quickly cutting the plastic clips on a face mask for easy removal.

of bloodborne pathogens during CPR. It is possible to slip the barrier mask under the face mask, attach the one-way mouthpiece or valve through the bars of the face mask and begin CPR within 5 to 10 seconds without removing the face mask.[2]

Decisions to remove a helmet and shoulder pads before initiating CPR should be based on the potential of injury to the cervical spine. **A coach should never remove the helmet from an athlete with a suspected cervical spine injury.** If it is reasonably certain that no injury has occurred to the cervical spine, both the helmet and shoulder pads can be quickly removed before initiating CPR. If injury to the cervical spine is a possibility, care must be taken to minimize movement of the head and neck while permitting CPR to be performed. The face mask should be dealt with as recommended earlier, and the jersey and shoulder pad strings and/or straps should be cut and the shoulder pads spread apart so that the chest may be compressed according to CPR guidelines. Although removal of the helmet and shoulder pads has been recommended by some, it seems that no matter how much care is taken, removal creates unnecessary movement of the cervical spine and delays initiation of CPR, neither of which is best for the injured athlete.[10]

If cervical neck injury is suspected yet the athlete is conscious and breathing and does not require CPR, the athlete should be transported with the helmet, chin strap, and shoulder pads in place. The face mask should be removed in case CPR becomes necessary.

### ABCs of CPR

The ABCs of CPR are easily remembered and indicate the sequential steps used for basic life support:

A–Airway opened
B–Breathing restored
C–Circulation restored

Frequently, when A is restored, B and C will resume spontaneously, and it is then unnecessary to perform these steps. In some instances, the restoration of A and B obviates the necessity for step C. When performing CPR on an adult victim, the following sequence should be followed.

### Opening the Airway

Open the airway by using the head-tilt/chin-lift method. Lift chin with one hand while pushing down on victim's forehead with the other, avoiding the use of excessive force. The tongue is the most common cause of respiratory obstruction; the forward lift of the jaw raises the tongue away from the back of the throat, thus clearing the airway. NOTE: On victims with suspected head or neck injuries, perform a modified jaw thrust maneuver by grasping each side of the lower jaw at the angles, thus displacing the lower mandible forward as the head is tilted backward. In executing this maneuver both elbows should rest on the same surface as that on which the victim is lying. Should the lips close, they can be opened by retracting the lower lip with a thumb. If breathing is still not restored, additional forward displacement of the jaw can be effected.

### Establishing Breathing

1. To determine if the victim is breathing, maintain the open airway, place your ear over the mouth, observe the chest, and look, listen, and feel for breath sounds.

2. If the victim is breathing and there is no evidence of trauma, roll the victim on his or her side into a recovery position.

3. If not breathing, with the hand that is on the athlete's forehead, pinch the nose shut, keeping the heel of the hand in place to hold the head back (if there is no neck injury) (Figure 7-3). Taking a deep breath, place your mouth over the athlete's mouth to provide an airtight seal and give two slow full breaths at a rate of 1½ to 2 seconds per inflation. Observe the chest rise and fall. Remove your mouth and listen for the air to escape through passive exhalation. If the airway is obstructed, reposition the victim's head and try again to ventilate. If still obstructed, give up to five abdominal thrusts followed by a finger sweep with the index finger to clear objects from the mouth. Be careful not to push the object further into the throat. Continue to repeat this sequence until ventilation occurs. NOTE: OSHA has mandated the use of barrier shields by coaches and athletic trainers to minimize the risk of transmitting bloodborne pathogens (Figure 7-4). These shields have a plastic or silicone sheet that spreads over the face and separates the coach from the athlete. Some models have a tubelike mouthpiece, which may help in situations in which the athlete is wearing a face mask.

### Establishing Circulation

1. To determine pulselessness, locate the Adam's apple with the index and middle fingers of the hand closest to the head. Then

**Figure 7-3**

Head-tilt/chin-lift technique for establishing an airway

**Figure 7-4**

A barrier mask protects the
coach from potential
exposure to bloodborne
spathogens.

**Figure 7-5**

With the middle and index
fingers of the hand closest to
the waist, the lower margin
of the victim's rib cage is
located. The fingers are then
run along the rib cage to the
notch where the ribs meet
the sternum. The middle
finger is placed on the notch
with the index finger next to
it on the lower end of the
sternum.

slide the fingers down into the groove on the side of the body
on which you are kneeling to locate the carotid artery. Palpate
the carotid pulse with one hand (allow 5 to 10 seconds) while
maintaining head tilt with the other.

2. Maintain open airway. Position yourself close to the side of the
   athlete's chest. With the middle and index fingers of the hand
   closest to the waist, locate the lower margin of the athlete's rib
   cage on the side next to you (Figure 7-5).

3. Run the fingers up along the rib cage to the xiphoid notch
   where the ribs meet the sternum.

4. Place the middle finger on the notch and the index finger next
   to it on the lower end of the sternum.

5. Next, the hand closest to the athlete's head is positioned on the
   lower half of the sternum next to the index finger of the first
   hand that located the notch; the heel of that hand is placed on
   the long axis of the sternum.

6. The first hand is then removed from the notch and placed on
   top of the hand on the sternum so that the heels of both hands
   are parallel and the fingers are directed straight away from the
   coach (Figure 7-6).

7. Fingers can be extended or interlaced, but they must be kept
   off the chest wall.

8. Elbows are kept in a locked position with arms straight and
   shoulders positioned over the hands, enabling the thrust to be
   straight down.

9. In a normal-sized adult, enough force must be applied to depress the sternum 1½ to 2 inches (4 to 5 cm). After depression, there must be complete release of the sternum to allow the heart to refill. The time of release should equal the time of compression. For one rescuer, compression must be given at the rate of 80 to 100 times per minute, maintaining a rate of fifteen chest compressions to two full breaths.

10. After four cycles of fifteen compressions and two breaths (15:2) or about 1 minute, recheck the pulse at the carotid artery (allow 5 seconds) while maintaining head tilt. If there is no pulse, continue the 15:2 cycle beginning with chest compressions.

**Every coach should be certified in CPR and should take a refresher examination at least once a year. It is wise to have all assistants certified as well.**[7]

### Obstructed Airway Management

An airway obstruction is a possibility in many sports activities; for example, an athlete may choke on a mouth guard, a broken piece of tooth, chewing gum, or even a chaw of tobacco. An unconscious athlete can have an obstructed airway when the tongue falls back in the throat, thus blocking the upper airway. Blood clots resulting from head, facial, or dental injuries may impede normal breathing, as may vomiting. When such emergencies arise, early recognition and prompt, knowledgeable action are necessary to avert a tragedy. When complete airway obstruction occurs, the individual is unable to speak, cough, or breathe. The athlete who is conscious will make a tremendous effort to breathe: The head is forced back, and the face initially is flushed and then becomes *cyanotic* (bluish color) as oxygen deprivation occurs. If partial airway obstruction is causing the choking, some air passage can be detected, but during a complete obstruction no air movement is discernible.

To relieve airway obstruction caused by foreign bodies, two maneuvers are recommended: (1) the Heimlich maneuver and (2) finger sweeps of the mouth and throat.[6]

**Heimlich maneuver**   As with CPR, the Heimlich maneuver (subdiaphragmatic abdominal thrusts) requires practice before proficiency is acquired. The two methods of obstructed airway management depend on whether the victim is in an erect position or has collapsed and is either unconscious or too heavy to lift. For the conscious victim, the standing Heimlich maneuver is performed until he or she is relieved. In cases of unconsciousness, five abdominal thrusts are applied, followed by a finger sweep with an attempt at ventilation.

*Method A*   Stand behind and to one side of the athlete. Place both arms around the waist just above the belt line, and permit the athlete's head, arms, and upper trunk to hang forward (Figure 7-7A). Grasp one of your fists with the other, placing the thumb side of the grasped fist

**Figure 7-6**

The heel of the headward hand is placed on the long axis of the lower half of the sternum next to the index finger of the first hand. The first hand is removed from the notch and placed on top of the hand on the sternum with fingers interlaced.

All coaches must have current CPR certification.

A

B

**Figure 7-7**

The Heimlich maneuver for an obstructed airway. A, Manual thrust maneuver for the conscious athlete. B, Manual thrust maneuver for the unconscious athlete.

immediately below the xiphoid process of the sternum, clear of the rib cage. Now sharply and forcefully thrust the fists into the abdomen, inward and upward, several times. This "hug" pushes up on the diaphragm, compressing the air in the lungs, creating forceful pressure against the blockage, and thus usually causing the obstruction to be promptly expelled. Repeat the maneuver until the victim is relieved or becomes unconscious. If the athlete loses consciousness, activate the EMS system, perform a finger sweep, open the airway, and try to ventilate. If the airway is still obstructed, reposition the head and try again. Then give up to five abdominal thrusts. Repeat this sequence as long as necessary.

*Method B*   If the athlete is on the ground or on the floor, place him or her on his or her back and straddle the hips, keeping your weight centered over your knees. Place the heel of your left hand against the back of your right hand and push sharply into the abdomen just above the umbilicus (note the position, Figure 7-7B). Repeat this maneuver up to

**Figure 7-8**

Finger sweeping of the
mouth is essential in
attempting to remove a
foreign object from a choking
victim.

five times, then repeat the finger sweep. Care must be taken in either of
these methods to avoid extreme force or applying force over the rib cage
because fractures of the ribs and damage to the organs can result.

**Finger sweeping**    If a foreign object such as a mouth guard is lodged
in the mouth or the throat and is visible, it may be possible to remove or
release it with your fingers. Care must be taken that the probing does not
drive the object deeper into the throat. It is usually impossible to open the
mouth of a conscious victim who is in distress, so the Heimlich maneuver should be put to use immediately. In the unconscious athlete, turn
the head either to the side or face up, open the mouth by grasping the
tongue and the lower jaw, hold them firmly between your thumb and
fingers, and lift—an action that pulls the tongue away from the back of
the throat and from the impediment. If this action is difficult to do, the
crossed finger method can usually be used effectively. The index finger of
your free hand (or if both hands are used, an assistant can probe) should
be inserted into one side of the mouth along the cheek deeply into the
throat; using a hooking maneuver, attempt to free the impediment, moving it into a position from which it can be removed (Figure 7-8). Attempt
to ventilate after each sweep until the airway is open. Once the object is
removed, if the athlete is not already breathing, an attempt is made to
ventilate him or her.

## Controlling Bleeding

An abnormal external or internal discharge of blood is called a *hemorrhage*. The hemorrhage may be venous, capillary, or arterial and may be
external or internal. Venous blood is characteristically dark red with a
continuous flow, capillary bleeding exudes from tissue and is a reddish
color, and arterial bleeding flows in spurts and is bright red. NOTE: The
coach must always be concerned with exposure to bloodborne pathogens
and other diseases when coming in contact with someone's blood or
other body fluids. It is essential to take *universal precautions* to minimize
this risk. Disposable latex gloves should be used routinely whenever the
athletic trainer comes in contact with blood or other body fluids. This
topic is discussed in detail in Chapter 8.2

External bleeding can usually
be managed by using direct
pressure, elevation, or
pressure points.

Techniques for Preventing
and Minimizing
Sport-Related Injuries

**Figure 7-9**

Direct pressure for the
control of bleeding is applied
with the hand over a sterile
gauze pad.

**Figure 7-10**

The two most common sites
for direct pressure are the
brachial artery and the
femoral artery.

## Controlling External Bleeding

External bleeding stems from open skin wounds such as abrasions, incisions, lacerations, punctures, or avulsions. The control of external bleeding includes the use of direct pressure, elevation, and pressure points.

**Direct pressure**   Pressure is directly applied directly over a wound with the hand over a sterile gauze pad. The pressure is applied firmly against the resistance of a bone (Figure 7-9).

**Elevation**   Elevation, in combination with direct pressure, provides an additional means for the reduction of external hemorrhage. Elevating a hemorrhaging part against gravity reduces hydrostatic blood pressure and facilitates venous and lymphatic drainage; consequently, elevating slows bleeding.[2]

**Pressure points**   When direct pressure combined with elevation fails to slow hemorrhage, the use of pressure points may be the method of choice. Eleven points on each side of the body have been identified for controlling external bleeding; the two most commonly used are the brachial artery in the upper limb and the femoral artery in the lower limb. The brachial artery is compressed against the medial aspect of the humerus, and the femoral artery is compressed as it is detected within the femoral triangle (Figure 7-10).

### Internal Hemorrhage

Internal hemorrhage is invisible to the eye unless manifested through some body opening or identified through x-ray studies or other diagnostic techniques. Its danger lies in the difficulty of diagnosis. When internal hemorrhaging occurs, either subcutaneously such as in a bruise or contusion, intramuscularly, or in joints, the athlete may be moved without danger in most instances. However, the detection of bleeding within a body cavity such as the skull, thorax, or abdomen is of the utmost importance because it could mean the difference between life and death. Because the symptoms are obscure, internal hemorrhage is difficult to diagnose properly. As a result of this difficulty, **athletes with internal injuries require hospitalization under complete and constant observation by a medical staff to determine the nature and extent of the injuries.** All severe hemorrhaging eventually results in shock and should therefore be treated on this premise. Even if there is no outward indication of shock, the athlete should be kept quiet and body heat should be maintained at a constant and suitable temperature (see the section on shock for the preferred body position).

### Managing Shock

With any injury shock is a possibility. But when severe bleeding, fractures, or internal injuries are present, the potential for shock increases. Shock occurs when a diminished amount of blood is available to the circulatory system. As a result, not enough oxygen-carrying blood cells are available to the tissues, particularly those of the nervous system. This situation occurs when the vascular system loses its capacity to hold the fluid portion of the blood because of dilation of the blood vessels within the body and disruption of the osmotic fluid balance. When shock occurs, a quantity of plasma is lost from the blood vessels to the tissue spaces of the body, leaving the blood cells within the vessels, thus causing stagnation and slowing the blood flow. This general collapse of the vascular system causes widespread tissue death, which eventually causes the death of the individual unless treatment is given.

Certain conditions such as extreme fatigue, exposure to extreme heat or cold, extreme dehydration and mineral loss, or illness predispose an athlete to shock. In a situation with potential for a shock condition, there are other signs by which the athletic trainer or coach should assess the possibility of the athlete's lapsing into a state of shock as an aftermath of the injury. The most important clue to potential shock is the recognition of a severe injury. It may happen that none of the usual signs of shock is present.

### Symptoms and Signs

The major signs of shock are moist, pale, cool, clammy skin; the pulse becomes weak and rapid; the respiratory rate increased and shallow; blood pressure decreases; and in severe situations there is urinary retention and fecal incontinence. If conscious, the athlete may display a disinterest in his or her surroundings or may display irritability, restlessness, or excitement. There may also be extreme thirst.[2]

### Management

Depending on the causative factor for the shock, the following emergency care should be given:

1. Maintain body temperature as close to normal as possible.
2. Elevate the feet and legs 8 to 12 inches for most situations. However, shock positioning varies according to the type of injury.[2] For example, for a neck injury, the athlete should be immobilized as found; for a head injury, his or her head and shoulders should be elevated; and for a leg fracture, his or her leg should be kept level and should be raised after splinting.

Shock can also be compounded or initially produced by the psychological reaction of the athlete to an injury situation. Fear or the sudden realization that a serious situation has occurred can result in shock. In the case of a psychological reaction to an injury, the athlete should be instructed to lie down and avoid viewing the injury. This athlete should be handled with patience and gentleness, but firmness as well. Spectators should be kept away from the injured athlete. Reassurance is of vital concern to the injured individual. The person should be given immediate comfort through the loosening of clothing. Nothing should be given by mouth until a physician has determined that no surgical procedures are indicated.

Signs of shock:
- Blood pressure is low
- Systolic pressure is usually below 90 mm Hg
- Pulse is rapid and very weak
- Athlete may be drowsy and appear sluggish
- Respiration is shallow and extremely rapid
- Pale, cool, clammy skin

Secondary assessment
consists of:
- History
- Observation
- Physical examination
- Special tests

Vital signs to observe:
- Pulse
- Respiration
- Blood pressure
- Temperature
- Skin color
- Pupils
- State of consciousness
- Weakness of movement
- Sensory changes

# CONDUCTING A SECONDARY ASSESSMENT

If the athlete has no life-threatening injuries, the coach should conduct a secondary assessment to survey the existing injury more precisely.

## Recognizing Vital Signs

Anyone providing emergency care has to be able to evaluate the existing physiological signs and symptoms of injury. Among these *vital signs* are heart rate, breathing rate, blood pressure, temperature, skin color, pupils of the eye, movement, the presence of pain, and level of consciousness. Although an athletic trainer must be able to assess in detail, and in some cases, accurately measure each of these vital signs, **it is perhaps more important for the coach to be able to recognize when one or more of the vital signs does not appear to be normal.** Table 7-1 provides a list of what is considered to be normal with each of these vital signs.

## On-Field Injury Inspection

Two phases of injury assessment take place during the secondary evaluation. The first involves the initial on-field injury inspection during which

---

**TABLE 7-1** Vital signs

| Sign | Description |
|---|---|
| Pulse | Normal pulse rate per minute for adults ranges between 60 and 80 beats and in children from 80 to 100 beats. Trained athletes usually have slower pulses. Pulse rate is measured at the carotid artery in the neck or the radial artery in the wrist (Figure 7-11). |
| Respiration | Normal breathing rate per minute is approximately 12 breaths in adults and 20 to 25 breaths in children. Breathing may be shallow (indicating shock), irregular, or gasping (indicating cardiac involvement). |
| Temperature | Normal body temperature is 98.6° F (37° C). Core temperature is most accurately measured in the rectum or at the tympanic membrane in the ear (Figure 7-12). |
| Skin color | Red skin may indicate heatstroke, high blood pressure, or elevated temperature. Pale, ashen, or white skin can mean insufficient circulation, shock, fright, hemorrhage, heat exhaustion, or insulin shock. Blue skin (cyanotic), primarily noted in lips and fingernails, usually means an airway obstruction or respiratory insufficiency. |
| Pupils | Pupils should be of equal size. Pupil should respond to light, resulting in constriction or dilation. Response is more critical than pupil size. |
| State of consciousness | Normally the athlete is alert, aware of the environment, and responds quickly to vocal stimulation. |
| Weakness of movement | Weakness of one side of the body compared to the other is not normal and may indicate nerve damage. |
| Sensory changes | Numbness, tingling, or complete loss of sensation is not normal. |
| Blood pressure | Normal systolic pressure for 15- to 20-year-old males ranges from 115 to 120 mm Hg. The diastolic pressure, on the other hand, usually ranges from 75 to 80 mm Hg. The normal blood pressure of females is usually 8 to 10 mm Hg lower than in males for both systolic and diastolic pressures. Blood pressure can only be measured using a blood pressure cuff (Figure 7-13). |

A                    B

**Figure 7-11**

Pulse rate taken at the A,
carotid artery, and B, radial
artery

**Figure 7-12**

Thermometer for measuring
tympanic membrane
temperature

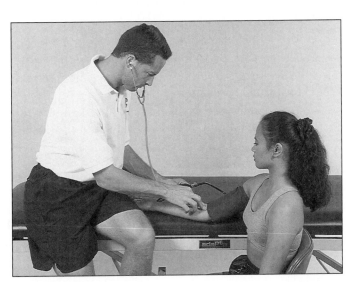

**Figure 7-13**

Blood pressure is measured
using a sphygmomanometer
and a stethoscope.

Techniques for Preventing
and Minimizing
Sport-Related Injuries

Some athletes normally have
irregular and unequal pupils.

The coach may do the on-
field inspection if there is no
athletic trainer.

7–2

___

*Critical Thinking* Exercise

A fencer comes into the training
room complaining of pain in his
shoulder that he has had for
about a week. He indicates that
he first hurt the shoulder when
lifting weights but did not think
it was a bad injury. During the
past week he has not been able
to lift because of pain. He has,
however, continued to fence
during practice but his shoulder
seems to be getting worse
instead of better.

? What evaluation scheme
should a coach use?

Decisions that can be made
from the secondary survey:
• Seriousness of injury
• Type of first aid required
• Whether injury warrants
  referral to a physician
• Type of transportation
  needed

early decisions are made relative to (1) the seriousness of the injury and
(2) how the injured athlete should be transported from the playing field.
Quite often this on-field inspection must be done by the coach when an
athletic trainer is not available. The more thorough off-field assessment is
usually done by an athletic trainer or physician, if necessary.

A logical process must be used to evaluate accurately the extent of a
musculoskeletal injury. Coaches must be aware of the major signs that reveal the site, nature, and above all, severity of the injury. Detection of
these signs can be facilitated, as is true with all trauma, by understanding
the mechanism or traumatic sequence and by methodically inspecting
the injury. Knowledge of the mechanism of an injury is extremely important in determining which area of the body is most affected.

In an attempt to understand the mechanism of injury, a brief history
of the complaint must be taken. The athlete is asked, if possible, about
the events leading up to the injury and how it occurred. The athlete is
further asked what was heard or felt when the injury took place. Such
sounds as a snap, crack, or pop at the moment of injury often indicate
bone fracture or injury to ligaments or tendons. The coach makes a visual
observation of the injured site, comparing it to the uninjured body part.
The initial visual examination can disclose obvious deformity, swelling,
and skin discoloration.

Finally, the region of the injury is gently palpated. Feeling, or palpating, a part can, in conjunction with visual and audible signs, indicate the
nature of the injury. Palpation is started away from the injury and gradually moved toward it. As the coach gently palpates the injury and surrounding structures, he or she can determine the extent of point tenderness, the extent of irritation (whether it is confined to soft tissue alone or
extends to the bony tissue), and deformities that may not be detected by
visual examination alone.

After the brief on-field injury inspection, the coach makes the following decisions regarding:

1. The seriousness of the injury
2. The type of first aid and immobilization necessary
3. Whether the injury warrants immediate referral to a physician
   for further assessment
4. The manner of transportation from the injury site to the
   sidelines, training room, or hospital

## Off-Field Assessment

A more thorough off-field evaluation is performed by either the athletic
trainer or a physician once the athlete has been removed from the site of
initial injury to a place of comfort and safety. **Although the coach is
not expected to have the expertise to do an in-depth injury evaluation, it is essential to make certain that medical personnel inform the coach of their findings.** This detailed assessment may be performed on the sidelines, in an emergency room, in the training room, or

in a sports medicine clinic. The evaluation scheme is divided into four broad categories: history, observation, physical examination, and special tests[5] (HOPS). There are numerous special tests that provide additional information about the extent of injuries.[5] The following discussion provides a brief overview of some of the steps and techniques that can be used in an off-field assessment.

### History

Obtaining as much information as possible about the injury is of major importance. Understanding how the injury occurred and listening to the complaints of the athlete and how key questions are answered can provide important clues to the exact nature of the injury. The examiner becomes a detective in pursuit of as much accurate information as possible, which will lead to a determination of the true nature of the injury. From the history the examiner develops strategies for further examination and possible immediate and follow-up management.

### Observation

Along with gaining knowledge and understanding of the athlete's major complaint from a history, general observation is also performed, often at the same time the history is taken. What is observed is usually affected by the athlete's major complaints.

### Palpation

The two areas of palpation are bony and soft tissue. As with all examination procedures, palpation must be performed systematically, starting with very light pressure followed by gradually deeper pressure and usually beginning away from the site of complaint, then gradually moving toward it.

### Special Tests

Special tests have been designed for almost every body region as means for detecting specific pathologies. They are often used to substantiate what has been learned from other testing. For example, special tests are commonly used to determine ligament stability, impingement signs, tightness of specific structures, muscle imbalance, and body alignment discrepancies. Special tests for various joints are discussed in Chapters 14 through 22.

## IMMEDIATE TREATMENT FOLLOWING ACUTE INJURY

Musculoskeletal injuries are extremely common in sports. The coach must be prepared to provide appropriate first aid immediately to control hemorrhage and associated swelling. **Every initial first-aid effort should be directed toward one primary goal—reducing the amount of swelling resulting from the injury.** If swelling can be controlled initially, the amount of time required for injury rehabilitation will be significantly reduced. Initial management of musculoskeletal injuries should include rest, ice, compression, and elevation (RICE).

RICE (rest, ice, compression, elevation) are essential in the emergency care of musculoskeletal injuries.

**Initial Management of Acute Injuries**

The appropriate technique for initial management of the acute musculoskeletal injury, regardless of where it occurs, is the following:

1. Apply a compression wrap directly over the injury. Wrapping should
   start distally and continue proximally. Tension should be firm and
   consistent. It may be helpful to wet the elastic wrap to facilitate the
   passage of cold from ice packs. A dry compression wrap should be left
   in place for at least 72 hours or until there is little chance of
   continued swelling.

2. Surround the injured area entirely with ice packs or bags and secure
   them in place. The ice should be left on for 20 minutes initially and
   then 1 hour off and 30 minutes on as much as possible over the next
   24 hours. During the following 48-hour period, ice should again be
   applied as often as possible.

3. The injured part should be elevated for most of the initial 72-hour
   period after injury. It is particularly important to keep the injury
   elevated while sleeping. This elevation also allows the damaged part
   to rest after the injury. The initial management of an injury is
   extremely important to reduce the length of time required for
   rehabilitation.

Focus Box 7-1 summarizes the specific technique for initial management
of acute injuries (Figure 7-14).

### Rest

Rest after any type of injury is an extremely important component of any
treatment program. Once a body part is injured, it immediately begins the
healing process. If the injured part is not rested and is subjected to external stresses and strains, the healing process never gets a chance to do
what it is supposed to do. Consequently the injured part does not heal,
and the time required for rehabilitation is markedly increased. The number of days necessary for resting varies with the severity of the injury.
Parts of the body that have experienced minor injury should be rested for
approximately 48 to 72 hours before a rehabilitation program is begun.

### Ice (Cold Application)

The initial treatment of acute injuries should use cold.[3] Therefore ice is used
for most conditions involving strains, sprains, and contusions. Ice is most
commonly used immediately after injury to decrease pain and promote local constriction of the vessels (vasoconstriction), thus controlling hemorrhage and edema. Cold applied to an acute injury lowers metabolism and
the tissue demands for oxygen, and reduces hypoxia. With ice treatments,
the athlete usually reports an uncomfortable sensation of cold, followed by
burning, then an aching sensation, and finally complete numbness.

A

B

C

**Figure 7-14**

RICE technique: A, A wet compression wrap should be applied over the horseshoe pad; B, Ice bags should be secured in place by a dry compression wrap; and C, The leg should be elevated during the initial treatment period.

Because subcutaneous (under the skin) fat conducts cold slowly, applications of cold for short periods are ineffective in cooling deeper tissues. For this reason, treatments of at least 20 minutes are recommended. Prolonged application of cold, however, can cause tissue damage.[3]

Ice packs should be applied to the area for at least 72 hours after an acute injury. With many injuries, regular ice treatments may be continued for several weeks.

For best results, ice packs (crushed ice and towel) should be applied over a compression wrap. Frozen gel packs should not be used directly against the skin, because they reach much lower temperatures than ice packs. A good rule of thumb is to apply a cold pack to a recent injury for a 20-minute period and repeat every 1 to 1½ hours throughout the waking day. Depending on the severity and site of the injury, cold may be applied intermittently for 1 to 72 hours. For example, a mild strain will probably require 1 day of 20-minute periods of cold application, whereas a severe knee or ankle sprain might need 3 to 7 days of intermittent cold. If in doubt about the severity of an injury, it is best to extend the time that ice is applied.[3]

## Compression

Immediate compression of an acute injury is perhaps more important than ice in controlling swelling. Placing external pressure on an injury assists in decreasing hemorrhage and hematoma formation by mechanically reducing the space available for swelling to accumulate. Fluid seepage into interstitial spaces is retarded by compression, and absorption is facilitated. However, application of compression to an anterior compartment syndrome or to certain injuries involving the head and neck is contraindicated.

Many types of compression are available. An elastic wrap that has been soaked in water and frozen in a refrigerator can provide both compression and cold when applied to a recent injury. Pads can be cut from felt or foam rubber to fit difficult-to-compress body areas. A horseshoe-shaped pad, for example, placed around the malleolus in combination with an elastic wrap and tape provides an excellent way to prevent or reduce ankle edema. Although cold is applied intermittently, compression should be maintained throughout the day and, if possible, throughout the night. Pressure buildup in the tissues may make it painful to leave a compression wrap in place for a long time. However, the wrap must be left in place even though there may be significant pain, because compression is so important in the control of swelling. The compression wrap should be left in place for at least 72 hours after an acute injury. In many chronic overuse problems, such as tendinitis, tenosynovitis, and particularly bursitis, the compression wrap should be worn until all swelling is almost entirely gone.

## Elevation

Along with cold and compression, elevation reduces internal bleeding. The injured part, particularly an extremity, should be elevated to elimi-

7–3

*Critical Thinking* Exercise

A field hockey player trips over an opponent's stick, turning her ankle inward, and falls to the turf, sustaining a grade 2 ankle sprain. She has immediate swelling and significant pain, and on examination, there appears to be some laxity in the ankle joint.

? What specifically should the coach do to most effectively control the initial swelling associated with this injury?

nate the effects of gravity on blood pooling in the extremities. Elevation assists the veins, which drain blood and other fluids from the injured area and return them to the central circulatory system. The greater the degree of elevation, the more effective the reduction in swelling. For example, in an ankle sprain the leg should be placed so that the ankle is virtually straight up in the air. The injured part should be elevated as much as possible during the first 72 hours.

## EMERGENCY SPLINTING

If a coach suspects that an athlete has a fracture, the rescue squad should be called immediately. Any suspected fracture should be splinted before the athlete is moved. Transporting a person with a fracture without proper immobilization can result in increased tissue damage, hemorrhage, and shock. The application of splints should be a simple process through the use of commercial emergency splints.[6] In most instances the coach does not have to improvise a splint because such devices are readily available in most sports settings.

A suspected fracture must be splinted before the athlete is moved.

Regardless of the type of splint used, the principles of good splinting remain the same. Two major concepts of splinting are (1) to splint from one joint above the fracture to one joint below the fracture and (2) to splint where the athlete lies. If at all possible, do not move the athlete until he or she has been splinted.

### Rapid Form Vacuum Immobilizers

The rapid form vacuum immobilizer is a new type of splint that is widely used by both EMTs and athletic trainers. It consists of styrofoam chips contained inside an airtight cloth sleeve that is pliable. It can be molded to the shape of any joint or angulated fracture using Velcro straps. A handheld pump sucks the air out of the sleeve, giving it a cardboardlike rigidity. This splint is most useful for injuries that are angulated and must be splinted in the position in which they are found (Figure 7-15A).

### Air Splints

An air splint is a clear plastic splint that is inflated with air around the affected part; it can be used for extremity splinting, but its use requires some special training. This splint provides support and moderate pressure to the body part and affords a clear view of the site for x-ray examination. The inflatable splint should not be used if it will alter a fracture deformity (Figure 7-15B).

### Splinting of Lower-Limb Fractures

Fractures of the ankle or leg require immobilization of the foot and knee. Any fracture involving the knee, thigh, or hip needs splinting of all the lower-limb joints and one side of the trunk.

### Splinting of Upper-Limb Fractures

Fractures around the shoulder complex are immobilized by a sling and swathe bandage, with the upper limb bound to the body securely.

**Figure 7-15**

A, Rapid form vacuum
immobilizer. B, Air splint

Upper-arm and elbow fractures must be splinted, with immobilization effected in a straight-arm position to lessen bone override. Lower-arm and wrist fractures should be splinted in a position of forearm flexion and should be supported by a sling. Hand and finger dislocations and fractures should be splinted with tongue depressors, gauze rolls, or aluminum splints.

### Splinting of the Spine and Pelvis

Injuries involving a possible spine or pelvic fracture are best splinted and moved using a spine board. Recently, a total body rapid form vacuum immobilizer has been developed for dealing with spinal injuries (Figure 7-16). The effectiveness of this piece of equipment as an immobilization device has yet to be determined.

## MOVING AND TRANSPORTING THE INJURED ATHLETE

Great caution must be taken
when transporting the
injured athlete.

Moving, lifting, and transporting the injured athlete must be executed using techniques that prevent further injury. Moving or transporting the

**Figure 7-16**

Rapid form total body
immobilizer

athlete improperly may cause more additional injuries than does any other emergency procedure.[1] There is no excuse for poor handling of the injured athlete. Planning should take into consideration all the possible transportation methods and the necessary equipment to execute them. Capable and well-trained personnel, spine boards, stretchers, and a rescue vehicle may be needed to transport the injured athlete.

## Suspected Spinal Injury

**When spinal injuries are suspected, the coach should immediately access the EMS and wait until the rescue squad arrives before attempting to move the athlete.** The only exception is in cases in which the athlete is not breathing and logrolling the athlete onto the back is required for CPR.

A suspected spinal injury requires extremely careful handling and is best left to properly trained paramedics, EMTs, or athletic trainers who are more skilled and have the proper equipment for such transport.[1] If such personnel are not available, moving should be done under the express direction of a physician, and a spine board should be used. One danger inherent in moving an athlete with a suspected spinal injury, in particular a cervical injury, is the tendency of the neck and head to turn because of the victim's inability to control his or her movements. Torque so induced creates a possibility of spinal cord or root damage when small fractures are present. The most important principle in transporting an individual on a spine board is to keep the head and neck in alignment with the long axis of the body. In such cases it is best to have one individual whose sole responsibility is to ensure and maintain proper positioning of the head and neck until the head is secured to a spine board.

### Placing the Athlete on a Spine Board

Once an injury to the neck has been recognized as severe, a physician and rescue squad should be summoned immediately. Once the rescue squad has been called the coach should assume the responsibility for providing primary emergency care that involves maintaining normal breathing, treating for shock, and keeping the athlete quiet and in the position

**Figure 7-17**

The athlete should be placed
on the spine board with the
head securely stabilized.

found until medical assistance arrives. Ideally, transportation should not
be attempted until the physician has examined the athlete and has given
permission to move him or her. Once the rescue squad arrives the coach
should do nothing more than play an assistive role in positioning the athlete on the spine board, carrying the athlete on the spine board to the rescue vehicle, and following the instructions of the EMTs. The athlete
should be transported while lying on his or her back with the curve of
the neck supported by a rolled-up towel or pad or encased in a stabilization collar. Neck stabilization must be maintained throughout transportation, first to the emergency vehicle, then to the hospital, and
throughout the hospital procedure. If stabilization is not continued, additional spinal cord damage and paralysis may ensue (Figure 7-17).

### Stretcher Carrying

Whenever a serious injury is suspected, the best and safest mode of transportation for a short distance is by stretcher. With each segment of the
body supported, the athlete is gently lifted and placed on the stretcher,
which is carried adequately by four assistants, two supporting the ends of
the stretcher and two supporting either side (Figure 7-18). Any person
with an injury serious enough to require the use of a stretcher must be
carefully examined before being moved.

When transporting a person with a limb injury, be certain the injury
is splinted properly before transport. Athletes with shoulder injuries are
more comfortably moved in a semi-sitting position, unless other injuries
preclude such positioning. If injury to the upper extremity is such that
flexion of the elbow is not possible, the individual should be transported
on a stretcher with the limb properly splinted and carried at the side and
with adequate padding placed between the arm and the body.

### Ambulatory Aid

Ambulatory aid (Figure 7-19) is support or assistance given to an injured
athlete who is able to walk. Before the athlete is allowed to walk, he
or she should be carefully scrutinized to make sure that the injuries are
minor. Whenever serious injuries are suspected, walking should be

**Figure 7-18**

Whenever a serious injury is
suspected, a stretcher is the
safest method for
transporting the athlete.

**Figure 7-19**

The ambulatory aid method
of transporting a mildly
injured athlete

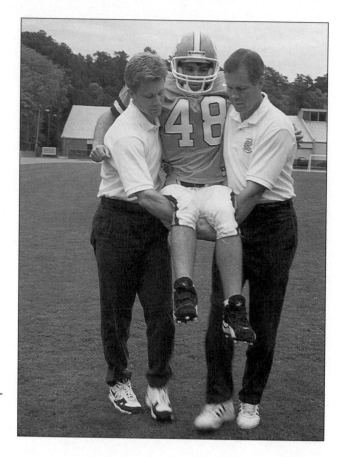

**Figure 7-20**

Manual conveyance method
for transporting a mildly
injured athlete

prohibited. Complete support should be given on both sides of the athlete by two individuals who are approximately the same height. The athlete's arms are draped over the assistants' shoulders, and their arms encircle his or her back.

## Manual Conveyance

Manual conveyance (Figure 7-20) may be used to move a mildly injured individual a greater distance than can be walked with ease. As with the use of ambulatory aid, any decision to carry the athlete must be made only after a complete examination to determine the existence of potentially serious conditions. The most convenient carry is performed by two assistants.

## Fitting and Using the Crutch or Cane

When an athlete has a lower-limb injury, weight bearing may be contraindicated. Situations of this type call for the use of a crutch or cane. Very often, the athlete is assigned one of these aids without proper fitting or instruction in its use. Improper fit and usage can place abnormal

**Figure 7-21**

The crutch must be properly
fitted to the athlete. A, The
crutch tips are placed 6
inches [15 cm] from the
outer margin of the shoe and
2 inches [5 cm] in front of
the shoe. B, The underarm
crutch brace is positioned 1
inch [2.5 cm] below the
anterior fold of the axilla.
C, The hand brace is placed
even with the athlete's hand,
with the elbow flexed
approximately 30 degrees.

stresses on various body parts. Constant pressure of the body weight on
the crutch's axillary pads can cause crutch palsy. This pressure on the axillary radial nerves and blood vessels can lead to temporary or even permanent numbness in the hands. Faulty mechanics in the use of crutches
or canes can produce chronic low back and/or hip strain.

### Fitting the Athlete

The adjustable, wooden crutch is well suited to the athlete (Figure 7-21).
For a correct fit the athlete should wear low-heeled shoes and stand with
good posture and the feet close together. The crutch length is determined
first by placing the tip 6 inches (15 cm) from the outer margin of the shoe
and 2 inches (5 cm) in front of the shoe. The underarm crutch brace is
positioned 1 inch (2.5 cm) below the anterior fold of the axilla. Next, the
hand brace is adjusted so that it is even with the athlete's hand and
the elbow is flexed at approximately a 30-degree angle. Fitting a cane to
the athlete is relatively easy. Measurement is taken from the superior aspect of the greater trochanter of the femur to the floor while the athlete
is wearing street shoes.

*Properly fitting a crutch or
cane is essential to avoid
placing abnormal stresses on
the body.*

### Walking with the Crutch or Cane

Many elements of crutch walking correspond with walking. The technique commonly used in sports injuries is the tripod method. In this
method, the athlete swings through the crutches without making any
surface contact with the injured limb or by partially bearing weight with
the injured limb. The following sequence is performed:

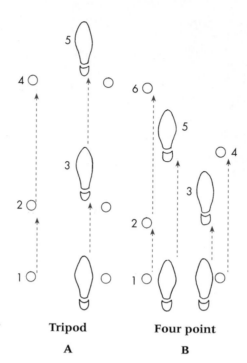

**Figure 7-22**

Crutch gait. A, Tripod
method. B, Four-point gait.

**Tripod**

**A**

**Four point**

**B**

1. The athlete stands on one foot with the affected foot completely elevated or partially bearing weight.
2. Placing the crutch tips 12 to 15 inches (30 to 37.5 cm) ahead of the feet, the athlete leans forward, straightens the elbows, pulls the upper crosspiece firmly against the side of the chest, and swings or steps between the stationary crutches (Figure 7-22). The athlete should avoid placing the major support in the axilla.
3. After moving through, the athlete recovers the crutches and again places the tips forward.

An alternate method is the four-point crutch gait. In this method, the athlete stands on both feet. One crutch is moved forward and the opposite foot is stepped forward. The crutch on the same side as the foot that moved forward moves just ahead of the foot. The opposite foot steps forward, followed by the crutch on the same side, and so on.

Once the athlete is able to move effectively on a level surface, negotiating stairs should be taught. As with level crutch walking, a tripod is maintained on stairs. In going upstairs, the unaffected support leg moves up one step while the body weight is supported by the hands. The full weight of the body is transferred to the support leg, followed by moving the crutch tips and affected leg to the step. In going downstairs, the crutch tips and the affected leg move down one step followed by the support leg. If a handrail is available, both crutches are held by the outside hand, and a similar pattern is followed as with the crutch on each side.

## COACH'S CORNER

The following checklist includes steps the coach must take in initial management and assessment of injury.

☐ Have an established emergency plan in place.

☐ Determine if the athlete is conscious or unconscious.

☐ If unconscious, access the emergency medical system.

☐ Conduct primary survey looking for life-threatening injuries (loss of breathing, bleeding, shock).

☐ Take appropriate measures to manage loss of breathing, bleeding, or shock until the rescue squad arrives. The rescue squad takes over injury management.

☐ If there is no loss of consciousness and no life-threatening injury conduct a secondary survey.

☐ Immobilize the injury if necessary.

☐ Determine how the athlete should be transported from the field.

☐ Notify the parents of injury if the athlete is a minor.

☐ Manage the injury using appropriate first aid measures (RICE).

☐ Fit the athlete with a crutch or cane if necessary.

☐ Refer the athlete to the team or family physician.

## SUMMARY

- An emergency is defined as "an unforeseen combination of circumstances and the resulting state that calls for immediate action." The prime concern of emergency aid is to maintain cardiovascular function and, indirectly, central nervous system function. All sports programs should have an emergency system that is activated any time an athlete is seriously injured.

- The coach must make a systematic assessment of the injured athlete to determine appropriate emergency care. A primary survey assesses and deals with life-threatening situations. Once stabilized, the secondary survey makes a more detailed assessment of the injury.

- The mnemonic for cardiopulmonary resuscitation is ABC: A—airway opened; B—breathing restored; C—circulation restored. To relieve an obstructed airway, the Heimlich maneuver and/or a finger sweep of the throat should be performed.

- Hemorrhage can occur externally and internally. External bleeding can be controlled by direct pressure, applying pressure at pressure points, and by elevation. Internal hemorrhage can occur subcutaneously, intramuscularly, or within a body cavity.

- Secondary assessment consists of four major areas: history, general observation, physical examination, and special tests. Special tests depend on the body site.

- Rest, ice, compression, and elevation (RICE) should be used for the immediate care of a musculoskeletal injury. Ice should be applied for at least 20 minutes every 1 to 1½ hours, and compression and elevation should be continuous for at least 72 hours following injury.

- Any suspected fracture should be splinted before the athlete is moved. Commercial rapid form vacuum immobilizers and air splints are most often used in an athletic training setting.

- Great care must be taken in moving the seriously injured athlete. The unconscious athlete must be handled as though he or she has a cervical fracture. Moving an athlete with a suspected serious neck injury must be performed only by persons specifically trained to do so. A spine board should be used, avoiding any movement of the cervical region.

- The coach should be responsible for the proper fitting and instruction in the use of crutches or a cane by an athlete with an injury to the lower extremity.

---

### *Solutions to Critical Thinking* Exercises

**7-1** Because of the mechanism of injury, it should be suspected that the athlete has a cervical neck injury. The head should be stabilized throughout. If the athlete is prone and breathing, do nothing until consciousness returns. An on-field exam should establish the athlete's unresponsiveness. Then the athlete should be carefully logrolled onto a spine board because CPR could be necessary at any time. The face mask should be removed in case CPR is required. The helmet and shoulder pads should be left in place. The athlete should then be transported to the emergency facility. Remember, in this situation the worst mistake the coach can make is not exercising enough caution.

**7-2** The coach should first take a subjective history from the injured athlete, followed by an objective examination that includes observation, palpation, special tests, tests for joint stability, and a functional performance evaluation.

**7-3** The ankle should be wrapped with a wet elastic compression wrap. Ice should be applied to both sides of the joint over the compression wrap and secured. The ankle should be elevated such that the leg is above 45 degrees at a minimum. The compression wrap, ice, and elevation should be maintained initially for at least 30 minutes but not longer than an hour. The coach should also make some determination as to whether a fracture is suspected and make the appropriate referral.

## REVIEW QUESTIONS AND CLASS ACTIVITIES

1. What considerations are important in a well-planned system for handling emergency situations?
2. Discuss the rules for managing and moving an unconscious athlete.
3. What are the life-threatening conditions that should be evaluated in the primary survey?
4. What are the ABCs of life support?
5. Identify the major steps in giving CPR and managing an obstructed airway. When may these procedures be used in a sports setting?

6. List the basic steps in assessing a musculoskeletal injury.
7. What techniques should be used to stop external hemorrhage?
8. What are the signs and symptoms of shock and how do you treat it?
9. What first-aid procedures are used to decrease hemorrhage, inflammation, and pain from a musculoskeletal injury?
10. Discuss the process for assessing an injury.
11. Describe the basic concepts of emergency splinting.
12. How should an athlete with a suspected spinal injury be transported?
13. What techniques can be used when transporting an athlete with a suspected musculoskeletal injury?
14. Explain how to properly fit crutches.

## REFERENCES

1. Almquist J: Spine injury management: a comprehensive plan for managing the cervical spine–injured football player, *Sports Med Update* 13(1):8, 1998.
2. Hafen BQ, Karren KJ: *First aid for colleges and universities,* Needham Heights, Mass, 1998, Allyn and Bacon.
3. Knight K: *Cryotherapy in sport injury management,* Champaign, Ill, 1995, Human Kinetics.
4. Knox KE, Kleiner DM: The efficiency of tools used to retract a football helmet face mask, *J Ath Train* 32(3):211, 1997.
5. Magee DL: *Orthopedic physical assessment,* Philadelphia, 1997, WB Saunders.
6. National Safey Council: *First aid and CPR,* Boston, 1999, Jones & Bartlett.
7. Ransone J, Dunn-Bennett LR: Assessment of first-aid knowledge and decision making of high school athletic coaches, *J Ath Train* 34(3): 267, 1999.
8. Roberts WO: Helmet removal in head and neck trauma, *Physician Sportsmed* 26(7): 77, 1998.
9. Starkey C, Ryan J: *Evaluation of orthopedic and athletic injuries,* Philadelphia, 1996, FA Davis.
10. Waninger KN: On-field management of potential cervical spine injury in helmeted football players: leave the helmet on, *Clin J Sportmed* 8(2):124, 1998.

## ANNOTATED BIBLIOGRAPHY

Hafen BQ, Karren KJ: *First aid for colleges and universities,* Needham Heights, Mass, 1998. Allyn and Bacon.

*A well-illustrated, simple approach to the treatment of emergency illness and injury.*

Leikin JB, Feldman BJ: *American Medical Association handbook of first aid and emergency care,* Philadelphia, 2000, Random House.

*Covering urgent emergency situations and the common injuries and ailments that occur in every family, this AMA guide takes the reader step-by-step through basic first-aid techniques, the* *medical symptoms to recognize before an emergency occurs, and what to do when one does.*

Magee DJ: *Orthopedic physical assessment,* Philadelphia, 1997, WB Saunders.

*An extremely well-illustrated book, with excellent depth of coverage. Its strength lies in its coverage of injuries commonly found during athletic training.*

National Safety Council: *First aid and CPR,* Boston, 1999, Jones and Bartlett.

*A complete and widely used first aid text that addresses all aspects of first aid and CPR.*

Techniques for Preventing
and Minimizing
Sport-Related Injuries

Starkey C, Ryan J: *Evaluation of orthopedic and athletic injuries,* Philadelphia, 1996, FA Davis.

*A detailed, well-illustrated text that addresses all aspects of injury assessment for the athletic trainer.*

## WEBSITES

American Red Cross: http://redcross. org/what.html

*The American Red Cross offers many emergency services and training. This site describes those services and introduces information about various training opportunities.*

American Heart Association: http:// www. amhrt.org

Cervical Spine Stabilization: http:// www. trauma.org/spine/cspine-stab. html

*Guidelines for evaluation of individuals with suspected cervical spine injury.*

National Safety Council: http:// www.nsc.org/

*The National Safety Council is a membership organization with resources on safety, health, and environmental topics, training, products, publications, news, and more.*

First Aid: http://www.mayohealth.org/ mayo/library/htm/firstaid.htm

*Website on first aid maintained by the Mayo Clinic.*

# Bloodborne Pathogens

*When you finish this chapter you will be able to:*

- Explain what bloodborne pathogens are and how they can infect coaches and athletes.
- Describe the transmission, symptoms and signs, and treatment of hepatitis B (HBV).
- Describe the transmission, symptoms, and signs of human immunodeficiency virus (HIV) infection.
- Describe how HIV is most often transmitted.
- List the pros and cons of sports participation of athletes with an HBV or HIV infection.
- Identify universal precautions as mandated by the Occupational Safety and Health Administration and how they apply to the coach.
- Discuss the various types of skin wounds.

I t has always been important for any health care provider to be concerned with maintaining an environment that is as clean and sterile as possible.[1,7] In our twenty-first century society, it has become critical for everyone in the population to take measures to prevent the spread of infectious diseases. Failure to do so may expose any individual to potentially life-threatening situations.

Because of the close physical contact that occurs through athletic participation, the potential for spread of infectious disease among coaches, athletes, and sports medicine personnel is of major concern. The coach must be aware of the potential dangers of exposure to blood or other infectious materials and take whatever measures are necessary to prevent contamination (Figure 8-1).

## WHAT ARE BLOODBORNE PATHOGENS?

Bloodborne pathogens:
- Hepatitis B (HBV)
- Human immuno-deficiency virus (HIV)

Mode of transmission:
- Human blood
- Semen
- Vaginal secretions
- Cerebrospinal fluid
- Synovial fluid

*Bloodborne pathogens* are pathogenic microorganisms that can potentially cause disease. They may be present in human blood and other bodily fluids including semen, vaginal secretions, cerebrospinal fluid, synovial fluid, and any other fluid contaminated with blood. The two most significant bloodborne pathogens include the hepatitis B virus (HBV) and the human immunodeficiency virus (HIV). A number of other bloodborne diseases exist, including hepatitis C, hepatitis D, and syphilis. Although HIV has been more widely addressed in the media, HBV has a higher possibility for spread.[10] HBV is stronger and more durable than HIV.[7] HBV

**Figure 8-1**

The coach must take
precautions to prevent
exposure and transmission of
bloodborne pathogens.

can be spread more easily via sharp objects, open wounds, or bodily fluids when compared to HIV.

## Hepatitis B Virus

HBV is a major cause of viral infection that results in swelling, soreness, and loss of normal function in the liver. The number of cases of HBV has risen dramatically during the last 10 years.[14]

### Signs of HBV

The signs in a person infected with HBV include flulike symptoms such as fatigue, weakness, nausea, abdominal pain, headache, fever, and possibly jaundice. It is possible that an individual infected with HBV will exhibit no signs or symptoms and may go undetected. In these individuals, the HBV antigen will always be present and thus the disease may be unknowingly transmitted to others through exposure to blood or other bodily fluids or by intimate contact.

An infected person's blood may test positive for the HBV antigen within 2 to 6 weeks after the symptoms develop. Approximately 85 percent of those infected recover within 6 to 8 weeks.

### Prevention

Good personal hygiene and avoiding high-risk activities are the best ways to avoid HBV.[7] HBV can survive for at least a week in dried blood or on contaminated surfaces and may be transmitted through contact with these surfaces. Caution must be taken to avoid contact with any blood or other fluid that potentially contains a bloodborne pathogen.

A vaccine is now available that can prevent contraction of HBV. The vaccine requires a series of three innoculations spread over a 6-month period. In 1991 the Occupational Safety and Health Administration (OSHA) mandated that vaccination against HBV must be made available by an employer at no cost to any individual who may be exposed to blood or other bodily fluids and may thus be at risk of contacting hepatitis B.[15] *All coaches, and any individual working in an allied health care*

OSHA: Occupational Safety
and Health Administration

*profession who may potentially come in contact with blood, should receive HBV immunization.*

## Human Immunodeficiency Virus

HIV infection is caused by a family of complex viruses that invade normal healthy cells, thus decreasing the effectiveness of the host cell in preventing disease. HIV is a viral infection that has the potential to eventually destroy the immune system. The rapid increase in the number of known individuals who are HIV positive is alarming. The World Health Organization has estimated that worldwide there were more than 10 to 12 million adult carriers of the virus, with 40 million as of the year 2000.[18]

### Symptoms and Signs of HIV

As with HBV, HIV is transmitted by exposure to infected blood or other bodily fluids or by intimate sexual contact. Symptoms of HIV include fatigue, weight loss, muscle or joint pain, painful or swollen glands, night sweats, and fever. HIV antibodies can be detected in a blood test within a year following exposure. Like people with HBV, people with HIV may be unaware that they have contracted the virus and may go as long as 8 to 10 years before developing any signs or symptoms. Unfortunately most individuals who test positive for HIV have a high probability of eventually developing acquired immunodeficiency syndrome (AIDS). Table 8-1 summarizes information on HBV and HIV.

AIDS: Acquired
immunodeficiency syndrome

### Acquired Immunodeficiency Syndrome

AIDS is an acronym for acquired immunodeficiency syndrome. A syndrome is a collection of signs and symptoms that are recognized as the effects of an infection. A person who has AIDS has no protection against even the simplest infections and thus is extremely vulnerable to developing a variety of illnesses, opportunistic infections, and/or cancers that

**TABLE 8-1** HBV and HIV transmission

| Disease | Symptoms & Signs | Mode of Transmission | Infectious Material |
|---------|------------------|----------------------|---------------------|
| Hepatitis B | Flulike, jaundice | Direct & indirect contact | Blood, saliva, semen, feces; also food, water, and other products |
| HIV | Fever, night sweats, weight loss, diarrhea, severe fatigue, swollen lymph nodes, lesions | Direct & indirect contact | Blood, semen, vaginal fluid |

cannot be stopped.[3] A positive HIV test cannot predict when the individual might show the symptoms of AIDS. Those individuals who develop AIDS generally die within 2 years after the symptoms appear.

### Management

Unlike HBV, there is no vaccine for HIV. Much research is being done to find a preventive vaccine and an effective treatment. Presently, it appears that certain combinations of various antiviral drugs, which have been labeled "cocktails," can slow replication of the virus and improve prospects for survival.

### Prevention

The best means for prevention is through education.[9] Coaches should take the responsibility of educating their athletes about HIV. Athletes must be made to understand that their greatest risk for contracting HIV is through intimate sexual contact with an infected partner and not through contact that occurs during athletic participation. Practicing safe sex is of major importance. (See Focus Box 8-1.) The athlete must choose nonpromiscuous sex partners and use condoms for vaginal or anal intercourse. Latex condoms provide a barrier against both HBV and HIV. Male condoms should have reservoir tips to reduce the chance of ejaculate being released from the sides of the condom. Condoms that are prelubricated are less likely to tear. Water-based, greaseless spermicides or lubricants should be avoided. If the condom tears, a vaginal spermicide should be used immediately. The condom should carefully be removed and discarded.[18]

> HIV is most often transmitted through intimate sexual contact.

> The use of latex condoms can reduce the chances of contracting HIV.

## DEALING WITH BLOODBORNE PATHOGENS IN ATHLETICS

In general the chances of transmitting HIV among athletes is low. There is minimal risk of on-field transmission of HIV from one player to another in sports.[16] One study involving professional football estimated the risk of

---

( 8-1 ) **Focus Box**

**HIV Risk Reduction**

- Avoid contact with others' bodily fluids, feces, and semen.
- Avoid sharing needles (e.g., injecting anabolic steroids or human growth hormones).
- Choose nonpromiscuous sex partners.
- Limit sex partners.
- Consistently use condoms.
- Avoid drugs that alter good judgment.
- Avoid sex with known HIV carriers.
- Get regular tests for sexually transmitted diseases (STDs).
- Practice good hygiene before and after sex.

8-2 **Focus Box**

**Risk Categories for Sports**[21]

- Greatest risk: Boxing, tae kwon do, wrestling, rugby
- Moderate risk: Basketball, field hockey, football, ice hockey, judo, soccer, team handball
- Lowest risk: Archery, badminton, baseball, bowling, canoeing/kayaking, cycling, diving, equestrian sports, fencing, figure skating, gymnastics, modern pentathalon, raquetball, rhythmic gymnastics, roller skating, rowing, shooting, softball, speed skating, skiing, swimming, synchronized swimming, table tennis, volleyball, water polo, weightlifting, yachting

transmission from player to player was less than one per one million games. In fact, at this writing there have been no validated reports of HIV transmission in sports.[13]

Sports that have a potentially higher risk for transmission are those that involve close physical contact and possible direct contact with the blood of another person.[21] Sports such as the martial arts, wrestling, and boxing have more theoretical potential for transmission.[13] (See Focus Box 8-2.)

### Policy Regulation

Athletes participating in organized sports are subject to procedures and policies relative to transmission of bloodborne pathogens.[11] The United States Olympic Committee (USOC), the National Collegiate Athletic Association (NCAA), the National Federation of State High School Athletic Associations, the National Basketball Association, the National Hockey League, the National Football League, and Major League Baseball have established policies to help prevent the transmission of bloodborne pathogens. They have also initiated programs to help educate athletes under their control.

All institutions should take the responsibility for educating their student-athletes about how bloodborne pathogens are transmitted. Efforts should also be made to educate the parents of high-school athletes.[4] Professional, collegiate, and high-school athletes should be made to understand that the real risk of contracting HBV or HIV is through their off-the-field activities, which may include unsafe sexual practices and sharing needles, particularly in the use of steroids. Athletes, perhaps more than other individuals in the population, think that they are immune and that infection will always happen to someone else.

Each institution should implement policies and procedures concerning bloodborne pathogens.[16] A recent survey of NCAA institutions found that a large number of health care providers at many colleges and universities demonstrated significant deficits in following the universal

8-1

*Critical Thinking* Exercise

A wrestler comes to his coach with concern about the possibility of contracting HIV from wrestling with a sweaty partner.

? What can the coach tell this athlete to help him ease his fear?

guidelines mandated by OSHA. In a sports medicine or other health care setting, following these universal precautions protects the athlete, the coach, and the health care providers.[12]

### HIV and Athletic Participation

There is no definitive answer as to whether asymptomatic HIV carriers should participate in sports.[6,19] Bodily fluid contact should obviously be avoided, and the participant should also avoid engaging in exhaustive exercise that may lead to an increased susceptibility to infection.[10]

The Americans with Disabilities Act of 1991 states that athletes infected with HIV cannot be discriminated against and may be excluded from participation only on a medically sound basis. Exclusion must be based on objective medical evidence that takes into consideration the risk of infection to others and of potential harm to the athlete and what means can be taken to reduce these risks.[13]

### Testing Athletes for HIV

HIV testing should not be used as a screening tool to determine if an athlete can participate in sports. Mandatory testing for HIV may not be allowed for legal reasons related to the Americans with Disabilities Act. In terms of importance, mandatory testing should be secondary to education to prevent transmission of HIV. Neither the NCAA nor the Centers for Disease Control and Prevention (CDC) recommends mandatory HIV testing for athletes.[16]

Athletes who engage in high-risk activities should be encouraged to seek voluntary anonymous testing for HIV. A blood test may detect the presence of the HIV virus within 3 months to 1 year following exposure. Testing therefore should occur at 6 weeks, at 3 months, and at 1 year after exposure.[18]

Many states have enacted laws that protect the confidentiality of the HIV-infected person. Coaches should be familiar with the laws of their state and make every effort to guard the confidentiality and anonymity of HIV testing for their athletes.[20]

## UNIVERSAL PRECAUTIONS IN AN ATHLETIC ENVIRONMENT

The guidelines instituted by OSHA were developed to protect the health care provider and the patient against bloodborne pathogens.[14] It is essential that every sports program develop and carry out a bloodborne pathogen exposure control plan. This plan should include counseling, education, volunteer testing, and the management of bodily fluids.[16]

OSHA's guidelines should be followed by anyone coming in contact with blood or other bodily fluids. Following are considerations specific to the sports arena.

### Preparing the Athlete

Before an athlete participates in practice or competition, all open skin wounds or lesions must be covered with a dressing that is fixed in place

For additional information on HIV and AIDS care, contact the Centers for Disease Control and Prevention (CDC) National AIDS Hotline: 1-800-342-2437.

Throughout the remainder of this text wherever there is a discussion of an injury or a technique of care that requires universal precautions the following icon will appear in the margin.

BIOHAZARD

**BIOHAZARD**

### *Critical Thinking* Exercise

A soccer player jumps to win a head ball and an opponent's head smashes the right eyebrow, creating a significant laceration. The athlete is conscious but is bleeding profusely from the wound.

**?** What techniques are most effective to control the bleeding, and what should be done to close the wound?

Latex gloves should be worn whenever the athletic trainer deals with blood or bodily fluids.

and does not allow for transmission to or from an athlete. An occlusive dressing lessens the chances of cross-contamination and also reduces chances of the wound reopening by keeping it moist and pliable.

### When Bleeding Occurs

As mandated by the NCAA and the USOC, open wounds or other skin lesions considered a risk for disease transmission should be provided with aggressive treatment.[17] Athletes with active bleeding must be removed from participation as soon as possible and only returned when it is deemed safe by the medical staff.[5] Uniforms containing blood must be evaluated for infectivity. A uniform that is saturated with blood must be removed and changed before the athlete can return to competition. All personnel managing potential infective wound exposures must follow universal precautions.[14]

### Personal Precautions

The coach or health care personnel working directly with bodily fluids on the field must make use of the appropriate protective equipment in all cases in which there is potential contact with bloodborne pathogens. Protective equipment includes disposable latex gloves, gowns, or aprons; masks and shields; eye protection; nonabsorbant gowns; and disposable mouthpieces for resuscitation devices.[14] *One-time use latex gloves must be used when handling any potentially infectious material.* Double gloving is suggested when there is heavy bleeding or when sharp instruments are used. Gloves are always carefully removed following their use (see Focus Box 8-3). In cases of emergency, heavy toweling may be used until gloves can be obtained.[1]

Hands and all skin surfaces that come in contact with blood or other bodily fluids should be washed immediately with soap and water or other antigermicidal agents.

First-aid kits must have protection for hands, face, and eyes and resuscitation mouthpieces. Kits should also make towelettes available for cleaning skin surfaces.[2]

---

8-3    *Focus Box*

---

**Glove Removal and Use (Figure 8-2)**

1. Avoid touching personal items when wearing contaminated gloves.
2. Remove first glove and turn inside out, beginning at the wrist and peeling off without touching skin.
3. Remove second glove making sure not to touch ungloved hand to soiled surfaces.
4. Discard gloves that have been used, discolored, torn, or punctured.
5. Wash hands immediately after glove removal.

**Figure 8-2**

Technique for removing
latex gloves

## Availability of Supplies and Equipment

In keeping with universal precautions, the sports program must have available chlorine bleach, antiseptics, proper receptacles for soiled equipment and uniforms, wound care bandages, and a designated container for sharps disposal such as needles, syringes, or scalpels.[5]

Biohazard warning labels should be fixed to regulated wastes, refrigerators containing blood, and other containers used to store or ship potentially infectious materials (Figure 8-3). The labels are fluorescent orange or red and should be affixed to containers. Red bags or containers should be used for disposal of potentially infected materials.

Universal precautions
minimize the risk of
exposure and transmission.

### Disinfectants

All contaminated surfaces, such as the field or court, should be cleaned immediately with a solution consisting of one part bleach to ten parts water (1:10) or with a disinfectant approved by the Environmental Protection Agency.[4] Disinfectants should inactivate the virus. Towels or other linens that have been contaminated should be bagged and separated from other laundry. Soiled linen is to be transported in red containers or bags that prevent soaking or leaking and are labeled with the biohazard warning labels (refer to Figure 8-3). Contaminated laundry should be washed in hot water (71°C for 25 minutes) using a detergent that deactivates the virus. Laundry done outside the institution should be taken to a facility that follows OSHA standards. Gloves must be worn during bagging and cleaning of contaminated laundry.

### Sharps

*Sharps* refers to sharp objects such as needles, razor blades, and scalpels. Extreme care should be taken when handling and disposing of sharps to minimize risk of puncturing or cutting the skin. OSHA mandates that

8–3

*Critical Thinking* Exercise

All institutions sponsoring athletic programs must initiate and carry out a bloodborne pathogen exposure control plan.

? What is the policy on universal precautions in an athletic environment as proposed by OSHA?

**Figure 8-3**

Soiled linens should be
placed in a leakproof bag
marked as a biohazard.

sharps be disposed of in a leakproof and puncture-resistant container.[4]
The container should be red and labeled as a biohazard (Figure 8-4).

### Protecting the Coach

It must be pointed out that OSHA guidelines for bloodborne pathogens
are intended to protect not only the coach, but also the athletic trainer
and other employees and not the athlete.[15] Coaches do not normally
come in contact with blood or other bodily fluids from an injured athlete,
so their risk is considerably reduced. It is the responsibility of the high
school, college, professional team, or clinic to ensure the safety of the
coach as a potential health care provider by instituting and annually
updating policies for education on the prevention of transmission of
bloodborne pathogens through contact with athletes. The institution
must provide the necessary supplies and equipment to carry out these
recommendations. The coach has the personal responsibility of adhering
to these policies and guidelines and enforcing them.

### Protecting the Athlete from Exposure

Several additional recommendations may further help protect the athlete. The USOC supports the required use of mouthpieces in those high-

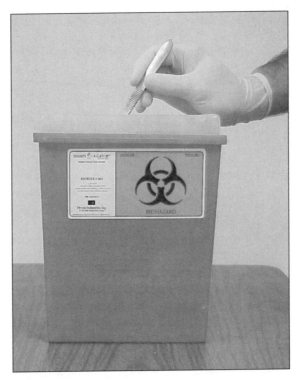

**Figure 8-4**

Sharps should be disposed of
in a red, puncture-resistant,
plastic container marked as a
biohazard.

risk sports listed in Focus Box 8-2. All athletes should shower immediately after practice or competition. Athletes who may be exposed to HIV
or HBV should be evaluated for immunization against HBV.

## POSTEXPOSURE PROCEDURES

Following a report of an exposure incident, the exposed individual
should have a confidential medical evaluation that includes documentation of the exposure route, identification of the source individual, a blood
test, counseling, and an evaluation of reported illness. Again, the laws
that pertain to reporting and notification of the test results relative to
confidentiality vary from state to state.[15]

## CARING FOR SKIN WOUNDS

Skin wounds are extremely common in sports. A wound is defined
as trauma to tissues that causes a break in the continuity of that tissue.[8]
The skin consists of two layers, the epidermis and the dermis. Because
of the soft, pliable nature of skin, it can be easily traumatized. Numerous mechanical forces can injure soft tissue. These forces produce friction or rubbing, scraping, compression or pressure, tearing, cutting, and
penetration, each of which can adversely affect the skin's integrity.
Wounds are classified according to the mechanical force that caused
them.

A

B

C

D

E

**Figure 8-5**

Wounds occurring in sports can present a serious problem of infection. A, Abrasion. B, Laceration. C, Puncture. D, Incision. E, Avulsion.

It is of the utmost importance to the well-being of the athlete that open wounds be cared for immediately. All wounds, even those that are relatively superficial, must be considered to be contaminated by microorganisms and therefore must be cleaned, medicated (when called for), and dressed. Dressing wounds requires a sterile environment to prevent infections.

Various types of wounds may be classified as follows (Figure 8-5):

*Abrasions* are common conditions in which the skin is scraped against a rough surface such as grass, artificial playing surface, floor, or mat. The top layer of skin wears away, exposing numerous blood capillaries. This exposure, with dirt and foreign materials scraping and penetrating the skin, increases the probability of infection unless the wound is properly debrided and cleansed.

*Lacerations,* also common in sports, occur when a sharp or pointed object tears the tissues, giving a wound the appearance of a jagged-edge cavity. As with abrasions, lacerations, present an environment conductive to severe infections. The same mechanism that causes a laceration also can lead to a skin avulsion, in which a piece of skin is ripped off.

*Incisions* are clean wounds that often appear where a blow has been delivered over a sharp bone or a bone that is poorly padded. They are not as serious as the other types of exposed wounds.

*Puncture wounds* can easily occur during physical activities and can be fatal. Direct penetration of tissues by a pointed object such as a track shoe spike can introduce the tetanus bacillus into the bloodstream, possibly making the athlete a victim of lockjaw. All puncture wounds and severe lacerations should be referred immediately to a physician.

*Avulsion wounds* occur when skin is torn from the body and are frequently associated with major bleeding. The avulsed tissue should be placed on moist gauze, preferabley saturated with saline solution. It is then put into a plastic bag, immersed in cold water, and taken along with the athlete to the hospital for reattachment.[8]

## Wound Infection

Tetanus is a bacterial infection that causes fever and convulsions. Tonic spasm of skeletal muscles is always a possibility for any nonimmunized athlete. The tetanus bacillus enters a wound as a spore and, depending on individual susceptibility, acts on the motor end plate of the central nervous system. After initial childhood immunization by tetanus vaccine, boosters should be given every 10 years.[8] An athlete not immunized should receive an injectin of tetanus immune globulin (Hyper-Tet) immediately after sustaining a skin wound. Focus Box 8-4 describes how to help reduce wound infections and Table 8-2 details the care of wounds.

**TABLE 8-2** Care of skin wounds

| Type of Wound | Action of Coach | Initial Care | Follow-up Care |
|---|---|---|---|
| Abrasion | 1. Provide initial care.<br><br>2. Wound seldom requires medical attention unless infected. | 1. Cleanse abraded area with soap and water; debride with brush.<br>2. Apply an antibiotic ointment to keep abraded surface moist. In sports it is not desirable for abrasions to acquire a scab. Place a nonadherent sterile pad (Telfa pad) over the ointment. | 1. Change dressing daily and look for signs of infection. |
| Laceration | 1. Cleanse around the wound. Avoid wiping more contaminating agents into the area.<br>2. Apply dry, sterile compress pad and refer to physician. | 1. Complete cleansing and suturing are accomplished by a physician; injections of tetanus vaccine may be required. | 1. Change dressing daily and look for signs of infection. |
| Puncture | 1. Cleanse around the wound. Avoid wiping more contaminating agents into the area.<br>2. Apply dry, sterile compress pad and refer to physician. | 1. Complete cleansing and injections of tetanus vaccine, if needed, are managed by a physician. | 1. Change dressing daily and look for signs of infection. |
| Incision | 1. Clean around wound.<br>2. Apply dry, sterile compress pad to control bleeding and refer to physician. | 1. Cleanse wound.<br>2. Suturing and injections of tetanus vaccine are managed by a physician, if needed. | 1. Change dressing daily and look for signs of infection. |
| Avulsion | 1. Clean around wound; save avulsed tissue.<br>2. Apply dry, sterile compress pad to control bleeding and refer to physician. | 1. Wound is cleansed thoroughly; avulsed skin is replaced and sutured by a physician; tetanus vaccine injection may be required. | 1. Change dressing daily and look for signs of infection. |

**Suggested Practices in Wound Care**

The following are suggested procedures to reduce the possibility of
wound infections.

1. Make sure all instruments used, such as scissors, tweezers, and swabs,
   are sterilized.
2. Wash hands thoroughly and put on latex gloves.
3. Clean a skin lesion using soap and water.
4. Place a nonmedicated dressing on a lesion if the athlete is to be sent
   for medical attention.
5. Avoid touching any parts of a sterile dressing that will come in contact
   with a wound.
6. Place medication on a pad rather than directly on a lesion.
7. Secure the dressing with tape or a wrap.
8. If necessary, follow the procedures described in this chapter for
   control of bleeding.

## COACH'S CORNER

The following is a checklist for the coach practicing universal precautions
in dealing with bloodborne pathogens.

☐ Make sure all open wounds or skin lesions are covered before
    practice or competition.
☐ Routinely use latex gloves when dealing with bleeding or wound
    care.
☐ Remove athletes with active bleeding from competition.
☐ Ensure that a uniform saturated with blood is removed and changed.
☐ Clean up blood spills with a disinfecting solution.
☐ Use the appropriate technique when removing gloves.
☐ Dispose of all soiled materials in a biohazard bag.
☐ Dispose of sharps in a biohazard container.
☐ Wash hands thoroughly after taking universal precautions.
☐ Report all exposure incidents.

## SUMMARY

- Bloodborne pathogens are microorganisms that can potentially cause
  disease and are present in human blood and other bodily fluids, including semen, vaginal secretions, synovial fluid, and any other fluid
  contaminated with blood. Hepatitis B virus (HBV) and human immunodeficiency virus (HIV) are bloodborne pathogens.

- A vaccine is available to prevent HBV. Currently no effective vaccine
  exists for treating HIV.

- An individual infected with HIV may develop acquired immunodeficiency syndrome (AIDS), which is fatal.

- The risks of contracting HBV or HIV may be minimized by avoiding exposure to blood and other bodily fluids and by practicing safe sex.

- The risk of an athlete being exposed to bloodborne pathogens on the field is minimal. Off-the-field activities involving risky sexual behaviors pose the greatest threat for transmission.

- Various national medical and sports organizations have established policies and procedures for dealing with bloodborne pathogens in the athletic population.

- The Occupational Safety and Health Administration (OSHA) has established rules and regulations that protect the health care employee.

- Universal precautions must be taken to avoid bloodborne pathogen exposure. All sports programs must carry out a plan for counseling, education, volunteer testing, and the management of exposure.

---

### Solutions to *Critical Thinking* Exercises

**8-1** Athletes must be made to understand that their greatest risk for contracting HIV is through intimate sexual contact with an infected partner and not through contact that occurs during athletic participation. It is highly unlikely that sweat carries HIV. However, this athlete should become concerned if his opponent begins bleeding; he should wait until the bleeding has been controlled and the wound securely covered before resuming physical contact.

**8-2** The coach must first take precautions to protect against the transmission of bloodborne pathogens. The wound should be cleaned with soap and water. Direct pressure should be applied to the wound over several layers of sterile gauze, which hopefully will absorb the bleeding. Ice may also be applied to help minimize the bleeding. The athlete, if not dizzy, should remain in a sitting position and should be referred to a physician for suturing. Sterile strips or a butterfly bandage may also be applied, although sutures generally leave a smaller scar. All blood-contaminated supplies should be disposed of in a clearly marked biohazard bag.

**8-3** Universal precautions should be practiced by anyone coming in contact with blood or other body fluids. This plan must include counseling, education, voluntary testing, and management of bodily fluids.

## REVIEW QUESTIONS AND CLASS ACTIVITIES

1. Define and identify the bloodborne pathogens.
2. Discuss HBV transmission, symptoms and signs, prevention, and treatment.
3. Discuss the pros and cons of allowing the participation of an athlete who is an HBV carrier.
4. Discuss HIV transmission, symptoms and signs, prevention, and treatment.
5. How is HIV transmitted and why is it eventually fatal at this time?
6. Should an athlete who tests positive for HBV or HIV be allowed to participate in sports?

7. How can an athlete avoid the risk of HIV infection?
8. Define OSHA and discuss its universal precautions for preventing exposure to bloodborne pathogens.
9. What precautions should a coach take when caring for a bleeding athlete on the field?
10. What are the different kinds of wounds that can occur and how should they be managed?

## REFERENCES

1. American Academy of Pediatrics: Human immunodeficiency virus [acquired immunodeficiency syndrome (AIDS) virus] in athletic settings, *Pediatrics* 88:640, 1991.
2. American Medical Association Department of HIV, Division of Health Science: *Digest of HIV/AIDS policy,* Chicago, 1993, American Medical Association.
3. American Medical Society for Sports Medicine and the American Academy for Sports Medicine: Human immunodeficiency virus (HIV) and bloodborne pathogens in sport, joint position statement, *Am J Sports Med* 23:510, 1995.
4. Arnold BL: A review of selected blood-borne pathogen position statements and federal regulations, *J Ath Train* 30(2):171, 1995.
5. Benson M: *2000–2001 NCAA sports medicine handbook,* Overland Park, Kan, 2000, NCAA.
6. Brown L, Dortman P: What is the risk of HIV infection in athletic competition? International Conference on AIDS 19939:PO-C21-3102, 1993.
7. Buxton BP et al: Prevention of hepatitis B virus in athletic training. *J Ath Train* 29(2):107, 1994.
8. Fincher LA: Wound care management, *Ath Ther Today* 4(1):11, 1999.
9. Hamann B: *Disease: identification, prevention, and control,* St Louis, 2000, Mosby.
10. Howe WB: The athlete with chronic illness. In Birrer RB, editor: *Sports medicine for the primary care physician,* ed 2, Boca Raton, Fla, 1994, CRC Press.
11. Landry GL: HIV infection and athletes, *Sports Med Digest* 15(4):1, 1993.
12. McGraw C, Dick R, Schneidewind K: Survey of NCAA institutions concerning HIV/AIDS policies and universal precautions, *Med Sci Sport Exer* 25:917, 1993.
13. Mitten MJ: HIV-positive athletes, *Physician Sportsmed* 22(10):63, 1994.
14. National Safety Council: *Bloodborne pathogens,* Boston, 1997, Jones and Bartlett.
15. OSHA: The OSHA bloodborne pathogens standard, *Federal Register* 55(235):64175, 1991.
16. Rogers KJ: Human immunodeficiency virus in sports. In Torg JS, Shephard RJ, editors: *Current therapy in sports medicine,* St. Louis, 1995, Mosby.
17. Sankaran G, editor: *HIV/AIDS in sport: impact, issues, and challenges,* Champaign, Ill, 1999, Human Kinetics.
18. Seltzer DG: Educating athletes on HIV disease and AIDS, *Physician Sportsmed* 21(1):109, 1993.
19. Stringer WW: HIV and aerobic exercise: current recommendations, *Sports med* 28(6):389, 1999.
20. Thomas CE: The HIV athlete: policy, obligations, and attitudes, *Sport Sci Rev* 5(2):12, 1996.
21. Zeiger T: *Management of bloodborne infections in sport,* Champaign, Ill, 1997, Human Kinetics.

**ANNOTATED BIBLIOGRAPHY**

Benson MA, editor: *National Collegiate Athletic Association 2000–2001 sports medicine handbook,* Overland Park, Kan, 2000, NCAA.

*A complete discussion of bloodborne pathogens and intercollegiate athletic policies and administration.*

Hall K et al, editors: *Bloodborne pathogens,* National Safety Council, Boston, 1997, Jones & Bartlett.

*A manual that presents OSHA's regulations specific to bloodborne pathogens.*

Hamann B: *Disease: identification, prevention, and control,* St Louis, 2000, Mosby.

*Designed for health educators; detailed coverage of AIDS and hepatitis.*

**WEBSITES**

Occupational Safety and Health Administration (OSHA): http://www.osha.gov

Department of Health and Human Services: http://www.os.dhhs.gov

HIV/AIDS Prevention: http://cdc.gov/nchstp/hiv_aids/dhap.htm

Centers for Disease Control and Prevention: http://www.cdc.gov

National Institute of Health: http://www.nih.gov

Bloodborne pathogens self-study module: http://www2.umdnj.edu/eohssweb/ bbp/intro.htm

*A self-study module that details work practice controls and current knowledge of HBV, HIV, and other bloodborne pathogens.*

# Psychological Aspects of Sports Injury

*When you finish this chapter you will be able to:*

- Discuss how athletes might respond psychologically to an injury.
- Describe the progressive reactions to injury, dependent on length of rehabilitation.
- Discuss predictors of injury and interventions.
- Identify stressors in the athlete's life.
- Discuss the concept of buffers for stress management.
- Discuss the importance of goal setting as a means of making the injured athlete compliant in the rehabilitation program.
- Identify the various considerations for the coach in managing the psychological impact of injury.
- Describe the decision-making process for returning the injured athlete to competition.

When the body is injured, it is likely that the mind is also affected. Research indicates that athletes who experience a negative psychological response to injury have a longer and more difficult period of rehabilitation.[10] Therefore, information regarding the effect that injury has on the athlete and the possible psychological care that can be given in the sport setting may facilitate the athlete's return to competition.[5]

As discussed in detail in Chapter 12, it is desirable to have an athletic trainer to oversee the rehabilitation process for the injured athlete. But if an athletic trainer is not available, the responsibility for dealing with the injured athlete falls on the shoulders of the coach. Certainly the coach can have a significant impact on the course of rehabilitation for the injured athlete (Figure 9-1). The manner in which the coach interacts with the injured athlete and how the athlete responds psychologically to injury collectively dictate the course of a rehabilitative program. The coach must pay attention to getting the mind, as well as the body, ready to return to competition.

## THE ATHLETE'S PSYCHOLOGICAL RESPONSE TO INJURY

Athletes don't all deal with injury in the same manner.[19] One athlete may view an injury as disastrous, another may view it as an opportunity to show courage, another athlete may relish the injury to prevent embar-

**Figure 9-1**

The coach must be aware of
the psychological impact that
his or her words or actions
have on the injured athlete.

rassment over poor performance, to provide an escape from a losing
team, or to discourage a domineering parent.[8]

Certain factors are commonly seen among athletes going through adjustment to injury and rehabilitation. Severity of injury usually determines length of rehabilitation.[11] Generally injuries may be classified as short term (less than 4 weeks), long term (greater than 4 weeks), chronic (recurring), or terminating (career ending) (Table 9-1). Regardless of severity of injury and the corresponding length of time required for rehabilitation, the injured athlete has to deal with a variety of emotions that may occur during three reactive phases of the injury and rehabilitation process. These reactive phases that the injured athlete typically goes through are: reaction to injury, reaction to rehabilitation, and reaction to return to competition or career termination.[11] It should be pointed out that all athletes do not necessarily have all reactions nor do all reactions fall precisely into the suggested sequence. Other factors that can influence reactions to injury and rehabilitation are the athletes' coping skills, past history of injury, social support, and personality traits.

With any type of injury, but particularly with those that require lengthy rehabilitation, athletes whose whole lives tend to revolve around a sport may have to make major adjustments in how they perceive themselves and come to terms with how they are perceived within their

Reactive phases
• reaction to injury
• reaction to rehabilitation
• reaction to return

Injury might mean major
changes in the way an
athlete behaves socially.

 9–1

***Critical Thinking*** Exercise

A volleyball player sprains the
medial collateral ligament in
her knee during a match.

**?** What emotional reactions
would you expect to see
throughout the initial injury,
rehabilitation, and return
phases of this short-term
injury?

**TABLE 9-1** Progressive reactions of injured athletes based on severity of injury and length of rehabilitation

| Length of rehabilitation | Reaction to injury | Reaction to rehabilitation | Reaction to return |
|---|---|---|---|
| Short (< 4 weeks) | shock relief | impatience optimism | eagerness anticipation |
| Long (> 4 weeks) | fear anger | loss of vigor irrational thoughts alienation | acknowledgment |
| Chronic (recurring) | anger frustration | dependence or independence, apprehension | confident or skeptical |
| Termination (career ending) | isolation grief process | loss of athletic identify | closure and renewal |

society. Therefore many athletes have difficulty controlling their emotions when they sustain an injury.

## PREDICTORS OF INJURY

### The Injury-Prone Athlete

Some athletes seem to have a pattern of injury, whereas others in exactly the same position with the same physical makeup are injury-free. It has been suggested that some psychological traits may predispose the athlete to repeated injury. No one particular personality type has been recognized as injury-prone. However, the individual who likes to take risks seems to represent the injury-prone athlete.[20] Other personality types that seem predisposed to injury are reserved, detached, or tender-minded players and/or apprehensive, over-protective, or easily distracted players.[20] These individuals usually also lack the ability to cope with the stress associated with the risks and their consequences. Other factors may also contribute to the likelihood of injury, such as attempting to reduce anxiety by being more aggressive or continuing to be injured because of fear of failure or guilt over unobtainable or unrealistic goals.[20]

*Injury-prone athletes are often risk-takers.*

### Stress and Risk of Injury

*Stress may be positive or negative.*

Much has been written about life stress events and the likelihood of illness. Stressors may be positive, such as making all-conference, or negative, such as not making the starting lineup or failing a drug test. Stressors that seem to predispose an athlete to injury are the negative stressors.[21]

Negative stressors lead to lack of attentional focus and muscle tension, which in turn leads to the stress-injury connection. Loss of attentional focus may cause the athlete to miss cues during a play that can set the stage for a possible injury. Muscle tension (bracing or guarding) leads to reduced flexibility, reduced motor coordination, and reduced muscle efficiency, setting the athlete up for a variety of injuries.

## INTERVENTIONS FOR STRESS REDUCTION

Unfortunately, many coaches do not have the interest in or ability to work with athletes who need help.[3] A screening device should be used to identify individuals who are experiencing some of life's situations that they are unprepared to handle. Obviously the coaching staff of a smaller team is more familiar with the athletes and their problems and can more effectively deal with them, but a larger team's staff should attempt to deal with the individual through the position coach or other available support personnel (i.e., counseling centers, sport psychologists, grief support groups, etc.).

### Using Buffers

In many instances athletes feel that their sport is the one positive thing in life that helps them get through times of extreme stress. Areas outside sports are often stressful and athletes tend to respond to interventions that are within their comfortable emotional framework. Buffers are techniques that allay the symptoms of stress but do not address the problem that originally caused the stress. Several buffers that may be beneficial in reducing the stress of injury and rehabilitation are: progressive relaxation with or without imagery, aerobic exercise, diet modifications (reduction of caffeine), treatment of sleep disorders, and time management programs. The use of buffers may be all the athlete needs to handle the stress of injury and rehabilitation.

#### Progressive Relaxation Techniques

Progressive relaxation techniques are most effective for athletes who tend to be stressed regarding an injury, who have problems sleeping, tension headaches, or general muscle bracing or tightness.[16] Relaxation training, with or without imagery, allows athletes to control feelings of stress and anxiety with a series of deep breathing, voluntary muscular contraction, and relaxation exercises. Relaxation and imagery are used by athletes to reduce the symptoms of anxiety associated with the reaction to injury and rehabilitation. Athletes who are coping well on their own should not be forced to spend extra time on relaxation training.

Jacobsen's progressive relaxation technique is thought to be effective because of the assumption that it is impossible to be nervous or tense when the muscles are relaxed.[16] The tenseness of the involuntary muscles and organs can be reduced when the contiguous skeletal muscles are relaxed. The muscles are tensed and relaxed so the athlete can become familiar with the feeling of the muscle in a relaxed state and in a tense state. The relaxation method involves the tensing and relaxing of muscles in a predetermined order. The arm and hand are done first because the difference in tense and relaxed muscles is more apparent in these muscle groups. The repetitions should be approximately 10 to 15 seconds for the tension segment and 15 to 20 seconds for the relaxation segment with about three repetitions for each muscle group. After the athlete is comfortable with the relaxation training then imagery can be introduced.

Techniques for Preventing
and Minimizing
Sport-Related Injuries

## Imagery

Imagery is the use of the senses to create or recreate an experience in the mind.[2] Visual images used in the rehabilitation process include visual rehearsal, emotive imagery rehearsal, and body rehearsal. Visual rehearsal uses both coping and mastery rehearsal. Coping rehearsal has athletes visually rehearse problems they feel may stand in their way to return to competition. They then rehearse how they will overcome these problems. Mastery rehearsal aids in gaining the confidence and motivational skills necessary. Athletes visualize their successful return to competition beginning with early practice drills continuing on to the game situation.

Emotive rehearsal aids the athlete in gaining confidence and security by visualizing scenes relating to positive feelings of enthusiasm, confidence, and pride; in other words, the emotional rewards of praise and success from participating well in competition.[4] Body rehearsal empirically helps athletes in the healing process. It is suggested that athletes visualize their bodies healing internally both during the rehabilitation procedures and throughout their daily activities.[13] To do this, athletes have to have a good understanding of the injury and of the type of healing occurring during the rehabilitation process.

Care should be taken to explain the healing and rehabilitative process clearly but not to overwhelm athletes with so much information that they become intimated and fearful. Educate athletes only to the amount of knowledge required. By the same token, don't hold back information athletes require for this imagery.

## GOAL SETTING AS A MOTIVATOR TO COMPLIANCE

Establishing progressive attainable goals is essential in rehabilitation.

Goal setting has been shown to be an effective motivator for compliance to rehabilitation of an athletic injury, as well as for reaching goals in a general sport setting.[6,17] Athletes have set goals since their first competition, usually starting at an early age. They set goals to run faster, jump higher, shoot straighter, throw longer, hit harder, and so on. These goals have all had one thing in common, they were not achieved with one burst of effort but came as the result of many short-term goals having been met before the achievement of the long-term goal. Focus Box 9-1 suggests nine factors that should be incorporated into goal setting for the athlete.[14]

In athletic rehabilitation athletes need to know exactly what the goal is and have a sense that it can be met. Telling an athlete that by a certain day the athlete should be partial weight bearing with crutches is neither specific nor measurable. It is more effective to say that by achieving a certain range of motion and strength level the foot can be placed on the ground with weight bearing and that the measurement of success is that the partial weight bearing is without pain. The goal must be a challenge but one that the athlete can reach with reasonable rehabilitation effort.[12] Goals that are easily reached have no reward in success. Goals must be personal and internally satisfying, not a goal imposed on the athlete by the coach. The setting of goals needs to be a joint venture between the

9–2

*Critical Thinking* Exercise

A softball player injures her throwing shoulder while sliding into second base. She has an injury that will likely require about three weeks to rehabilitate.

? What type of imagery technique might she engage in during rehabilitation that may help facilitate her return to activity?

9-1

### *Focus Box*

**Nine factors to incorporate into goal setting for the athlete**

- Set specific and measurable goals
- Use positive versus negative language
- Goals should be challenging but realistic
- Set a reasonable timetable
- Integrate short-, medium-, and long-term goals
- Link outcome to process
- Internalize goals
- Monitor and evaluate goals
- Link sport goals to life goals

athlete and the coach to be successful.[7] The athlete has to take responsibility for the progress of the injury and be responsible for doing the necessary rehabilitation.

Goal setting incorporates a multitude of other motivating factors that intuitively appear to increase the odds of compliance by reducing the stress associated with injury rehabilitation. These buffers incorporated within the goal setting paradigm are: positive reinforcement when goals are met, time management for incorporating goals into a lifestyle, a feeling of social support when goals are set with the coach, feelings of increased self-efficacy when goals are achieved, etc. Goals are easily understood by athletes, are concrete concepts, are active events, and have been a natural part of their sport that requires no additional time commitment.[3] Goals can be set daily for a sense of accomplishment, weekly for a sense of progress, and monthly or yearly for long-term achievement.

## CONSIDERATIONS FOR THE COACH IN MANAGING THE PSYCHOLOGICAL IMPACT OF INJURY

The coach is often the first person an athlete interacts with after injury. When athletes are injured they should be shown that the coach cares for the athlete as a person and not just as a part of the team. Their perception of the coach makes a difference in recovery time and effort. First they have to respect the coach as a person before they can trust the coach in the rehabilitative setting. Successful communication between the coach and the athlete is essential for effective rehabilitation. Taking an interest in athletes before injuries have occurred enables the coach to know the athletes' personalities and work with them in helping to build their confidence.

Active listening is one of the coach's most important skills. The coach must learn to listen to the athlete beyond the complaining. The coach should listen for fear, anger, depression, or anxiety in the athlete and his

9-3

### *Critical Thinking* Exercise

The coach is discussing goals for rehabilitation with an injured soccer player.

 How should these goals be set and what can be done to help the athlete feel successful in her rehabilitation program?

or her voice. With *fear,* the athlete may be wondering what the pain means in terms of function and if he or she will be accepted by peers. *Anger* is often a feeling of being victimized by the injury and the unfairness of it. In *depression,* the athlete may have an overwhelming feeling of hopelessness or loneliness. With *anxiety* the athlete wonders how he or she can survive the injury and what will happen if he or she cannot return to full competition.[11]

Body language is important as well. The coach who continues to work on paperwork while talking to the athlete is sending a noncaring message. The coach needs to be concerned, and should look athletes in the eye with a genuine interest in their problems. This will go a long way toward gaining confidence and respect.

It is important for the coach to consider the athlete as an individual instead of as "the sprained ankle." If the injury is the only consideration, the athlete becomes just an injury and not a person. As a result the attitude projected to the athlete is just that, and the coach is perceived as caring for the athlete superficially.

The relationship between the coach and the athlete should be one of person to person. When the athlete is treated as an equal the relationship is improved, and it helps the athlete accept responsibility for his or her own rehabilitation. With injury athletes lose control over their physical efforts. They go from 4 to 5 hours a day of practice or competition to no activity. They are in a temporary lifestyle change. Their feelings affect the success or failure of the rehabilitation process. The coach must establish rapport and a sense of genuine concern and caring for the athlete, who is not fooled by superficial concern.

Neglecting injured athletes or giving them the perception that they are "outcasts" also can contribute to injury and reinjury. Coaches who foster this attitude are saying to the players that they have no self-worth if they are injured. Some coaches go so far as to prevent team contact until injured players are ready to return or to belittle them in front of their peers, believing that this will make the athlete want to get back to competition quicker. This tactic may work with some players with minor injuries but only causes major adjustment difficulties for athletes who suffer severe injury.

Some coaches refuse to talk to the athlete or tell others that the athlete really doesn't want to play or isn't tough enough. The coach and athlete experience frustration with the injury. During this period either the athletic staff shows its concern for the athlete and in return wins the athlete's loyalty and dedication, or they undermine the athlete's trust, setting up for a let down when the athlete gets in the position of controlling the outcome of a contest and may underperform out of spite.

During an injury evaluation the coach should allow the athlete to provide as much input about his or her injury as possible. Paraphrasing or restating the information to the athlete is invaluable to the coach who is unsure of the mechanism of injury or its results. Statements such as "I see" or "Go ahead" or simple silence to allow athletes to fully express themselves are of value. Important information can be gained by asking at the end of gathering subjective information "What have I not asked you or do I need to know about this injury?" Then give the athlete input in to the decision of where to go from here.

The coach is often the person who effectively explains the injury to the athlete. Care should be taken to explain the situation to the athlete in understandable terms. In most cases the simplest explanation acceptable to the athlete is the best. Athletes must have injuries explained to them to their satisfaction. Disseminating injury information appropriate to athletes' emotional and intellectual level can be a real challenge. The rate and degree of acceptance are not the same with all athletes. Severity of injury is certainly important, but the athlete's perception of that severity is what matters in the rehabilitation process.[11] Thus the physiological must be interrelated with the psychological.

The amount of stress associated with playing a sport and the meaning the sport has to the athlete can affect the athlete's compliance to rehabilitation.[1] The athlete has a more successful rehabilitation when engaged fully in the activity of rehabilitation, much as the athlete has a more successful sport career when more interest and involvement are put into the sport. Stress can be a deterrent to engaging in rehabilitation. Several techniques the coach can use (relaxation, imagery, cognitive restructuring, thought stopping) may lessen the stressful reaction to injury. Often a change in an athlete's perception concerning injury and rehabilitation can affect outcome.

Returning to competition is another area in which the coach can help the athlete. Often the perception of the athlete is either that he or she is ready to return and not being allowed to or that he or she is being forced to return before ready. The coach can assist the athlete to make a decision based on the facts and not clouded by emotions.

The coach can be of great help when athletes are unable or unwilling to continue to participate in their sport. Frequently the athlete's identity is intertwined with the sport played.[15] The transition into a completely different culture can be a traumatic experience. It is stressful to enter a culture and not know one's place or identity in that culture. To not know what the game is and what the rules are is frustrating to the injured athlete.

## RETURN TO COMPETITION

Perhaps the most difficult aspect of the rehabilitative process is making a decision as to when it is safe to return to competition. Certainly the athletic trainer or team physician is well prepared to make such a decision. Unfortunately, untrained personnel, such as fellow teammates, parents, and coaches sometimes assume this responsibility when no athletic trainer is present. This situation has the potential to result in poor medical care and leaves the coach vulnerable to legal action as a result of negligence. Courts expect competent medical care to be provided to athletes.

The phrase "you have to play with pain" has been interpreted literally to mean that the athlete has to play through an injury. The difference is that some injuries may be mild and only somewhat painful, resulting in no reinjury in competition, whereas a more severe injury is made worse by continuing to compete. The competitive athlete may be more "body aware" than the general public and therefore more apt to respond to injury with the use of rest, ice, compression, and elevation (RICE) to promote healing. The general public, on the other hand, is more likely to respond to the pain of injury than consider the healing process.[18] Therefore the athlete may want to return to competition in spite of pain whereas the nonathlete may want the pain to be treated before any activity is undertaken.

The athlete who continues to play with an unhealed or poorly rehabilitated injury constantly reduces the chances of a healthy life of activity. The athlete has to live past the few years of competition. Most athletes, however, have difficulty seeing past the present season or at best have the goal of participating in their sport until they can no longer compete, regardless of the consequences. The rewards of competition and the admiration of others take sports out of perspective and retard a healthy attitude toward sports. The attitude of some athletes is "Give it up for the sport" because "I'm invincible." Lack of this attitude is viewed by some as weakness or not being a team player. These athletes have difficulty adjusting to an injury, especially a career-ending one.

One research study found that coaches were likely to return players on the basis of status and game situation, whereas the athletic trainer's decisions were more likely to be dictated by the status of the athlete's injury.[9] Athletes who feel that a missed practice or game will relegate them to the bench for the year or those who have been encouraged to play no matter what are candidates for injury and reinjury, thus they only reinforce the decision of the coach to play someone else. Usually what happens, however, is that athletes with unhealed injuries perform poorly because they are not at full strength. The athlete with 4.5 speed who can run only a 5.0 illustrates to the coach that the athlete is not ready for competition. This also illustrates to the athlete that more time and effort are necessary to get ready to return.

The treatment of athletic injury and rehabilitation is more than just physical, emotional, and psychological aspects of the individual. The impact of the environment, the support of the athletic community, and the culture in which the athlete resides at the time of injury combine to influence the course the athlete takes from injury, through rehabilitation, to return to competition. Treating the athlete's physical injury and attending to the additional factors that influence the injured athlete are the challenges that face the coach.

## COACH'S CORNER

The following is a checklist of things the coach can do to address the psychological aspects of dealing with an injured athlete.

☐ Establish a rapport and a sense of genuine concern and caring for the athlete.

☐ Earn the athlete's trust.

☐ Establish good open communication with the athlete.

☐ Take a personal interest in athletes before an injury occurs.

☐ Be a good active listener.

☐ Look the athlete in the eye with genuine interest and use good body language.

☐ Don't neglect or ignore the injured athlete.

☐ Facilitate continuing social support by teammates.

☐ Provide as much information about his or her injury as possible.

☐ Make sure the athlete is included in the decision-making process.

## SUMMARY

- Following injury to the athlete the coach must pay attention to getting the mind, as well as the body, ready to return to competition.

- Athletes don't all respond to an injury in the same manner.

- Regardless of the severity of injury and the corresponding length of time required for rehabilitation, the injured athlete has to deal with a variety of emotions that may occur during three reactive phases of the injury and rehabilitation process: reaction to injury, reaction to rehabilitation, and reaction to return to competition or career termination.

- No one personality type has been recognized as injury-prone.

- Negative stressors seem to predispose an athlete to injury.

- Interventions for stress reduction include the use of buffers, progressive relaxation, and imagery.

- Setting appropriate goals is an effective motivator for compliance to rehabilitation of an athletic injury.

- The way the coach interacts with the injured athlete, both in what is said and perceived actions, has a major impact on the course of injury rehabilitation.

- Decisions for returning the injured athlete to play should be based on the status of the athlete's injury.

### Solutions to Critical Thinking Exercises

**9-1** Initially the athlete experiences shock and relief, followed by impatience and optimism during the rehabilitation phase, and finally eagerness and anticipation during the return phase.

**9-2** Mastery rehearsal aids in gaining confidence and motivational skills. Athletes visualize their successful return to competition beginning with early practice drills continuing on to the game situation.

**9-3** The athlete needs to know exactly what the goal is and have a sense that it can be met. Setting a progressive series of attainable goals is critical so that the athlete does not become frustrated.

## REVIEW QUESTIONS AND CLASS ACTIVITIES

1. How might an athlete possibly respond psychologically to an injury?
2. Identify the sequence of possible emotions associated with the three reactive phases of the injury process for short-term, long-term, chronic, and career-ending injuries.
3. What are some of the personality characteristics of an individual who is likely to be injury-prone?
4. What is the difference between negative and positive stress and which is more likely to cause injury?
5. What are buffers and how can they be used for stress management?
6. How are the techniques of imagery used in a rehabilitation program?
7. What are the primary considerations in setting appropriate goals for the injured athlete to achieve during the rehabilitation program?
8. Generate a list of the things that the coach should and should not do in managing the psychological impact of injury on the athlete.
9. What factors should come into consideration in the decision-making process for returning the injured athlete to competition?

## REFERENCES

1. Andersen MB, Williams JM: A model of stress and athletic injury: predictions and prevention, *J Sport Exerc Physiol* 10:294, 1988.
2. Block N: *Imagery,* Boston, 1981, MIT Press.
3. Brewer BW et al: Perceptions of psychological interventions in the context of sport injury rehabilitation, *Sport Psychologist* 8:176, 1994.
4. Coote D, Tenenbaum G: Can emotive imagery aid in tolerating exertion efficiently? *J Sports Med Phys Fitness* 38(4):344, 1998.
5. Crossman J, Jamieson J: Differences in perceptions of seriousness and disrupting effects of athlete injury as viewed by athletes and their trainer, *Percept Motor Skills* 61:1131, 1985.
6. Danish S: Psychological aspects in the care and treatment of athletic injuries. In Vineger PE, Hoerner EF, editors: *Sports injuries: the un-thwarted epidemic,* ed 2, Boston, 1986, PSG.
7. DePalma MT, DePalma B: The use of instruction and the behavioral approach to facilitate injury rehabilitation, *Ath Train* 24:217, 1989.
8. Evans L, Hardy L: Sport injury and grief response: a review, *J Sport Exerc Psychol* 17:227, 1995.
9. Flint FA, Weiss MR: Returning injured athletes to competition: a role and ethical dilemma, *Canadian J Sport Sci* 17:34, 1992.
10. Ford IW, Gordon S: Guidelines for using sport psychology in rehabilitation, *Ath Ther Today* 3(3):41, 1998.
11. Gieck J, Hedgpeth E: Psychological considerations for rehabilitation of the injured athlete. In Prentice W: *Rehabilitation techniques in sports medicine,* Boston, 1999, WCB/McGraw-Hill.
12. Gilbourne D, Taylor AH: From theory to practice: the integration

of goal perspective theory and life development approaches within an injury-specific goal-setting program, *J Appl Sport Psychol* 10(1): 124, 1998.

13. Green LB: Imagery in the rehabilitation of injured athletes. *Sport Psychologist* 6:416, 1992.

14. Heil J: *Psychology of sport injury,* Champaign, Ill, 1993, Human Kinetics.

15. Holmes TH, Rahe RH: The social readjustment rating scale. *J Psychosom Res* 11:213, 1976.

16. Jacobsen E: Variation of specific muscles contracting during muscle imagination, *Am J Physiol* 96:101, 1931.

17. Locke EA, Latham GP: The application of goal setting to sport, *J Sport Psychol* 7:205, 1985.

18. Norris C: *Psychological aspects of sports injury: diagnosis and management for physiotherapists,* London, 1993, Butterworth Heinemann.

19. Rotella RJ: Psychological care of the injured athlete. In Kuland D, editor: *The injured athlete,* ed 2, Philadelphia, 1985, Lippincott.

20. Sanderson FH: Psychology and injury prone athletes, *Br J Sports Med* 11:56, 1992.

21. Vinokur A, Selzer ML: Desirable versus undesirable life events: their relationship to stress and distress, *J Personality Social Psychol* 32:329, 1975.

## ANNOTATED BIBLIOGRAPHY

Taylor J, Taylor S: *Psychological approaches to sports injury rehabilitation,* Gaithersburg, Md, 1997, Aspen Publishers.

*This text specifically addresses how to deal with injury rehabilitation from a psychological perspective.*

Weinberg RS, Gould D: *Foundations of sport and exercise psychology,* Champaign, Ill, 1999, Human Kinetics.

*Discusses the techniques that a coach should incorporate for contributing to the success of an athlete.*

Williams JM: *Applied sport psychology: personal growth to peak performance,* Mountain View, Calif, 1997, Mayfield Publishing.

*Leading sports psychologists have done an excellent job of presenting both the "whys" and "how tos" of the intervention techniques in sport psychology.*

## WEBSITES

Association for the Advancement of Applied Sport Psychology: http:// spot.colorado.Edu/~aaasp/ sportpsy.html

*Emphasis on the role of psychological factors in sport and exercise.*

NASPSPA North American Society for Psychology of Sport and Physical Activity: www.naspspa.org/

Sport Psychology Oversite: http:// www.personal.umich.edu/~bing/ oversite/sportpsych.html

*A comprehensive list of links to sites that focus on mental training and performance enhancement.*

Mind Games: Applied Sport Psychology For Every Athlete: http://www. drrelax.com

*A new, web-based system of individualized psychological training.*

Human Kinetics: Psychology of Exercise and Sport: http://www.e-sportpsych. com

*News, associations, conferences, open jobs, products, etc.*

Sport Psychology for Athletes: http:// www. drrelax.com/baseball.htm

*The use of psychological training and preparation.*

## Chapter 10

# Environmental Factors

*When you finish this chapter you will be able to:*

- Describe the physiology of hyperthermia and the clinical signs of heat stress and how they can be prevented.
- Identify the causes of hypothermia and the major cold disorders and how they may be prevented.
- Explain how an athlete should be protected from exposure to the sun.
- Describe precautions that should be taken in an electrical storm.

E nvironmental stress can adversely affect an athlete's performance and, in some instances, can pose a serious health threat. The environmental categories that coaches, athletic trainers, and sports physicians need to pay attention to are hyperthermia, hypothermia, exposure to the sun, and electrical storms.

## HYPERTHERMIA

A major concern in sports is the problem of hyperthermia. Over the years, particularly among football players, there have been a number of deaths caused by hyperthermia.[1] It is vitally important that the coaching staff have knowledge about temperature and humidity factors to assist them in planning practice. The coach must clearly understand when environmental heat and humidity are at a dangerous level and act accordingly. In addition, the clinical signs of heat stress must be recognized and managed properly.

### Heat Stress

Regardless of the level of physical conditioning, extreme caution must be taken when exercising in hot, humid weather. Prolonged exposure to extreme heat can result in heat illness.[8] Heat stress is certainly preventable, but each year many athletes suffer illness and, occasionally, death from some heat-related cause.[15] Athletes who exercise in hot, humid en-

Heat can be gained or lost through:
- Metabolic heat production
- Conductive heat exchange
- Convective heat exchange
- Radiant heat exchange
- Evaporative heat loss

vironments are particularly vulnerable to heat stress. The physiological processes in the body can continue to function only as long as body temperature is maintained within a normal range.[14] Maintenance of normal temperature in a hot environment depends on the ability of the body to dissipate heat. Body temperature can be affected by five factors: metabolic heat production, conductive heat exchange, convective heat exchange, radiant heat exchange, and evaporative heat loss.

### Metabolic Heat Production

Normal metabolic function in the body results in the production and radiation of heat. Consequently, metabolism always causes an increase in body heat depending on the intensity of the physical activity. The higher the metabolic rate, the more heat produced. *may achieve a temp. of 109 degree (f)*

### Conductive Heat Exchange

Physical contact with other objects can result in either heat loss or heat gain. A football player competing on astroturf on a sunny August afternoon experiences an increase in body temperature simply by standing on the turf.

### Convective Heat Exchange

Body heat can be either lost or gained depending on the temperature of the circulating medium. A cool breeze always tends to cool the body by removing heat from the body surface. Conversely, if the temperature of the circulating air is higher than the temperature of the skin, there is a gain in body heat.

### Radiant Heat Exchange

Radiant heat from sunshine causes an increase in body temperature. Obviously, the effects of radiation are much greater in the sunshine than in the shade. However, on a cloudy day a person's body also emits radiant heat energy, and this radiation may also result in either heat loss or heat gain. During exercise the body attempts to dissipate heat produced by metabolism by dilating superficial arterial and venous vessels, thus channeling blood to the capillaries in the skin.

### Evaporative Heat Loss

Sweat glands in the skin allow water to be transported to the surface where it evaporates, taking large quantities of heat with it. When the temperature and radiant heat of the environment become higher than body temperature, loss of body heat becomes highly dependent on the process of sweat evaporation. The sweat must evaporate for heat to be dissipated. But the air must be relatively free of water for evaporation to occur. Heat loss through evaporation is severely impaired when the relative humidity reaches 65 percent and virtually stops when the humidity reaches 75 percent.

## Monitoring the Heat Index

The coach must exercise common sense when overseeing the health care of athletes training or competing in the heat. Obviously, when the combination of heat, humidity, and bright sunshine is present, extra caution is warranted. The universal *wet bulb globe temperature (WBGT) index* provides the coach with an objective means for determining necessary precautions for practice and competition in hot weather.[12] The index incorporates readings from several different thermometers. The dry bulb temperature (DBT) is recorded from a standard mercury thermometer. The wet bulb temperature (WBT) uses a wet wick or piece of gauze wrapped around the end of a thermometer that is swung around in the air. Globe temperature (GT) measures the sun's radiation and uses a black metal casing around the end of the thermometer. Once the three readings have been taken, the following formula is used to calculate the WBGT index:

$$WBGT = 0.1 \times DBT + 0.7 \times WBT + GT \times 0.2$$

Using this formula yields an index on which recommendations relative to outdoor activity are based (Table 10-1).

The DBT and WBT can be easily measured using either of two instruments, a physiodyne (Figure 10-1A) or a sling psychrometer (Figure 10-1B). Both instruments calculate the difference between DBT and WBT, which is relative humidity. Either instrument is relatively inexpensive and easy to use.

## Heat Illnesses

It should be obvious that heat-related problems have the greatest chance of occurring on days when the sun is bright and the temperature and relative humidity are high. But it is certainly true that various forms of heat illness, including heat cramps, heat exhaustion, or heatstroke, can occur whenever the body's ability to dissipate heat is impaired.

**TABLE 10-1** WGBT index and recommendations for fluid replacement and work/rest periods

| Heat Category | WBGT°F | Easy Work Work/Rest* | Easy Work Water Per Hour | Moderate Work Work/Rest* | Moderate Work Water Per Hour | Hard Work Work/Rest* | Hard Work Water Per Hour |
|---|---|---|---|---|---|---|---|
| 1 | 78–81.9 | No limit | 1/2 qt. | No limit | 3/4 qt. | 40/20 min | 3/4 qt. |
| 2 | 82–84.9 | No limit | 1/2 qt. | 50/10 min | 3/4 qt. | 30/30 min | 1 qt. |
| 3 | 85–87.9 | No limit | 3/4 qt. | 40/20 min | 3/4 qt. | 30/30 min | 1 qt. |
| 4 | 88–89.9 | No limit | 3/4 qt. | 30/30 min | 3/4 qt. | 20/40 min | 1 qt. |
| 5 | >90 | 50/10 min | 1 qt. | 20/40 min | 1 qt. | 10/50 min | 1 qt. |

*Rest means minimal physical activity (sitting or standing) and should be accomplished in the shade if possible.

**Figure 10-1**

A, A physiodyne, or B, a sling psychrometer may be used to determine the WBGT heat index.

### Heat Cramps

Heat cramps are extremely painful muscle spasms that occur most commonly in the calf and abdomen, although any muscle can be involved (Table 10-2). *The occurrence of heat cramps is related primarily to excessive loss of water and, to a lesser extent, loss of electrolytes. Electrolytes* are ions (sodium, chloride, potassium, magnesium, and calcium) that are essential elements in muscle contraction.[6]

Profuse sweating involves losses of large amounts of water and small quantities of electrolytes, thus destroying the balance in concentration of these elements within the body. This imbalance ultimately results in painful muscle contractions and cramps. The person most likely to get heat cramps is one who is in fairly good condition who simply overexerts in the heat.

**Treatment**   Heat cramps may be prevented by adequate replacement of fluids. Ingestion of salt tablets is not recommended. The immediate treatment for heat cramps is ingestion of large quantities of fluid and mild stretching with ice massage of the muscle in spasm.[10] An athlete who experiences heat cramps will generally not be able to return to practice or competition for the remainder of the day because cramping is likely to reoccur.

### Heat Exhaustion

Heat exhaustion results from inadequate replacement of fluids lost through sweating (Table 10-2). Clinically, the victim of heat exhaustion

*Heat cramps occur because of some imbalance between water and electrolytes.*

*Heat exhaustion results from dehydration.*

**TABLE 10-2** Heat disorders: treatment and prevention

| Disorder | Cause | Clinical Features and Diagnosis | Treatment | Prevention |
|---|---|---|---|---|
| Heat cramps | Hard work in heat; sweating heavily; imbalance between water and electrolytes | Muscle twitching and cramps, usually after midday; spasms in arms, legs, abdomen | Ingesting large amounts of water, mild stretching, and ice massage of affected muscle | Acclimatize athlete properly; provide large quantities of water; increase intake of calcium, sodium, and potassium slightly |
| Heat exhaustion | Prolonged sweating; inadequate replacement of body fluid losses; diarrhea; intestinal infection | Excessive thirst, dry tongue and mouth; weight loss; fatigue; weakness; incoordination; mental dullness; small urine volume; slightly elevated body temperature; high serum protein and sodium; reduced swelling | Bed rest in cool room, IV fluids if drinking is impaired; increase fluid intake to 6 to 8 l/day; sponge with cool water; keep record of body weight; keep fluid balance record; provide semiliquid food until salination is normal | Supply adequate water and other liquids<br><br>Provide adequate rest and opportunity for cooling |
| Heatstroke | Thermoregulatory failure of sudden onset | Abrupt onset, preceded by headache, vertigo, and fatigue, flushed skin; relatively less sweating than seen with heat exhaustion; pulse rate increases rapidly and may reach 160 to 180; respiration increases; blood pressure seldom rises; temperature rises rapidly to 105° or 106° F (40° to 41° C); athlete feels as if he or she is burning up; diarrhea, vomiting; circulatory collapse may produce death; can lead to permanent brain damage | Heroic measures to reduce temperature must be taken immediately (e.g., sponge cool water and air fan over body, massage limbs); remove to hospital as soon as possible | Ensure proper acclimatization, proper hydration<br><br>Educate those supervising activities conducted in the heat<br><br>Adapt activities to environment<br><br>Screen participants with past history of heat illness for malignant hyperthermia |

collapses and manifests profuse sweating, pale skin, mildly elevated temperature (102°F), dizziness, hyperventilation, and rapid pulse.

It is sometimes possible to spot athletes who are having problems with heat exhaustion. They may begin to develop heat cramps. They may become disoriented and light-headed, and their physical performance will not be up to their usual standards when fluid replacement has not been adequate. In general, persons in poor physical condition who attempt to exercise in the heat are most likely to get heat exhaustion.

**Treatment**   Immediate treatment of heat exhaustion requires ingestion and eventually intravenous replacement of large quantities of fluids. It is essential to obtain a rectal temperature to differentiate heat exhaustion from heatstroke. In heat exhaustion the rectal temperature will be around 102° F. If possible, the athlete should be placed in a cool environment, although it is more critical to replace fluids.[11]

### Heatstroke

Unlike heat cramps and heat exhaustion, heatstroke is a serious, life-threatening emergency (Table 10-2). The specific cause of heatstroke is unknown; however, it is clinically characterized by sudden collapse with loss of consciousness; flushed, hot skin; less sweating than is seen with heat exhaustion; shallow breathing; a rapid, strong pulse; and most important, a core temperature of 106° F or higher. Basically heatstroke is a breakdown of the thermoregulatory mechanism caused by excessively high body temperature; the body loses the ability to dissipate heat through sweating.[7]

Heatstroke can occur suddenly and without warning. The athlete does not usually experience signs of heat cramps or heat exhaustion. The possibility of death from heatstroke can be significantly reduced if body temperature is lowered to normal within 45 minutes. The longer the body temperature is elevated to 106° F or higher, the higher the mortality rate.

**Treatment**   *It is imperative that the victim be transported to a hospital as quickly as possible.* Every first-aid effort should be directed to lowering body temperature. Get the athlete into a cool environment. Strip all clothing off the athlete, sponge him or her down with cool water, and fan with a towel. Do not immerse the athlete in cold water. The replacement of fluid is not critical in initial first aid.[17]

### Preventing Heat Illness

*The coach needs to understand that heat illness is preventable.* Exercising common sense and caution will keep heat illnesses from occurring.[18] The following suggestions should be considered when planning a practice or competitive program during hot weather.

### Fluid Replacement

During hot weather athletes need to continually rehydrate by replacing fluids lost through evaporation of sweat (Figure 10-2). Unfortunately

Heatstroke is a life-threatening emergency.

***Critical Thinking*** Exercise

A high school football coach in southern Louisiana is concerned about the likelihood that several of his players will suffer heat-related illness during preseason football practice the first 2 weeks of August.

**?**  What intervention strategies can the coach implement to help the athletes avoid heat-related illnesses?

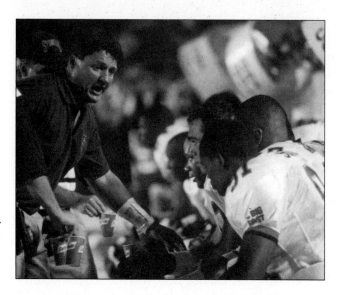

**Figure 10-2**

Athletes must have unlimited
access to water or sports
drinks, especially in hot
weather.

The prevention of
hyperthermia involves:
• Gradual acclimatization
• Identification of susceptible
  individuals
• Lightweight uniforms
• Routine weight record
  keeping
• Unrestricted fluid
  replacement

dehydration occurs frequently during physical activity because athletes do not ingest enough fluid to match sweat loss even though unlimited fluids are readily available.[14] In fact, seldom is more than 50 percent of this fluid loss replaced. Ideally, fluid replacement should match sweat loss. Fluid is most effectively replaced at regular intervals of about 15 minutes.

The problem in fluid replacement is how rapidly the fluid can be eliminated from the stomach into the intestine, from which it can enter the bloodstream. Water is absorbed rapidly from the intestine. Beverages containing 6 percent carbohydrate (glucose) are absorbed at about the same rate as water as long as there is normal hydration.[13] Cold drinks (45° to 55° F [7.2° to 12.8° C]) tend to empty more rapidly from the stomach than do warmer drinks; they are not more likely to induce cramps, nor do they offer any particular threat to a normal heart.

Athletes can tell if they are appropriately hydrated by paying attention to the color and volume of their urine. Within 60 minutes of exercise, a nearly clear urine of normal to above-normal output indicates that the athlete is appropriately hydrated.

**Sports drinks**   A number of sports drinks are available that may be used in fluid replacement (see Chapter 5). The sports drinks maximize carbohydrate content.

Ingestion of drinks containing 6 percent glucose and electrolytes is most useful for replenishing fluids and electrolytes before and after activity in the heat.[7] The drinks are also beneficial for replacing glucose in activities lasting longer than 1 hour.

### Gradual Acclimatization

Gradual acclimatization is probably the single most effective method of avoiding heat stress. Acclimatization should involve not only becoming accustomed to heat but also becoming acclimatized to exercising in hot temperatures.[4] A good preseason conditioning program—started well before the advent of the competitive season and carefully graded as to intensity—is recommended. During the first 5 or 6 days, an 80 percent acclimatization can be achieved on the basis of a 2-hour practice period in the morning and a 2-hour practice period in the afternoon. Each practice should be broken down into 20 minutes of work alternated with 20 minutes of rest in the shade.

### Identifying Susceptible Individuals

Athletes with a large muscle mass are particularly prone to heat illness.[18] Heat victims also tend to be overweight. In addition, a considerable loss of fluid makes the athlete highly susceptible to heat illness. Although slight differences exist, the same precautionary measures apply to both males and females.

### Keeping Weight Records

Careful weight records of all players must be kept. Weights should be measured both before and after practice for at least the first 2 weeks of practice. If a sudden increase in temperature and/or humidity occurs during the season, weight should be recorded again for a time. A loss of 3 to 5 percent of body weight reduces blood volume and could lead to a health threat.[11] The athlete should be held out of practice until normal body weight has been regained.

### Uniforms

Uniforms should be selected on the basis of temperature and humidity. Initial practices should be conducted in light-colored, short-sleeved T-shirts, shorts, and socks, moving gradually into short-sleeved net jerseys, lightweight pants, and socks as acclimatization proceeds. All early-season practices and games should be conducted in lightweight uniforms. Because of the specialized equipment worn by the players, football requires particular consideration. In hot, humid environments, the helmet should be removed as often as possible.

## HYPOTHERMIA

Cold weather is a frequent adjunct to many outdoor sports in which the sport itself does not require heavy protective clothing; consequently, the weather becomes a pertinent factor in injury susceptibility.[3] In most instances, the activity itself enables the athlete to increase the metabolic rate sufficiently for normal physiological functioning and to dissipate the resulting heat and perspiration through the usual physiological mechanisms. An athlete may fail to warm up sufficiently or may become chilled because of relative inactivity for varying periods demanded by the particular sport, either during competition or training. Consequently, the athlete is predisposed to hypothermia.

Low temperatures alone can pose some problems, but when such temperatures are further accentuated by wind, the chill factor becomes critical (Figure 10-3.)[16] A third factor, dampness or wetness, further

Many sports played in cold weather do not require heavy protective clothing; thus, weather becomes a factor in injury susceptibility.

Low temperatures accentuated by wind and dampness can pose major problems for athletes.

Techniques for Preventing
and Minimizing
Sport-Related Injuries

**Figure 10-3**

Low temperatures can pose
serious problems for the
athlete, but windchill could
be a critical factor.

increases the risk of hypothermia. Air at a temperature of 50° F is relatively comfortable, but water at the same temperature is intolerable. Certainly the combination of cold, wind, and dampness creates an environment that easily predisposes the athlete to hypothermia.

As muscular fatigue builds up during strenuous physical activity in cold weather, the rate of exercise begins to drop and may reach a level at which the body heat loss to the environment exceeds the metabolic heat protection, resulting in definite impairment of neuromuscular responses and exhaustion. A relatively small drop in body core temperature can induce shivering sufficient to materially affect the athlete's neuromuscular coordination. Shivering ceases below a body temperature of 85° to 90° F (29.4° to 32.2° C). Death is imminent if the core temperature rises to 107° F (41.6° C) or drops to between 77° and 85° F (25° to 29° C).

Cold injuries in sports
include:
• Frostnip
• Frostbite

## Cold Disorders

Athletes need to replace fluids when working out in a cold environment as much as they do in a hot environment.[9] Because dehydration reduces blood volume, less fluid is available for warming the tissues. Athletes performing in a cold environment should be weighed before and after practice, especially in the first 2 weeks of the season.[3] Severe overexposure to a cold climate occurs less often than hyperthermia does in a warm climate; however, it is still a major risk of winter sports, long-distance running in cold weather, and swimming in cold water.[9]

### Frostnip

Frostnip involves ears, nose, cheeks, chin, fingers, and toes. It commonly occurs during a high wind, severe cold, or both. The skin initially appears very firm, with cold, painless areas that may peel or blister in 24 to 72 hours. Affected areas can be treated early by firm, sustained pressure of the hand (without rubbing), by blowing hot breath on the spot, or if the injury is to the fingertips, by placing them in the armpits.

### Frostbite

Superficial frostbite involves only the skin and subcutaneous tissue. The skin appears pale, hard, cold, and waxy. Palpating the injured area reveals a sense of hardness but with yielding of the underlying deeper tissue structures. When rewarming, the superficial frostbite at first feels numb, then stings and burns. Later the area may produce blisters and be painful for a number of weeks.[9]

Deep frostbite is a serious injury indicating that tissues are frozen. This medical emergency requires immediate hospitalization. As with frostnip and superficial frostbite, the tissue is initially cold, hard, pale or white, and numb. Rapid rewarming is required, including hot drinks, heating pads, or hot water bottles that are 100° to 110° F (38° to 43° C).[9] During rewarming the tissue becomes blotchy, red, swollen, and extremely painful. Later the injury may become gangrenous, causing a loss of tissue.

## Prevention

Apparel for competitors must be geared to the weather. The clothing should not restrict movement, should be as lightweight as possible, and should consist of material that permits the free passage of body heat and sweat that otherwise accumulates on the skin or the clothing and provide a chilling effect when activity ceases. The athlete should routinely dress in thin layers of clothing that can easily be added or removed to prevent sweating as the temperature decreases or increases. To prevent chilling, warm-up suits should be worn before exercise, during activity breaks or rest periods, and at the termination of exercise.[3]

## OVEREXPOSURE TO SUN

Athletes, along with coaches, athletic trainers, and other support staff, frequently spend a great deal of time outdoors in direct sunlight. Applying sunscreens to protect these individuals from overexposure to ultraviolet radiation (UVR) is seldom done.

SPF stands for sun protection
factor.

10-2

*Critical Thinking* Exercise

A track athlete is competing in
a day-long outdoor track meet.
She is extremely concerned
about getting sunburned and
has liberally applied sunscreen
with an SPF of 30 during the
early morning. It is a very hot,
sunny day and she is sweating
heavily. She is worried that her
sunscreen has worn off and asks
the coach for more sunscreen.
The coach hands her sunscreen
with an SPF of 15, and the
athlete complains that it is not
strong enough to protect her.

? What can the coach tell the
athlete to assure her that she
will be well protected by the
sunscreen she has been given?

## Long-Term Effects on Skin

The most serious effects of long-term UVR exposure are premature aging
of the skin and skin cancer.[5] Lightly pigmented individuals are more susceptible. Premature aging of the skin is characterized by dryness, crack-
ing, and a decrease in the elasticity of the skin. Skin cancer is the most
common malignant tumor found in humans and has been epidemiolog-
ically and clinically associated with exposure to UVR. Fortunately the rate
of cure exceeds 95 percent with early detection and treatment.[5]

## Using Sunscreens

Sunscreens applied to the skin can help prevent many of the damaging
effects of UVR.[5] A sunscreen's effectiveness in absorbing the sunburn-
inducing radiation is expressed as the sun protection factor (SPF). An SPF
of 6 indicates that an athlete can be exposed to UVR six times longer than
without a sunscreen before the skin will begin to turn red. Higher numbers provide greater protection. However, athletes who have a family or
personal history of skin cancer may experience significant damage to the
skin even when wearing an SPF 15 sunscreen. Therefore, these individuals should wear an SPF 30 sunscreen.

Sunscreen should be worn regularly by athletes, coaches, and athletic
trainers who spend time outside. This caution is particularly relevant for
individuals with fair complexions, light hair, or blue eyes or those whose
skin burns easily. People with dark complexions should also wear sunscreens to prevent sun damage.

Sunscreens are needed most between the months of March and No-
vember but should be used year-round. Sunscreens are needed most between 10 A.M. and 4 P.M. and should be applied 15 to 30 minutes before
sun exposure. Although clothing and hats provide some protection from
the sun, they are not a substitute for sunscreens (a typical white cotton
T-shirt provides an SPF of only 5). Reflected sunlight from water, sand,
and snow may effectively increase sun exposure and risk of burning.

## ELECTRICAL STORMS

Research indicates that lightning is the number two cause of death by
weather phenomena, accounting for 110 deaths per year.[19] Each institution should designate a chain of command to establish who should monitor both the weather forecast and changing weather, and to determine
who makes the decision to remove a team from the practice field. Persons
who can hear thunder or see lightning are in immediate danger and
should seek a protective safe shelter in an indoor facility at once. An indoor facility is recommended as the safest protective shelter. However, if
an indoor facility is not available, an automobile is a relatively safe alternative. If neither of these is available, the following guidelines are recommended. Avoid standing under large trees and telephone poles. If the
only alternative is in trees, choose a small grove of trees in a wooded area
that is not on a hill. As a last alternative, find a ditch, ravine, or valley. In

all instances outdoors, assume a crouched position. Avoid standing water and metal objects at all times (metal bleachers, metal cleats, umbrellas, etc.)[2]

The most dangerous storms give little or no warning; thunder and lightning are not heard or seen. Lightning is always accompanied by thunder, although 20 percent to 40 percent of thunder cannot be heard because of atmospheric disturbances. The **flash-to-bang method** provides an estimate of how far away lightning is occurring.[2] From the time lightning is sighted, the number of seconds until the bang occurs is counted and divided by five to calcuate the number of miles away the lightning is occurring. When the flash-to-bang count is at 30 seconds there is inherent danger and conditions should be closely monitored. When the count is 15 seconds everyone should leave the field immediately and seek safe shelter.[2]

At times, the only natural forewarning that precedes a strike is feeling the hair stand on end and skin tingle. At this point, the person is in imminent danger of being struck by lightning and should drop to the ground and assume a crouched position immediately. The person should not lie flat. Should a ground strike occur nearby, lying flat increases the body's surface area that is exposed to the current traveling through the ground.[19]

The National Severe Storms Service recommends that 30 minutes should pass after the last sound of thunder is heard or lightning strike is seen before resuming play. This is sufficient time to allow the storm to pass and move out of lightning strike range. The perilous misconception that it is possible to see lightning coming and have time to act before it strikes could prove to be fatal. In reality, the lightning that can be seen flashing is actually the return stroke flashing upward from the ground to the cloud, not downward. When the lightning strike is seen, it already has hit.

> **flash-to-bang method**
> Estimates how far away lightning is occurring.

## COACH'S CORNER

The following checklist includes basic guidelines that should be followed during an electrical storm.

- ☐ In situations in which thunder or lightning may be present and you feel your hair stand on end and skin tingle, immediately assume a crouched position: Drop to your knees, place your hands and arms on your legs, and lower your head. Do not lie flat.

- ☐ If thunder and/or lightning can be heard or seen, stop activity and seek protective shelter immediately. An indoor facility is recommended as the safest protective shelter. However, if an indoor facility is not available, an automobile is a relatively safe alternative. If neither of these options is available, you should avoid standing under large trees and telephone poles. If the only alternative is a tree, choose a small tree in a wooded area that is not on a hill. As a last alternative, find a ravine or valley. In all instances outdoors, assume the aforementioned crouched position.

☐ Avoid standing water and metal objects at all times (e.g., metal bleachers, metal cleats, umbrellas, etc.).

☐ Allow 30 minutes to pass after the last sound of thunder or lightning strike before resuming play.

## SUMMARY

- Environmental stress can adversely affect an athlete's performance and pose a serious health problem.

- Regardless of the athletes' level of physical conditioning, coaches must take extreme caution when conducting exercises in hot, humid weather. Prolonged exposure to extreme heat can result in heat cramps, heat exhaustion, or heatstroke.

- Heat illness is preventable. Exercising common sense and caution will keep heat illnesses from occurring. Coaches can prevent heat illness by encouraging adequate fluid replacement, acclimatizing athletes gradually, identifying susceptible individuals, keeping weight records, and selecting appropriate uniforms.

- Hypothermia is most likely to occur in a cool, damp, windy environment. Extreme cold exposure can cause conditions such as frostnip and frostbite.

- Athletes, coaches, and athletic trainers should be protected from overexposure to ultraviolet radiation (UVR) by the routine application of sunscreens.

- Thirty minutes should be allowed to pass after the last sound of thunder is heard or last lightning strike is seen before play is resumed.

### 10-3

**Critical Thinking** Exercise

A lacrosse team is practicing on a remote field with no indoor facility in close proximity. The weather is rapidly worsening, with the sky becoming dark and the wind blowing harder. Twenty minutes are left in the practice session and the coach is hoping to finish practice before it begins to rain. Suddenly, there is a bolt of lightning and an immediate burst of thunder.

**?** How should the coach manage this extremely dangerous situation?

---

### Solutions to Critical Thinking Exercises

**10-1** The coach should understand that heat-related illnesses are preventable. The athletes should come into preseason practice at least partially acclimatized to working in a hot, humid environment and during the first week of practice should become fully acclimatized. Temperature and humidity readings should be monitored and practice should be modified according to conditions. Practice uniforms should maximize evaporation and minimize heat absorption to the greatest extent possible. Weight records should be maintained to identify individuals who are becoming dehydrated. Most important, the athletes must keep themselves hydrated by constantly drinking large quantities of water both during and between practice sessions.

**10-2** The sun protection factor (SPF) indicates the sunscreen's effectiveness in absorbing the sunburn-inducing radiation. An SPF of 15 indicates that an athlete can be exposed to UVR fifteen times longer than without a sunscreen before the skin begins to turn red. Therefore the athlete needs to understand that a higher SPF doesn't indicate a greater degree of protection. She must simply apply the SPF 15 sunscreen twice as often as necessary with an SPF 30 sunscreen.

**10-3** As soon as lightning is observed, the coach should immediately end practice and get the athletes under cover. If an indoor facility is not available, an automobile is a relatively safe alternative. The athletes should avoid standing under large trees or telephone poles. As a last alternative, athletes should assume a crouched position in a ditch or ravine. Athletes should avoid any standing water or metal objects around the fields.

## REVIEW QUESTIONS AND CLASS ACTIVITIES

1. How do temperature and humidity cause heat illnesses?
2. Describe the symptoms and signs of the most common heat disorders.
3. What steps should be taken to avoid heat illnesses?
4. How is heat lost from the body to produce hypothermia?
5. Identify the physiological basis for the body's susceptibility to a cold disorder.
6. What should athletes do to prevent heat loss?
7. How should athletes protect themselves from the effects of ultraviolet radiation?
8. What precautions can be taken to minimize injury during an electrical storm?

## REFERENCES

1. Armstrong LE, Epstein Y, Greenleaf JE: ACSM position stand: heat and cold illnesses during distance running, *Med Sci Sports Exerc* 28(12):i–x, 1997.
2. Bennett B: A model lightning safety policy for athletics, *J Ath Train* 32(3):251, 1997.
3. Bodine KL: Avoiding hypothermia: caution, forethought, and preparation, *Sports Med Alert* 6(1):6, 2000.
4. Dabinett J: Preparing for competition in hot and humid environments, *Sports Exerc Injury* 4(1):10, 1998.
5. Davis M: Ultraviolet therapy. In Prentice W, editor: *Therapeutic modalities in sports medicine,* Dubuque, 1999, WCB/McGraw-Hill.
6. Eichner ER: Heat cramps: salt is simplest, most effective antidote, *Sports Med Digest* 21(8):88, 1999.
7. Epstein Y et al: Exertional heat stroke: a case series, *Med Sci Sports Exerc* 31(2):224, 1999.
8. Gutierrez G: Solar injury and heat illness, *Physician Sportsmed* 23(7):43, 1995.
9. Kanzenbach TL, Dexter WW: Cold injuries: protecting your patients from the dangers of hypothermia and frostbite, *Postgrad Med* 105(1):72, 1999.
10. Kay D, Marino FE: Fluid ingestion and exercise hyperthermia: implications for performance, thermoregulation, metabolism and the development of fatigue, *J Sports Sci* 18(2):71, 2000.
11. Knochel JP: Management of heat conditions, *Ath Ther Today* 1(4):30, 1996.
12. McCann DJ, Adams WC: Wet bulb globe temperature index and performance in competitive distance runners, *Med Sci Sports Exerc* 29(7):955, 1997.
13. Montain SJ, Maughan RJ, Sawka MN: Fluid replacement strategies for exercise in hot weather, *Ath Ther Today* 1(4):24, 1996.
14. Murray R: Dehydration, hyperthermia, and athletes: science and practice, *J Ath Train* 31(3):248, 1996.
15. *NCAA Sports Medicine Handbook 2000–2001,* Indianapolis, In, 2000, National Collegiate Athletic Association.
16. Sallis R, Chassay CM: Recognizing and treating common cold-induced injury in outdoor sports, *Med Sci Sports Exerc* 31(10):1367, 1999.
17. Sandor RP: Heat illness: on-site diagnosis and cooling, *Physician Sportsmed* 25(6):35, 1997.
18. Sparling PB, Millard-Stafford M: Keeping sports participants safe in hot weather, *Physician Sportsmed* 27(7):27, 1999.
19. Walsh K, Hanley M, Graner S: A survey of lightning policy in selected division I colleges, *J Ath Train* 32(3):206, 1997.

## ANNOTATED BIBLIOGRAPHY

*NCAA Sports Medicine Handbook 2000–2001,* Indianapolis, In, 2000, National Collegiate Athletic Association.

*Contains guidelines and recommendations for preventing heat illness and hypohydration, cold stress, and for lightning safety.*

Strauss RH, editor: *Sports medicine,* Philadelphia, 1996, WB Saunders.

*Provides four pertinent chapters on the subject of environmental disorders that can affect the athlete.*

### WEBSITES

National Lightning Safety Institute (NLSI): http://www.lightningsafety.com/

*National Lightning Safety Institute provides consulting, education, training, and expert witness relating to lightning hazard mitigation.*

FEMA: Extreme Heat Fact Sheet: http://www.fema.gov/library/heatf.htm

*Fact Sheet: Extreme Heat. Doing too much on a hot day, spending too much time in the sun, or staying too long in an overheated place can cause heat-related illnesses.*

OnHealth: Heath Illness (Heat Exhaustion, Heatstroke, Heat Cramps): http://www. onhealth. com/conditions/resource/conditions/item

*Prolonged or intense exposure to hot temperatures can cause heat-related illnesses, such as heat exhaustion, heat cramps, and heatstroke (also known as sunstroke).*

Excite Health Home: Sunburn: http://adam.excite.com/info/?id-003227

Excite Health Home: Hypothermia: http://adam.excite.com/info/?id-000038

A Hypothermia Treatment Technology WebSite: http://www.hypothermia-ca.com

OA Guide to Hypothermia & Cold Weather Injuries: http://www.princeton.edu/~rcurtis/ hypocold.html

Chapter

## 11

# Bandaging and Taping Techniques

*When you finish this chapter you will be able to:*

- Explain the need for and demonstrate the application of elastic bandages.
- Demonstrate site preparation for taping.
- Know the various types of tape that can be used.
- Understand what you are trying to accomplish by the application of a specific taping technique.
- Demonstrate basic skills in the use of taping for a variety of body parts.

B andaging and taping techniques are used routinely by coaches, athletic trainers, and athletes.[5] They may be used to accomplish a variety of specific objectives including:

- Providing compression to minimize swelling in the initial management of injury
- Reducing the chances of injury by applying tape prophylactically before an injury occurs
- Providing additional support to an injured structure

Correctly and effectively applying a bandage or a "tape job" to a specific body part is a skill usually left to the athletic trainer. It is true that athletic trainers have been instructed in and generally become highly proficient in applying a variety of bandaging and taping techniques to accomplish the objectives listed. If an athletic trainer is not available the responsibility for taping the athletes on a particular team will likely fall on the coach.

Certainly bandaging and taping skills are not difficult. They can be mastered by anyone willing to spend time practicing and learning what works best in a given situation.[7] Of course certain taping and bandaging techniques are more advanced and should be used only by those with some advanced experience. However, there are some very basic techniques that a coach can easily apply with only a little training.

Anyone can master taping and bandaging with practice.

## ELASTIC BANDAGES

Elastic bandages can be applied for a variety of purposes. They are most often used for compression of an acute injury to limit the amount of swelling that occurs (Figure 11-1). They may also be used to secure a dressing for a wound, or to hold a pad or an ice bag in place. An elastic bandage is also useful in providing support to injured soft tissue structures. Elastic wraps are active bandages; they let the athlete move without restriction.

Elastic bandages are generally made of two-ply cotton yarns, reinforced with heat-resistant elastic rubber threads that are often made of latex. (Athletes that may have allergies to latex should be warned.) The bandages come in a variety of widths and lengths and should be selected according to the body part to be bandaged. The sizes most frequently used are the 2-, 3-, 4-, and 6-inch widths by either 5- or 6-yard length. The 4- and 6-inch bandages are usually also available in double lengths of 10 yards.

### Application

The elastic bandage must be applied in a specific manner to achieve the purpose of the wrap. When a roller bandage is to be placed on a body part, the roll should be held in the preferred hand with the loose end extending from the bottom of the roll. The back surface of the loose end is placed on the part and held in position by the other hand. The bandage is then unrolled and passed around the injured area. As the hand pulls

Elastic Bandages
- apply firm even pressure
- wrap distal to proximal

**Figure 11-1**

Technique for using an elastic wrap

Techniques for Preventing
and Minimizing
Sport-Related Injuries

**Figure 11-2**

Ankle and foot spica

Check circulation after
applying an elastic wrap.

---

**spica** (spy ka)
A figure-eight bandage, with
one of the two loops being
larger.

---

the material from the roll, it also standardizes the bandage pressure and
guides the bandage in the proper direction. To anchor and stabilize the
bandage, a number of turns, one on top of the other, are made. Circling
a body part requires the operator to alternate the bandage roll from one
hand to the other and back again.

For maximum benefit from an elastic bandage, it should be applied
uniformly and firmly but not too tightly. Excessive or unequal pressure
can hinder the normal blood flow within the body part. The following
points should be considered when using the roller bandage:

- Wrapping should always begin distally and move proximally.
- A body part should be wrapped in the position of maximum muscle
  contraction to ensure unhampered movement and circulation.
- It is better to use a large number of turns with moderate tension than
  a limited number of turns applied too tightly.
- Each turn of the bandage should be overlapped by at least one half of
  the overlying wrap to prevent the separation of the material while
  engaged in activity. Separation of the bandage turns tends to pinch
  and irritate the skin.

When limbs are wrapped, fingers and toes should be checked often for
signs of circulation impairment. Abnormally cold or cyanotic (bluish) fingers or toes are signs of excessive bandage pressure.

## Elastic Bandaging Techniques

### Ankle and Foot Spica

The ankle and foot **spica** bandage (Figure 11-2) is used in sports for the
compression of new injuries and for holding wound dressings in place.

**Materials needed**   Depending on the size of the ankle and foot, a
2- or 3-inch (5 to 7.5 cm) wrap is used.

**Position of the athlete**   The athlete sits with ankle and foot extended over a table.

**Procedure**

1. An anchor is placed around the foot near the metatarsal arch.
2. The elastic bandage is brought across the instep and around the
   heel and returned to the starting point.
3. The procedure is repeated several times, with each succeeding
   revolution progressing upward on the foot and the ankle.
4. Each spica overlaps approximately three fourths of the preceding
   layer.

### Lower Leg Spiral Bandage

The spiral bandage (Figure 11-3) is widely used in sports for covering a
large area of a cylindrical part.

**Materials needed**   Depending on the size of the area, a 3- or 4-inch
(7.5 to 10 cm) wrap is required.

**Figure 11-3**

Spiral bandage

**Position of the athlete**   If the wrap is for the lower limb, the athlete bears weight on the opposite leg.

**Procedure**

1. The elastic bandage is anchored at the smallest circumference of the limb and is wrapped upward in a spiral against gravity.

2. To prevent the bandage from slipping down on a moving extremity, two pieces of tape should be folded lengthwise and placed on the bandage at either side of the limb or tape adherent can be sprayed on the part.

3. After the bandage is anchored, it is carried upward in consecutive spiral turns, each overlapping the other by at least $^1/_2$ inch.

4. The bandage is terminated by locking it with circular turns, which are then firmly secured by tape.

Groin Support

The following procedure is used to support a groin strain and hip adductor strains (Figure 11-4).

**Materials needed**   One roll of extra-long 6-inch (15 cm) elastic bandage, a roll of 1½-inch (3.8 cm) adhesive tape, and nonsterile cotton.

**Position of the athlete**   The athlete stands on a table with weight placed on the uninjured leg. The affected limb is relaxed and internally rotated.

**Procedure**

1. A piece of nonsterile cotton or a felt pad may be placed over the injured site to provide additional compression and support.

 11-1

**Critical Thinking** Exercise

A baseball player strains his right groin while running the bases.

? Which elastic wrap should be applied when the athlete returns to his sport and why?

**Figure 11-4**

Elastic groin support

***Critical Thinking*** Exercise

A wrestler sustains a left
shoulder point injury.

**?** The coach cuts a sponge
rubber doughnut to protect the
shoulder point from further
injury. How is the doughnut
held in place?

2. The end of the elastic bandage is started at the upper part of the
inner aspect of the thigh and is carried posteriorly around the
thigh. Then it is brought across the lower abdomen and over the
crest of the ilium on the opposite side of the body.

3. The wrap is continued around the back, repeating the same
pattern and securing the wrap end with 1½-inch (3.8 cm)
adhesive tape.

**Note**  Variations of this method can be seen in Figure 11-5, used to
support injured hip flexors.

Shoulder Spica

The shoulder spica (Figure 11-6) is used mainly for the retention of
wound dressings and for moderate muscular support.

**Figure 11-5**

Hip spica for hip flexors

**Materials needed**   One roll of extra-long 4- to 6-inch (10 to 15 cm) elastic wrap, 1½-inch adhesive tape, and padding for axilla.

**Position of the athlete**   Athlete stands with side toward the operator.

**Procedure**

1. The axilla must be well padded to prevent skin irritation and constriction of blood vessels.

2. The bandage is anchored by one turn around the affected upper arm.

3. After anchoring the bandage around the arm on the injured side, the wrap is carried around the back under the unaffected arm and across the chest to the injured shoulder.

4. The affected arm is again encircled by the bandage, which continues around the back. Every figure-eight pattern moves progressively upward with an overlap of at least half of the previous underlying wrap.

Elbow Figure Eight

The elbow figure-eight bandage (Figure 11-7) can be used to secure a dressing in the antecubital fossa or to restrain full extension in hyperextension injuries. When it is reversed, it can be used on the posterior aspect of the elbow.

**Materials needed**   One 3-inch elastic roll and 1½-inch adhesive tape.

**Position of the athlete**   Athlete flexes elbow between 45 degrees and 90 degrees, depending on the restriction of movement required.

**Procedure**

1. Anchor the bandage by encircling the lower arm.

2. Bring the roll obliquely upward over the posterior aspect of the elbow.

3. Carry the roll obliquely upward, crossing the antecubital fossa; then pass once again completely around the upper arm and return to the beginning position by again crossing the antecubital fossa.

4. Continue the procedure as described, but for every new sequence move upward toward the elbow one half the width of the underlying wrap.

**Figure 11-6**

Elastic shoulder spica

**Figure 11-7**

Elastic elbow figure-eight bandage

**Figure 11-8**

Hand and wrist figure-eight

### Hand and Wrist Figure Eight

A figure-eight bandage (Figure 11-8) can be used for mild wrist and hand support and for holding dressings in place.

**Materials needed**   One 2-inch bandage.

**Position of the athlete**   Athlete positions elbow at a 45-degree angle.

**Procedure**

1. The anchor is executed with one or two turns around the palm of the hand.

2. The roll is carried obliquely across the anterior or posterior portion of the hand, depending on the position of the wound, to the wrist, which it circles once, then it is returned to the primary anchor.

3. As many figures as needed are applied.

## NONELASTIC AND ELASTIC ADHESIVE TAPING

### Nonelastic White Adhesive Tape

Nonelastic white adhesive tape has great adaptability for use in sports because of its uniform adhering qualities, lightness, and the relative strength of the backing materials.[8] All of these qualities are of value both in securing wound dressings in place and in providing support and protection to injured areas.[3] This tape comes in a variety of sizes; 1-, 1½, and 2-inch widths are commonly used in sports medicine. When nonelastic white adhesive tape is purchased, factors such as cost, grade of backing, quality of adhesive, and properties of unwinding should be considered.

### Tape Grade

When purchasing white adhesive tape, consider:
• Grade of backing
• Quality of adhesive
• Winding tension

Nonelastic white adhesive tape is most often graded according to the number of longitudinal and vertical fibers per inch of backing material. The heavier and more costly tape contains eighty-five or more longitudinal fibers and sixty-five vertical fibers per square inch. The lighter, less expensive grade has sixty-five or fewer longitudinal fibers and forty-five vertical fibers.[2]

### Adhesive Properties

The tape should adhere readily when applied and should maintain this adherence in the presence of profuse perspiration and activity. Besides sticking well, the adhesive must contain as few skin irritants as possible and must be easily removed without leaving a residue or pulling away the superficial skin.

### Winding Tension

The winding tension of a tape roll is important to the operator. If tape is to be applied for protection and support, there must be even and constant unwinding tension. In most cases a proper wind needs little additional tension to provide sufficient tightness.

## Elastic Adhesive Tape

Elastic adhesive tape is often used in sports medicine. Because of its conforming qualities, stretch tape is used for small, angular body parts, such as the feet, wrist, hands, and fingers. As with nonelastic white adhesive tape, elastic adhesive tape comes in a variety of widths; 1-, 2-, 3-, and 4-inch widths are typical.

## Storing Adhesive Tape

When storing tape, take the following steps:

- Store in a cool place
- Stack so that the tape rests on its flat top or bottom to avoid distortion

*Store tape in a cool place, and stack it flat.*

## Preparation for Taping

Special attention must be given when applying tape directly to the skin.[10] Focus Box 11-1 gives a list of supplies needed for proper taping. Perspiration, oil, and dirt prevent tape from adhering to the skin. Whenever tape is used, the skin surface should be cleaned with soap and water to remove all dirt and oil. Also, hair should be shaved to prevent additional irritation when the tape is removed (Figure 11-9A). A quick-drying tape adherent spray can be used to help the tape adhere to the skin although it is not absolutely necessary (Figure 11-9B). Also, at certain points such as over bony prominences the tape can produce friction blisters. Extra foam or gauze pads (heel and lace pads) with a small amount of lubricant can help to minimize the occurrence of blisters (Figure 11-9C).

*Skin surface should be cleansed and hair should be shaved before applying tape.*

Taping directly on skin provides maximum support. However, applying tape day after day can lead to skin irritation. A roll of foam that is thin, porous, extremely lightweight, and resilient called "underwrap" or "prewrap" easily conforms to the contours of the part to be taped and protects the skin to some degree. Underwrap material should be applied only one layer thick (Figure 11-9D).[6]

## Proper Taping Technique

The correct tape width depends on the area to be covered. The more acute the angles, the narrower the tape must be to fit the many contours. For example, the fingers and toes usually require ½- or 1-inch (1.25 or

11-3

***Critical Thinking*** Exercise

A freshman football player has a chronically weak ankle that he has sprained several times. He wants to have the ankle taped before games and practices but has never had it taped before.

? What can the coach do to minimize the occurrence of blisters and ensure that the tape provides support?

**Taping Supplies**

Effective taping requires the availability of numerous supplies:

1. Razor for hair removal
2. Soap for cleaning skin
3. Alcohol for removal of oil from skin
4. Adhesive spray for tape adherent
5. Prewrap material for skin protection
6. Heel and lace pads
7. White adhesive tape (linen-backed tape) ($^1/_2$-inch, 1-inch, $1^1/_2$-inch, and 2-inch)
8. Adhesive and stretch tape (1-inch, 2-inch, 3-inch, and 4-inch)
9. Felt and foam padding material
10. Tape scissors
11. Tape cutters
12. Elastic bandages (2-inch, 3-inch, 4-inch, and 6-inch)

**Figure 11-9**

Taping preparation. A, Shaving.
B, Applying tape adherent
spray. C, Placing heel and
lace pads. D, Applying one
layer of underwrap.
E, Applying anchor strips.

A

B

C

D

E

A

B

**Figure 11-10**

Technique for tearing
adhesive tape

2.5 cm) tape; the ankles require 1½-inch (3.75 cm) tape; and the larger
skin areas such as thighs and back can accommodate 2- to 3-inch (5 to
7.5 cm) tape with ease.[9]

## Tearing Tape

With some practice nonelastic white adhesive tape can be easily torn by
hand. Tearing elastic tape is more difficult and it is usually necessary to
cut it with scissors. Various techniques can be used in tearing tape (Figure 11-10).[10] The following is a suggested procedure:

1. Hold the tape roll in the preferred hand with the index finger
   hooked through the center of the tape roll and the thumb
   pressing its outer edge.
2. With the other hand, grasp the loose end between the thumb
   and index finger.
3. With both hands in place, pull both ends of the tape so that it is
   tight. Next, make a quick, scissorslike move to tear the tape. In
   tearing tape the movement of one hand is away from the body
   and the other hand toward the body. Remember, do not try to
   bend or twist the tape to tear it.

When tearing is properly executed, the torn edges of the nonelastic
white adhesive tape are relatively straight, without curves, twists, or
loose threads sticking out. Once the first thread is torn, the rest of the
tape tears easily. Learning to tear tape effectively from many different positions is essential for speed and efficiency.[5]

## Removing Adhesive Tape

Tape usually can be removed from the skin by hand, by tape scissors or
tape cutters, or by chemical solvents.[1]

### Manual Removal

When pulling tape from the body, be careful not to tear or irritate the
skin. Tape must not be wrenched in an outward direction from the skin

**Figure 11-11**

Removing adhesive tape

but should be pulled in a direct line with the body (Figure 11-11). Remember to remove the skin carefully from the tape and not to peel the tape from the skin. One hand gently pulls the tape in one direction, and the opposite hand gently presses the skin away from the tape.

### Use of Tape Scissors or Cutters

The characteristic tape scissors or cutters have a blunt nose that slips underneath the tape smoothly without gouging the skin. Take care to avoid cutting the tape too near the site of the injury, lest the scissors aggravate the condition. If possible cut on the uninjured side.

### Using "Tape Remover"

Tape remover is an alcohol-based liquid that is useful for removing adherent residue from the skin. It works best when scrubbing the area with a towel or cloth. Some individuals have a skin sensitivity to this chemical that produces a reaction. Everyone should wash the tape remover off using soap and water.

## COMMON TAPING TECHNIQUES

### Arch

Taping the arch supports the entire plantar aspect of the foot (Figure 11-12).

**Materials needed**   One roll of 1-inch (2.5 cm) and one roll of 1½-inch (3.8 cm) tape and tape adherent.

**Position of the athlete**   The athlete lies face downward on a table with the foot to be taped extending approximately 6 inches (15 cm) over the edge of the table.

**Procedure**

1.  Place an anchor strip around the ball of the foot (1).

2. Starting at the third metatarsal head, take the tape around the

**Figure 11-12**

Arch taping technique

heel from the lateral side and meet the strip where it began (2 and 3).

3. The next strip starts near the second metatarsal head and finishes on the fourth metatarsal head (4).

4. The last strip begins on the fourth metatarsal head and finishes on the fifth (5). The technique, when completed, forms a fanshaped pattern covering the metatarsal region (6).

5. Lock strips (7 through 11) using 1¹/₂-inch (3.8 cm) tape and encircling the complete arch.

### Great Toe

This procedure is used for taping a sprained great toe (Figure 11-13).

**Materials needed**   One roll of 1-inch (2.5 cm) tape and tape adherent.
**Position of the athlete**   The athlete assumes a sitting position.
**Procedure**

1. The greatest support is given to the joint by a half-figure-eight taping (1 through 3). Start the series at an acute angle on the top of the foot and swing down between the great and first toes, first encircling the great toe and then coming up, over, and across the starting point. Repeat this process, starting each series separately.

2. After the required number of half-figure-eight strips are in position, place one lock piece around the ball of the foot (4).

### Toes

**Materials needed**   One roll of ¹/₂- to 1-inch (1.25 to 2.5 cm) tape, ¹/₈-inch (0.3 cm) sponge rubber, and tape adherent.

**Figure 11-13**

Taping for a sprained great toe

**Figure 11-14**

Taping for fracture of a toe

If the athlete has sensitive skin, thoroughly clean the area to be wrapped.

**Position of the athlete**   The athlete assumes a sitting position.
**Procedure**

1. Cut a ⅛-inch (0.3 cm) sponge rubber wedge and place it between the affected toe and a healthy one.
2. Wrap two or three strips of tape around the toes (Figure 11-14). This technique splints a fractured toe with a nonfractured one.

Ankle

Ankle taping applied directly to the athlete's skin affords the greatest support; however, when applied and removed daily, skin irritation occurs.[4] To avoid this problem, apply an underwrap material. Before taping, follow these procedures:[1]

1. Shave all the hair off the foot and ankle.
2. Apply a coating of tape adherent to protect the skin and offer an adhering base. note: It may be advisable to avoid the use of a tape adherent, especially if the athlete has a history of developing tape blisters. In cases of skin sensitivity, the ankle surface should be thoroughly cleansed of dirt and oil and an underwrap material applied; or tape directly to the skin.
3. Apply a gauze pad coated with friction-proofing material such as grease over the instep and to the back of the heel.
4. If underwrap is used, apply a single layer. The tape anchors extend beyond the underwrap and adhere directly to the skin.
5. Do not apply tape if skin is cold or hot from a therapeutic treatment.

The closed basket weave, or Gibney, technique (Figure 11-15) offers strong tape support and is primarily used in athletic training for newly sprained or chronically weak ankles.[4]

   **Materials needed**   One roll of 1½-inch (3.8 cm) tape and tape adherent.

   **Position of the athlete**   The athlete sits on a table with the leg extended and the foot held at a 90-degree angle.
   **Procedure**

1. Place an anchor around the ankle approximately 5 or 6 inches (12.5 to 15 cm) above the malleolus, just below the belly of the gastrocnemius muscle, and a second anchor around the instep directly over the styloid process of the fifth metatarsal (1 and 2).
2. Apply the first strip posteriorly to the malleolus and attach it to the ankle strips (3). NOTE: When applying strips, pull the foot into eversion for an inversion strain and into a neutral position for an eversion strain.
3. Start the first Gibney directly under the malleolus and attach it to the foot anchor (4).

**Figure 11-15**

Closed basket weave
ankle taping

4. In an alternating series, place three strips and three Gibneys on the ankle with each piece of tape overlapping at least half of the preceding strip (5 through 8).

5. After applying the basket weave series, continue the Gibney strips up the ankle, thus giving circular support (9 through 15).

6. For arch support, apply two or three circular strips lateral to medial (16 and 17).

7. After completing the conventional basket weave, apply two or three heel locks to ensure maximum stability (18 and 19).

Achilles Tendon

Achilles tendon taping (Figure 11-16) is designed to prevent the Achilles tendon from overstretching.

**Materials needed**    One roll of 3-inch (7.5 cm) elastic tape, one roll of 1½-inch (3.8 cm) linen tape, and tape adherent.

**Position of the athlete**    The athlete kneels or lies face down, with the affected foot hanging relaxed over the edge of the table.

**Procedure**

1. Apply two anchors with 1½-inch (3.8 cm) tape, one circling the leg loosely approximately 7 to 9 inches (17.5 to 22.5 cm) above the malleoli and the other encircling the ball of the foot (1 and 2).

**Figure 11-16**

Achilles tendon taping

**Figure 11-17**

Taping for shin splints

2. Cut two strips of 3-inch (7.5 cm) elastic tape approximately 8 to 10 inches (20 to 25 cm) long. Moderately stretch the first strip from the ball of the athlete's foot along its plantar aspect up to the leg anchor (3). The second elastic strip (4) follows the course of the first, but cut it and split it down the middle lengthwise. Wrap the cut ends around the lower leg to form a lock. CAUTION: Keep the wrapped ends above the level of the strain.

3. Complete the series by placing two or three lock strips of elastic tape (5 through 7) loosely around the arch and five or six strips (8 through 13) around the athlete's lower leg.

**Notes**

1. Locking too tightly around the lower leg and foot tends to restrict the normal action of the Achilles tendon and create more tissue irritation.

2. A variation to this method is to use three 2-inch-wide (5 cm) elastic strips in place of strips 3 and 4. Apply the first strip at the plantar surface of the first metatarsal head and end it on the lateral side of the leg anchor. Apply the second strip at the plantar surface of the fifth metatarsal head and end it on the medial side of the leg anchor. Center the third strip between the other two strips and end it at the posterior aspect of the calf. Wrap strips of 3-inch (7.5 cm) elastic tape around the forefoot and lower calf to close them off.

Medial Shin Splints

Taping can afford some relief of the symptoms of shin splints (Figure 11-17).

**Materials needed**  One roll of 1½-inch (3.8 cm) linen or elastic tape and adherent.

**Position of the athlete**   The athlete sits on a table with the knee bent and the foot flat on the table. The purpose of this position is to fully relax the muscles of the lower leg.

**Procedure**

1. Apply two anchor tape strips, the first to the anterolateral aspect of the ankle and lower leg and the second to the posterolateral aspect of the midcalf (1 and 2).

2. Starting at the lowest end of the first anchor, run a strip of tape to the back of the lower leg, spiraling it over the shin to attach on the lower end of the second anchor strip. Apply three strips of tape in this manner, with each progressively moving upward on the leg. As each strip comes across the previous strip, make an effort to pull the muscle toward the tibia (3 strips).

3. After applying seven pieces of tape, lock their ends with one or two cross-strips (10 and 11).

4. After completing the procedure, you may apply an elastic wrap in a spiral fashion.

**Note**   A variation to this method is to place a ½-inch (1.25 cm) thickness of felt 1 inch wide by 6 inches long (2.5 by 15 cm) on the medial border of the tibia secured by underwrap. Beginning distally, use 6-inch (15 cm) strips of white tape to hold the pad in place and provide support. The strips do not encircle the leg but are completely covered by elastic tape or a 3-inch (7.5 cm) elastic bandage.

### Knee

Athletes with unstable knees, like those with ankle instabilities, should never use tape and bracing as a replacement for proper exercise rehabilitation. If properly applied, taping can help protect the knee and aid in the rehabilitation process (Figure 11-18).

**Materials needed**   One roll of 2-inch (5 cm) linen tape, one roll of 3-inch (7.5 cm) elastic tape, a 1-inch (2.5 cm) heel lift, and skin adherent.

**Position of the athlete**   The athlete stands on a 3-foot (90 cm) table with the injured knee held in a moderately relaxed position by a 1-inch (2.5 cm) heel lift. The hair is completely removed from an area 6 inches (15 cm) above to 6 inches (15 cm) below the patella.

**Procedure**

1. Lightly encircle the thigh and leg at the hairline with a 3-inch (7.5 cm) elastic anchor strip (1 and 2).

2. Precut 12 elastic tape strips, each approximately 9 inches (22.5 cm) long. Stretching them to their utmost, apply them to the knee as indicated in Figure 11-18 (3 through 14).

3. Apply a series of three strips of 2-inch (5 cm) linen tape (15 through 22). Some individuals find it advantageous to complete a knee taping by wrapping loosely with an elastic wrap, thus

**Figure 11-18**

Taping for injuries to the ligaments of the knee

**Figure 11-19**

Hamstring taping

providing an added precaution against the tape's coming loose
from perspiration.

**Caution**   Tape must not constrict patella.

Hamstring Support

It is extremely difficult to relieve injured hamstring muscles completely
by any wrapping or taping technique, but some stabilization can be afforded by each. The hamstring taping technique (Figure 11-19) is designed to stabilize the moderately to severely contused or torn hamstring
muscles, enabling the athlete to continue to compete.

**Materials needed**   One roll of 2- or 1½-inch (5 or 3.8 cm) tape, skin
toughener, and a roll of 3-inch (7.5 cm) elastic tape or a 6-inch (15 cm)
elastic wrap.

**Position of the athlete**   The athlete lies face downward or may stand
on the table, with the affected limb flexed at approximately a 15-degree
angle at the knee, so the hamstring muscle is relaxed and shortened.

**Procedure**

1. Apply this taping similarly to the quadriceps technique. Place an
   anchor strip on either side of the thigh (1 and 2), and then
   crisscross strips, approximately 9 inches (22.5 cm) in length,
   diagonally upward on the posterior aspect of the thigh, forming
   an X (3 through 11).

2. After the hamstring area is covered with a series of crisscrosses,
   apply a longitudinal lock on either side of the thigh (12 and 13).

3. Place 3-inch (7.5 cm) elastic tape or a 6-inch (15 cm) elastic
   wrap around the thigh if needed to hold the crisscross taping in
   place.

Elbow

Tape the elbow as follows to prevent hyperextension (Figure 11-20).

**Materials needed**   One roll of 1½-inch (3.8 cm) tape, tape adherent, and 2-inch (5 cm) elastic bandage.

**Position of the athlete**   The athlete stands with the affected elbow
flexed at 90 degrees.

**Procedure**

1. Apply two anchor strips loosely around the arm, approximately
   2 inches (25 cm) to each side of the curve of the elbow
   (antecubital fossa) (1 and 2).

2. Construct a checkrein by cutting a 10-inch (25 cm) and a 4-inch
   (10 cm) strip of tape and laying the 4-inch (10 cm) strip against
   the center of the 10-inch (25 cm) strip, blanking out that
   portion. Next place the checkrein so that it spans the two anchor
   strips with the blanked-out side facing downward. Leave
   checkrein extended 1 to 2 inches past anchor strips on both
   ends. This allows anchoring of the checkreins with circular strips
   to secure against slippage (3 and 4).

3. Place five additional 10-inch (25 cm) strips of tape over the basic checkrein.

4. Finish the procedure by securing the checkrein with three lock strips on each end (5 through 10). A figure-eight elastic wrap applied over the taping will prevent the tape from slipping because of perspiration.

### Wrist

Wrist taping (Figure 11-21) stablizes and protects badly injured wrists.

**Materials needed**   One roll of 1-inch (2.5 cm) tape and tape adherent.

**Position of the athlete**   The athlete stands with the affected hand flexed toward the injured side and the fingers moderately spread to increase the breadth of the wrist for the protection of nerves and blood vessels.

**Procedure**

1. Apply one anchor strip around the wrist approximately 3 inches (7.5 cm) from the hand (1); wrap another anchor strip around the spread hand (2).

2. With the wrist bent toward the side of the injury, run a strip of tape from the anchor strip near the little finger obliquely across the wrist joint to the wrist anchor strip. Run another strip from the anchor strip on the index finger side across the wrist joint to the wrist anchor. This forms a crisscross over the wrist joint (3 and 4). Apply a series of four or five crisscrosses, depending on the extent of splinting needed (5 through 8).

3. Apply two or three series of figure-eight tapings over the crisscross taping (9 through 11). Start by encircling the wrist once, carry a strip over the back of the hand obliquely, encircling the hand twice, and then carry another strip obliquely upward across the back of the hand to where the figure-eight started. Repeat this procedure to ensure a strong, stabilizing taping.

### Thumb

Sprained thumb taping (Figure 11-22) is designed to give both protection for the muscle and joint and support to the thumb.

**Materials needed**   One roll of 1-inch (2.5 cm) tape and tape adherent.

**Position of the athlete**   The athlete should hold the injured thumb in a relaxed neutral position.

**Procedure**

1. Place an anchor strip loosely around the wrist and another around the distal end of the thumb (1 and 2).

2. From the anchor at the tip of the thumb to the anchor around the wrist, apply four splint strips in a series on the side of greater injury (dorsal or palmar side) (3 through 5) and hold them in place with one lock strip around the wrist and one encircling the tip of the thumb (6 and 7).

**Figure 11-20**

Taping to restrict elbow motion

**Figure 11-21**

Wrist taping technique

**Figure 11-22**

Taping for a sprained thumb

3. Add three thumb spicas. Start the first spica on the radial side at the base of the thumb and carry it under the thumb, completely encircling it, and then cross the starting point. The strip should continue around the wrist and finish at the starting point. Each of the subsequent spica strips should overlap the preceding strip by at least ⅔ inch (1.7 cm) and move downward on the thumb (8 and 9). The thumb spica with tape provides an excellent means of protection during recovery from an injury.

Finger and Thumb Checkreins

The sprained finger or thumb may require the additional protection afforded by a restraining checkrein (Figure 11-23).

**Materials needed**   One roll of 1-inch (2.5 cm) tape.

**Position of the athlete**   The athlete spreads the injured fingers widely but within a range that is free of pain.

**Procedure**

1. Bring a strip of 1-inch (2.5 cm) tape around the middle phalanx of the injured finger over to the adjacent finger and around it also. The tape left between the two fingers, which are spread apart, is called the checkrein.

2. Add strength with a lock strip around the center of the checkrein.

## COACH'S CORNER

The following is a checklist for the coach applying adhesive tape to an injured body part.

☐ If the part to be taped is a joint, place it in the position in which it is to be stabilized. If the part is muscle, make the necessary allowance for contraction and expansion.

☐ Overlap the tape at least half the width of the tape below. Unless tape is overlapped sufficiently, the active athlete will separate it, exposing the underlying skin to irritation.

☐ Avoid continuous taping. Tape continuously wrapped around a part may cause constriction. It is suggested that one turn be made at a time and that each encirclement be torn to overlap the starting end by approximately 1 inch. This rule is particularly true of white adhesive tape.

☐ Keep the tape roll in the hand whenever possible. By learning to keep the tape roll in the hand, seldom putting it down, and by learning to tear the tape, an operator can develop taping speed and accuracy.

☐ Smooth and mold the tape as it is laid on the skin. To save additional time, tape strips should be smoothed and molded to the body part as they are put in place; this is done by stroking the top with the fingers, palms, and heels of both hands.

☐ Allow tape to fit the natural contour of the skin. Each strip of tape must be placed with a particular purpose in mind. Linen-backed tape is not sufficiently elastic to bend around acute angles but must be allowed to fall as it may, fitting naturally to the body contours. Failing to allow this fit creates wrinkles and gaps that can result in skin irritations.

☐ Start taping with an anchor piece and finish by applying a lock strip. Commence taping, if possible, by sticking the tape to an anchor piece that encircles the part. This placement affords a good medium for the stabilization of succeeding tape strips so that they will not be affected by the movement of the part.

☐ Where maximum support is desired, tape directly over skin. In cases of sensitive skin, prewrap may be used as a tape base. With pre-wrap, some movement can be expected between the skin and the base.

☐ Do not apply tape if skin is hot or cold from a therapeutic treatment.

**Figure 11-23**

Finger and thumb checkreins

## SUMMARY

• Elastic bandages, when properly applied, can contribute to recovery from sport injuries.

- Elastic bandages must be applied uniformly, firmly but not so tightly as to impede circulation.

- Historically, taping has been an important aspect of athletic training. Sports tape is used in a variety of ways—as a means of holding a wound dressing in place, as support, and as protection against musculoskeletal injuries.

- For supporting and protecting musculoskeletal injuries, two types of tape are currently used—nonelastic white adhesive and elastic adhesive.

- Tape must be stored in a cool place and must be stacked on the flat side of each roll.

- The skin of the athlete must be carefully prepared before tape is applied.

- The skin should first be carefully cleaned; then all hair should be removed.

- An adherent may be applied, followed by an underwrap material, if needed, to help avoid skin irritation.

- Tape must be applied in a manner that provides the least amount of irritation and the maximum support.

- All tape applications require great care that the proper materials are used, that the proper position of the athlete is ensured, and that procedures are carefully followed.

*Solutions to Critical Thinking* Exercises

**11-1** The coach applies a 6-inch (15 cm) elastic wrap as a hip adductor restraint. This technique is designed to prevent the groin from being overstretched and the hip adductors reinjured.

**11-2** The coach applies tape and a 4-inch (10 cm) elastic shoulder spica to hold the doughnut in place.

**11-3** First the ankle should be shaved. Then a tape adherent spray should be applied. Heel and lace pads with a small amount of lubricant should be applied over bony prominences. One layer of underwrap can be applied. Tape should be applied with even pressure leaving no gaps.

## REVIEW QUESTIONS AND CLASS ACTIVITIES

1. What are elastic bandages used for? How do you apply them?
2. Observe the athletic trainer bandaging and taping in the training room.
3. What types of tape are available? What is the purpose of each type? What qualities should you look for in selecting tape?
4. How should you prepare an area to be taped?
5. How should you tear tape?
6. How should you remove tape from an area? Demonstrate the various methods and cutters that can be used to remove tape.
7. What are some general rules for tape application and why should you follow them?

8. What are some common taping procedures?

9. Bring the different types of tape to class. Discuss their uses and the qualities to look for in purchasing tape. Have the class practice tearing tape and preparing an area for taping.

10. Take each joint or body part and demonstrate the common taping procedures used to give support to that area. Have the students pair up and practice these taping jobs on each other. Discuss the advantages and disadvantages of using tape as a supportive device.

## REFERENCES

1. Alt W, Lohrer H, Gollhofer A: Functional properties of adhesive ankle taping: neuromuscular and mechanical effects before and after exercise, *Foot Ankle Int* 20(4):238, 1999.

2. Austin K: *Taping techniques,* Chicago, 1994, Mosby-Wolfe.

3. Callaghan MJ: Role of ankle taping and bracing in the athlete, *Br J Sports Med* 31(2):102, 1997.

4. Heit EJ, Lephart SM, Rozzi SL: The effect of ankle bracing and taping on joint position sense in the stable ankle, *J Sport Rehab* 5(3):206, 1996.

5. Jones K: Athletic taping and bracing. In Sallis RE, Massamino F, editors: *Essentials of sport medicine,* St Louis, MO, 1996, Mosby–Year Book.

6. Manfroy PP, Ashton-Miller JA, Wojtys EM: The effect of exercise, prewrap, and athletic tape on the maximal active and passive ankle resistance to ankle inversion, *Am J Sports Med* 25(2):156, 1997.

7. Perrin DH: *Athletic taping and bracing,* Champaign, Ill, 1995, Human Kinetics.

8. Sports Medicine Council of British Columbia: *Manual of athletic taping,* Philadelphia, 1995, FA Davis.

9. *Sports taping basics: lower body,* Champaign, Ill, 1996, Human Kinetics.

10. *Sports taping basics: upper body,* Champaign, Ill, 1996, Human Kinetics.

## ANNOTATED BIBLIOGRAPHY

Arnheim D, Prentice W: *Principles of athletic training,* Boston, 2000, McGraw-Hill.

    *Contains a comprehensive chapter on a variety of taping and bandaging skills with complete descriptions of techniques.*

Perrin DH: *Athletic taping and bracing,* Champaign, Ill, 1995, Human Kinetics.

    *Discusses specific injuries; gives step-by-step instructions for applying tape, braces, wraps, and orthotics; and presents stretching and strengthening exercises that reduce the chances of reinjury.*

Sports Medicine Council of British Columbia: *Manual of athletic taping,* Philadelphia, 1995, FA Davis.

    *Guidelines for taping and wrapping athletes' joints and limbs to both prevent and manage injuries. Chapters include: injury recognition; anatomy and taping techniques for the ankle, foot, knee, wrist, hand, elbow, and muscles and tendons; and resources.*

First aider, Gardner, Kan, Cramer Products.

    *Published seven times throughout the school year, this periodical contains useful taping and bandaging techniques that have been submitted by readers.*

*Sports Medicine Guide,* Mueller Sports Medicine, 1 Quench Dr, Prairie du Sac, WI, 53578.

    *Published four times a year, this quarterly often presents, along with discussions on specific injuries, many innovative taping and bandaging techniques.*

**WEBSITES**

Properties of Athletic Tape: http://
www.stanford.edu/~rwbragg/
tape.html

Cramer Sports Medicine: http://www.
cramersportsmed.com/

Mueller Sports Medicine—Retail
Tape and Wrap: http://www.
muellersportsmed.com/
retailtapeandwrap.htm

Johnson & Johnson: http://www.
jnj.com/

# Basics of Injury Rehabilitation

*When you finish this chapter you will be able to:*

- Explain the philosophy of the rehabilitative process in a sports medicine environment.
- Identify the individual short-term and long-term goals of a rehabilitation program.
- Describe the criteria and the decision-making process for determining when the injured athlete may return to full activity.
- Discuss how a coach might use therapeutic modalities in a rehabilitation program.

The athletic trainer is responsible for design, implementation, and supervision of the rehabilitation program.

The long-term goal is to return the injured athlete to practice or competition as quickly and safely as possible.

Sports medicine rehabilitation = aggressiveness.

# PHILOSOPHY OF ATHLETIC INJURY REHABILITATION

Although coaches make every effort to create a safe playing environment and prevent injuries, the nature of athletic participation dictates that injuries will eventually occur. Fortunately, few of the injuries that occur in an athletic setting are life threatening. The majority of the injuries are not serious and lend themselves to rapid rehabilitation. Long-term rehabilitation programs require the supervision of a highly trained professional to be safe and effective. In an athletic setting, the coach should rely on the athletic trainer to assume the primary responsibility for design, implementation, and supervision of the rehabilitation program for the injured athlete. The coach, in the absence of an athletic trainer, is responsible for design, implementation, and supervision of the rehabilitation program for the injured athlete.

The competitive nature of athletics necessitates an aggressive approach to rehabilitation. Because of the short competitive season in most sports, the injured athlete does not have the luxury of simply sitting around and doing nothing until the injury heals. *The goal of the injured athlete is to return to activity as soon as safely possible.*[9] Consequently, the tendency is to try to push the athlete to return. Unfortunately there is a thin line between not pushing the athlete hard enough or fast enough and being overly aggressive. In either case, a mistake in judgment on the part of the person overseeing the rehabilitation program may hinder the athlete's return to activity.

## GOALS OF A REHABILITATION PROGRAM

Designing an effective rehabilitation program is simple if several basic components are addressed. These basic components may also be considered as the short-term goals of a rehabilitation program and should include: (1) providing correct immediate first aid and management following injury to limit or control swelling; (2) reducing or minimizing pain; (3) restoring full range of motion; (4) restoring or increasing muscular strength, endurance, and power; (5) reestablishing neuromuscular control; (6) improving balance; (7) maintaining cardiorespiratory fitness; and (8) incorporating appropriate functional progressions.[8] *The long-term goal is almost invariably to return the injured athlete to practice or competition as quickly and safely as possible.*

### Providing Correct First Aid and Controlling Swelling

As discussed in detail in Chapter 7, the process of rehabilitation begins immediately after injury. Initial first-aid and management techniques are perhaps the most critical part of any rehabilitation program. How the injury is managed initially has a significant impact on the course of the rehabilitative process.[2] Everything that is done in first-aid management of any injury should be directed toward controlling the swelling.[1] To control and significantly limit the amount of swelling, the RICE principle—rest, ice, compression, and elevation—should be applied (Figure 12-1). Each factor plays a critical role in limiting swelling, and all these elements should be used simultaneously (see Chapter 7).

### Controlling Pain

When an injury occurs, the athlete experiences some degree of pain. The extent of the pain is determined in part by the severity of the injury, by the athlete's individual response to and perception of pain, and by the circumstances under which the injury occurred. The coach can effectively control acute pain by using the RICE technique immediately after injury.[7] In addition, using appropriate therapeutic modalities such as ice, heat, or electrical stimulating currents can help modulate pain throughout the rehabilitation process.[10]

***Critical Thinking*** Exercise

A soccer player has been diagnosed as having a grade 2 sprain of the MCL in her knee. The team physician has referred the athlete to the coach, who is charged with the responsibility of overseeing the rehabilitation program.

**?** What are the short-term goals of a rehabilitation program, and how can the coach best achieve these?

***Critical Thinking*** Exercise

A runner complains of anterior knee pain. She has greatly cut back on the distance of her training runs and indicates that she has been taking antiinflammatory medication to help her continue to train. However, she is frustrated because her knee seems to be getting worse instead of better.

**?** What can the coach recommend to most effectively help her deal with her knee pain?

**Figure 12-1**

The RICE technique should be used immediately following injury to limit swelling.

**Figure 12-2**

Stretching techniques are
used with tight
musculotendinous structures
to improve range of motion.

Components of a
rehabilitation program:
• Controlling swelling
• Reducing pain
• Restoring full range of
  motion
• Restoring muscle strength,
  endurance, power
• Reestablishing
  neuromuscular control
• Regaining balance
• Maintaining cardio-
  respiratory fitness
• Incorporating functional
  progressions

Controlling swelling:
• Rest
• Ice
• Compression
• Elevation

Limited range of movement
= stretching.

## Restoring Range of Motion

Injury to a joint is always followed by some associated loss of motion.
That loss of movement may be caused by resistance of the muscle and its
tendon to stretch, by contracture of the ligaments and capsule around a
joint, or by some combination of the two. The athlete should engage in
stretching activities designed to improve flexibility (Figure 12-2).

## Restoring Muscular Strength, Endurance, and Power

Muscular strength, endurance, and power are among the most essential
factors in restoring the function of a body part to preinjury status (see
Chapter 4). Isometric, progressive resistance (isotonic), isokinetic, and
plyometric exercises can benefit rehabilitation.[5] A major goal in performing strengthening exercises is to work through a full, pain-free range of
motion.

### Isometric Exercise

Isometric exercises are commonly performed in the early phase of rehabilitation when a joint is immobilized for a time. They are useful in cases
in which using resistance training through a full range of motion may
make the injury worse. Isometrics increase static strength and assist in
decreasing the amount of atrophy. Isometrics also can lessen swelling by
causing a muscle pumping action to remove fluid and edema.

### Progressive Resistance Exercise

Progressive resistance exercise (PRE) is the most commonly used
strengthening technique in a rehabilitation program. PRE may be done
with free weights, exercise machines, or rubber tubing (Figure 12-3).
Progressive resistance exercise uses isotonic contractions in which force is
generated against resistance while the muscle is changing in length. In a
rehabilitation program, both eccentric (shortening) and concentric
(lengthening) strengthening exercises should be used.

**Figure 12-3**

Progressive resistance
exercise using isotonic
contractions is the most
widely used rehabilitative
strengthening technique.

### Isokinetic Exercise

Isokinetic exercise is commonly used in the rehabilitative process.[8] It is most often incorporated during the later phases of a rehabilitation program. Isokinetics use a fixed speed with accommodating resistance to provide maximal resistance throughout the range of motion (Figure 12-4). The speed of movement can be altered in isokinetic exercise. Isokinetic measures are commonly used as criteria for return of the athlete to functional activity following injury.

Strengthening exercises:
• Isometrics
• Progressive resistance
  exercise
• Isokinetics
• Plyometrics

### Plyometric Exercise

Plyometric exercises are most often incorporated into the later stages of a rehabilitation program. Plyometrics use a quick stretch of a muscle to facilitate a subsequent concentric contraction. Plyometric exercises are useful in restoring or developing the athlete's ability to produce dynamic movements associated with muscular power (Figure 12-5). The ability to

**Figure 12-4**

Isokinetic exercise is most
often used in the later stages
of rehabilitation.

**Figure 12-5**

Plyometric exercise focuses on improving dynamic, power movements.

Neuromuscular control produces coordinated movements.

**Figure 12-6**

Reestablishing neuromuscular control and balance are critical components in regaining functional performance capabilities.

generate force very rapidly is a key to successful performance in many sport activities. It is critical to address the element of muscular power in rehabilitation programs for the injured athlete.

## Reestablishing Neuromuscular Control

Neuromuscular control is the mind's attempt to teach the body conscious control of a specific movement. Neuromuscular control relies on the central nervous system to interpret and integrate proprioceptive and kinesthetic information and then to control individual muscles and joints to produce coordinated movement.[11] Following injury and subsequent rest and immobilization, the central nervous system "forgets" how to put this information together. Regaining neuromuscular control means regaining the ability to follow some previously established sensory pattern. Strengthening exercises, particularly those that tend to be more functional, are essential for reestablishing neuromuscular control.[11]

## Regaining Balance

The ability to balance and maintain postural stability is essential to reacquiring athletic skills.[3] A rehabilitation program must include functional exercises that incorporate balance training to prepare the athlete for return to activity (Figure 12-6). Failure to address balance problems may predispose the athlete to reinjury.[4]

## Maintaining Cardiorespiratory Fitness

Maintaining cardiorespiratory fitness is perhaps the single most neglected component of a rehabilitation program. An athlete spends a considerable amount of time preparing the cardiorespiratory system to handle the increased demands made upon it during a competitive season. When injury occurs and the athlete is forced to miss training time, levels of cardiorespiratory fitness may decrease rapidly. Thus the coach must design or substitute alternative activities that allow the athlete to maintain existing levels of cardiorespiratory fitness as early as possible in the rehabilitation period (Figure 12-7).[6]

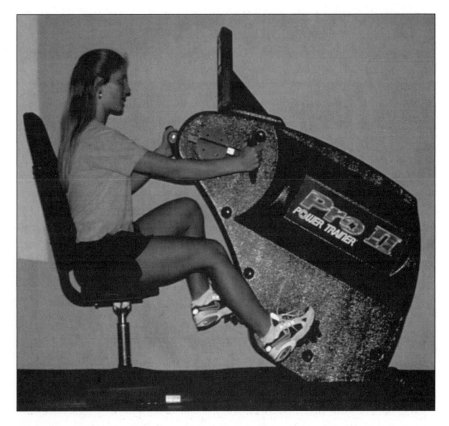

**Figure 12-7**

Every rehabilitation program
must include some exercise
designed to maintain
cardiorespiratory fitness.

Depending on the nature of the injury, several possible activities can help the athlete maintain fitness levels. A lower extremity injury necessitates non-weight-bearing activities. Pool activities provide an excellent means for injury rehabilitation. Cycling also can positively stress the cardiorespiratory system.

Balance = postural stability.

All exercise rehabilitation must be conducted as part of a carefully designed plan.

## Functional Progressions

The purpose of any rehabilitation program is to restore normal function following injury. Functional progressions involve a series of gradually progressive activities designed to prepare the individual for return to a specific sport (Focus Box 12-1).[11] Those skills necessary for successful participation in a given sport are broken down into component parts, and the athlete gradually reacquires those skills within the limitations of his or her own individual progress.[12] Every new activity introduced must be carefully monitored by the coach to determine the athlete's ability to perform and his or her physical tolerance. If an activity does not produce additional pain or swelling, the level should be advanced; new activities should be introduced as quickly as possible.

Functional progressions will gradually assist the injured athlete in achieving normal pain-free range of motion, in restoring adequate

*Critical Thinking* Exercise

Following an ankle sprain, a
basketball player is placed in
an ankle immobilizer and given
crutches with instructions to
begin with totally non-weight-
bearing movement and
progress to full weight-bearing
movement without crutches as
soon as possible. After 4 days
the athlete is out of the
immobilizer and can walk
without crutches but still has a
significant limp.

? What should the coach do
to help the athlete regain a
normal gait pattern, and why is
it important to do so as soon as
possible?

Functional progressions
incorporate sport-specific
skills into the rehabilitation
program.

12-1 **Focus Box**

**Return to running following lower extremity injury functional
progression:**

- Walking
- Jogging on track with walking of curves
- Jogging full track
- Running on track with jogging of curves
- Running full track
- Running for fitness—2 to 3 miles three times per week
- Lunges—90 degree, pivot, 180 degree
- Sprints—"W", triangle, 6 second, 20 yd, 40 yd, 120 yd
- Acceleration/deceleration runs
- Shuffle slides progressing to shuffle run
- Carioca

strength levels, and in regaining neuromuscular control throughout the
rehabilitation program.

Functional Testing

Functional testing uses functional progression drills for the purpose of assessing the athlete's ability to perform a specific activity (Figure 12-8).
Functional testing involves the performance of a single maximal effort to
give the coach some idea of how close the athlete is to a full return to activity. For years coaches have used a variety of functional tests to assess
the athlete's progress, including agility runs (e.g., figure eights, shuttle
runs, cariocas), side stepping, vertical jumps, hopping for time or distance, and co-contraction tests.[11]

**Figure 12-8**

Performance on functional
tests can determine the
capability of the athlete to
return to full activity.

# USING THERAPEUTIC MODALITIES

Most athletic trainers routinely incorporate the use of therapeutic modalities including cold (cryotherapy), heat (thermotherapy), ultrasound, electrotherapy, massage, traction, and intermittent compression into their rehabilitation programs. Athletic trainers have had formal classroom instruction and supervised clinical experience in using various therapeutic modalities and in many states are licensed to do so.[10]

In the absence of an athletic trainer, a coach might choose to use simple inexpensive therapeutic modalities such as cold, heat, or perhaps massage to treat an injured athlete; using other modalities is usually beyond the scope of a coach's expertise. The coach must be aware of and follow the laws that specifically dictate how certain therapeutic modalities can be used.[10]

## Ice Packs (Bags)

Ice packs are most often used for minimizing swelling and for analgesia immediately following injury. Flaked or crushed ice can be encased in a wet towel and placed on the part to be treated. An ice pack made by placing crushed or chipped ice in a self-sealing plastic bag may also be used. Both types of ice packs can easily mold to the contour of the part. When the plastic packs are used, a wet towel should be placed between the skin and the pack. Besides toweling, an elastic wrap should be available and should be used to hold the pack firmly in place. Usually an elastic bandage compression wrap and elevation are used with an ice pack. These packs are safely used for 20 minutes.[10]

## Hot Packs

Hot packs are most often used post-acutely (after swelling has stopped) to increase blood and lymphatic flow and facilitate reabsorption of the by-products of the injury process into the lymphatic system. Heat may also be used for its analgesic and relaxation effects. Caution should be exercised in using heat too early following injury. Cold should be used for at least 72 hours post injury before using any type of heat.

Commercial moist heat packs, sometimes called *hydrocollator packs,* contain silicate gel in a cotton pad, which is immersed in thermostatically controlled hot water at a temperature of 160° F. Each pad retains water and a relatively constant heat level for a 20- to 30-minute treatment period. A minimum of six layers of toweling or commercial terry cloth are used between the packs and the skin. The athlete should not lie on top of the hot pack.

## Massage

Massage is defined as the systematic manipulation of the soft tissues of the body. The movements of gliding, compressing, stretching, percussing, and vibrating are regulated to produce specific responses in the athlete. Massage causes mechanical, physiological, and psychological responses.[10]

Mechanical responses to massage occur as a direct result of the graded pressures and movements of the hand on the body. Such actions encourage venous and lymphatic drainage and mildly stretch superficial and scar tissue. Connective tissue can be effectively stretched by friction massage, which helps prevent rigidity in scar formation. Massage can increase circulation and, as a result, increase metabolism and aid in the removal of metabolites such as lactic acid. It also helps to remove edema by increasing circulation at and around the injury site, assisting in the normal venous blood return to the heart. Relaxation can be induced by slow, superficial stroking of the skin that is beneficial for tense, anxious athletes who may require gentle hands-on treatment.[10]

## CRITERIA FOR FULL RECOVERY

All exercise rehabilitation plans must determine what is meant by complete recovery from an injury. Often it means that the athlete is fully reconditioned and has achieved full range of movement, strength, neuromuscular control, cardiovascular fitness, and sport-specific functional skills. Besides physical well-being, the athlete must also have regained full confidence to return to his or her sport. Specific criteria for a return to full activity after rehabilitation are determined to a large extent by the nature and severity of the specific injury, but also depend on the philosophy and judgment of both the physician and the coach (Focus Box 12-2).[7]

The decision to release an athlete recovering from injury to a full return to athletic activity is the final stage of the rehabilitation/recovery process. The decision should be carefully considered by each member of the sports medicine team involved in the rehabilitation process. The team physician should be ultimately responsible for deciding that the athlete is ready to return to practice and/or competition. That decision should be based on collective input from the coach, the athletic trainer, and the athlete.

**COACH'S CORNER**

The following is a checklist for the coach who is deciding what components to address in designing an injury rehabilitation program.

- ☐ Provide correct immediate first aid and management following injury to limit or control swelling.
- ☐ Reduce or minimize pain.
- ☐ Restore full range of motion.
- ☐ Reestablish neuromuscular control.
- ☐ Restore or increase muscular strength, endurance, and power.
- ☐ Improve balance.
- ☐ Maintain cardiorespiratory fitness.
- ☐ Incorporate appropriate functional progressions.

**12-2** **Focus Box**

**Full Return to Activity**

In considering the athlete's return to activity, the following concerns should be addressed:

- *Physiological healing constraints.* Has rehabilitation progressed to the later stages of the healing process?
- *Pain status.* Has pain disappeared, or is the athlete able to play within his or her own levels of pain tolerance?
- *Swelling.* Is there still a chance that swelling may be exacerbated by a return to activity?
- *Range of motion.* Is range of motion adequate to allow the athlete to perform both effectively and with minimized risk of reinjury?
- *Strength.* Is strength, endurance, or power great enough to protect the injured structure from reinjury?
- *Neuromuscular control/proprioception/kinesthesia.* Has the athlete "relearned" how to use the injured body part?
- *Cardiorespiratory fitness.* Has the athlete been able to maintain cardiorespiratory fitness at or near the level necessary for competition?
- *Sport-specific demands.* Are the demands of the sport or a specific position such that the athlete will not be at risk of reinjury?
- *Functional testing.* Does performance on appropriate functional tests indicate that the extent of recovery is sufficient to allow successful performance?
- *Prophylactic strapping, bracing, padding.* Are any additional supports necessary for the injured athlete to return to activity?
- *Responsibility of the athlete.* Is the athlete capable of listening to his or her body and of knowing enough not to put himself or herself in a potential reinjury situation?
- *Predisposition to injury.* Is this athlete prone to reinjury or a new injury when not 100 percent?
- *Psychological factors.* Is the athlete capable of returning to activity and competing at a high level without fear of reinjury?
- *Athlete education and preventive maintenance program.* Does the athlete understand the importance of continuing to engage in conditioning exercises that can greatly reduce the chances of reinjury?

## SUMMARY

- The rehabilitation philosophy in sports medicine is an aggressive one, with the ultimate goal being to return the injured athlete to full activity as quickly and safely as possible.

- Short-term goals of a rehabilitation program are: (1) providing correct immediate first aid and management following injury to limit or control swelling; (2) reducing or minimizing pain; (3) restoring full range of motion; (4) restoring or increasing muscular strength, endurance, and power; (5) reestablishing neuromuscular control; (6) improving balance; (7) maintaining cardiorespiratory fitness; and (8) incorporating appropriate functional progressions.

- The athlete should be permitted to fully return to activity when he or she is fully reconditioned and has achieved full range of movement, strength, neuromuscular control, cardiovascular fitness, and sport-specific functional skills. Besides physical well-being, the athlete must also have regained full confidence to return to his or her sport.

---

### *Solutions to Critical Thinking* Exercises

**12-1** In sports medicine, the short-term goals in any rehabilitation program should include controlling pain, regaining range of motion, regaining strength, reestablishing neuromuscular control, and maintaining levels of cardiorespiratory fitness. The approach to rehabilitation should be aggressive. Decisions as to when and how to alter and progress specific components within a rehabilitation program should be based on, and are limited by, the healing process. The long-term goal is to return the athlete to full activity as soon as safely possible.

**12-2** Anterior knee pain can result from many different causes. However, strengthening of the quadriceps can often be quite helpful. If full-range-of-motion strengthening exercises increase pain, the athlete should begin with isometric exercises done at different points in the range and should progress to full-range concentric and eccentric resistance exercise as tolerated. Exercises such as minisquats,

stepping exercises, or leg presses are excellent exercises for strengthening quadriceps and tend to be more functional than are exercises done on an exercise machine.

**12-3** Following injury and subsequent rest and immobilization, it is not unusual for the athlete to "forget" how to walk. The coach must help the athlete relearn neuromuscular control, which means regaining the ability to follow some previously established motor and sensory pattern by regaining conscious control of a specific movement until that movement becomes automatic. Strengthening exercises, particularly those that tend to be more functional, are essential for reestablishing neuromuscular control. Addressing neuromuscular control is critical throughout the recovery process but may be most critical during the early stages of rehabilitation to avoid reinjury or even overuse injuries to additional structures.

## REVIEW QUESTIONS AND CLASS ACTIVITIES

1. Explain the role of the coach in a rehabilitation program.
2. Describe the techniques for controlling swelling following injury.
3. Why it is important to modulate pain during a rehabilitation program?
4. How is range of motion restored after an injury?
5. Compare the use of isometric, progressive resistance, isokinetic, and plyometric exercises in rehabilitation.
6. How is neuromuscular control related to movement?
7. Why must an athlete condition the body generally while an injury heals?
8. How and when should functional progressions be incorporated into the rehabilitation program?

9. Describe how to determine if an athlete is ready to return to activity following injury.

10. What modalities should a coach use in treating the athlete and for what should they be used?

## REFERENCES

1. Arnheim D, Prentice W: *Principles of athletic training,* ed 10, NY, 2000, McGraw-Hill.

2. Buschbacher R, Braddom R: *Sports medicine and rehabilitation: a sport specific approach,* Philadelphia, 1994, Hanley & Belfus.

3. Guskiewicz K, Perrin D: Research and clinical applications of assessing balance, *J Sport Rehab* 5(1):45, 1996.

4. Irrgang J, Whitney S, Cox E: Balance and proprioceptive training for rehabilitation of the lower extremity, *J Sport Rehab* 3(1):68, 1994.

5. Kisner C, Colby A: *Therapeutic exercise: foundations and techniques,* Philadelphia, 1996, FA Davis.

6. Magnusson P, McHugh M: Current concepts on rehabilitation in sports medicine. In Nicholas J, Hirschman E: *The lower extremity and spine in sports medicine,* St Louis, 1995, Mosby.

7. Malone T, editor: *Orthopedic and sports physical therapy,* St Louis, 1996, Mosby–Year Book.

8. Perrin D: *Isokinetic exercise and assessment,* Champaign, Ill, 1993, Human Kinetics.

9. Prentice W: *Rehabilitation techniques in sports medicine,* Dubuque, Iowa, 1999, WC Brown/McGraw-Hill.

10. Prentice W: *Therapeutic modalities in sports medicine,* Dubuque, Iowa, 1999, WC Brown/McGraw-Hill.

11. Tippett S, Voight M: *Functional progressions for sport rehabilitation,* Champaign, Ill, 1995, Human Kinetics.

12. Zachazewski J, Magee D, Quillen S: *Athletic injuries and rehabilitation,* Philadelphia, 1996, WB Saunders.

## ANNOTATED BIBLIOGRAPHY

Buschbacher R, Braddom R: *Sports medicine and rehabilitation; a sport specific approach,* Philadelphia, 1994, Hanley & Belfus.

*Discusses the rehabilitation of injuries that occur in specific sports.*

Prentice W: *Rehabilitation techniques in sports medicine,* ed 3, Dubuque, Iowa, 1999, WC Brown/McGraw-Hill.

*A comprehensive text dealing with all aspects of rehabilitation used in a sports medicine setting.*

Tippett S, Voight M: *Functional progressions for sport rehabilitation,* Champaign, Ill, 1995, Human Kinetics.

*Presents scientific principles and practical applications for using functional exercise to rehabilitate athletic injuries.*

**WEBSITES**

Cramer First Aider: http://www.ccsd.k12.wy.us/CCHS_web/sptmed/fstaider.htm

National Athletic Trainers' Association: http://www.nata.org

*Accesses rehabilitation in the athletic training journals.*

The Physician and Sportsmedicine: http://www.physsportmed.com

*Search back issues and access the ones specifically geared toward weight training and rehabilitation.*

Archives of Physical Medicine and Rehabilitation: http://www.archives-pmr.org/

The AOSSN Online Media Kit: http://www.sportsmed.org/k/kd.htm

Journal of Sport Rehabilitation: http://www.esportmed.com/journals/journal.cfm?id=JSR

# PART

## 3

# RECOGNITION AND MANAGEMENT
# OF SPECIFIC INJURIES
# AND CONDITIONS

# Recognizing Different Sports Injuries

*When you finish this chapter you will be able to:*

- Differentiate between acute and chronic injury.
- Describe acute traumatic injuries, including fractures, dislocations and subluxations, contusions, ligament sprains, muscle strains, muscle soreness, and nerve injuries.
- Describe chronic overuse injuries involving tendinitis, tenosynovitis, bursitis, osteoarthritis, and myofascial trigger points.
- Explain the various phases of the healing process.

N o matter how much attention is directed toward the general principles of injury prevention, the nature of participation in sports dictates that sooner or later injury will occur. Generally injuries that occur in an athletic setting may be classified as either acute or chronic. Acute injuries are caused by trauma; chronic injuries can result from overuse as occurs with the repetitive dynamics of running, throwing, or jumping. In this chapter we discuss the more common traumatic and overuse injuries that are likely be seen by the coach.

## ACUTE (TRAUMATIC) INJURIES

### Fractures

Acute injuries = trauma
Chronic injuries = overuse

Fractures (broken bones) occur as a result of extreme stresses and strains placed on bones. Before discussing fractures, a brief discussion of bone anatomy is necessary.[9] The gross structure of the long bones includes the diaphysis, epiphysis, articular cartilage, and periosteum (Figure 13-1). The *diaphysis* is the main shaft of the bone. It is hollow, cylindrical, and covered by compact bone. The *epiphysis* is located at the ends of long bones. It is the growth area of the bone in adolescents. The ends of long bones are covered with a layer of *articular cartilage* that covers the joint surfaces of the epiphysis. This cartilage provides protection during movement and cushions jars and blows to the joint. A dense, white, fibrous membrane, the *periosteum*, covers long bones except at joint surfaces. Interlacing with the periosteum are fibers from the muscle tendons.

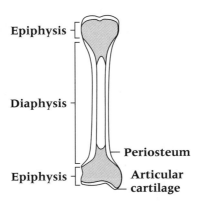

Epiphysis

Diaphysis

Epiphysis

Periosteum

Articular cartilage

**Figure 13-1**

The gross structure of the long bones includes the diaphysis, epiphysis, articular cartilage, and periosteum.

Throughout the periosteum on its inner layer exist countless blood vessels and **osteoblasts** (bone-forming cells). The blood vessels provide nutrition to the bone, and the osteoblasts provide bone growth and repair.

Fractures generally can be classified as either closed or open.[9] A **closed fracture** is one in which there is little or no movement or displacement of the broken bones. Conversely, in an **open fracture** there is enough displacement of the fractured ends that the bone actually breaks through surrounding tissues, including the skin. An open fracture increases the possibility of infection. Both types of fractures can be serious if not managed properly. Signs and symptoms of a fracture include obvious deformity, point tenderness, swelling, and pain on active and passive movement. The only definitive technique for determining if a fracture exists is to have it x-rayed.

Several different kinds of fractures can occur (Figure 13-2). Long bones can be stressed or forced to fail by tension, compression, bending, twisting (torsion), and shear.[7] These forces, either singly or in combination, can cause a variety of fractures. For example, spiral fractures are caused by twisting, whereas oblique fractures are caused by the combined forces of axial compression, bending, and torsion. Transverse fractures occur because of bending (Figure 13-3). Along with the type of stress, the amount of force must be considered. The more complex the fracture, the more energy is required. External energy can be used to deform and then actually fracture bone. Some energy can be dispersed to soft tissue adjacent to the bone.[3]

### Healing of a Fracture

In most instances the fracture of a bone requires immobilization for some period in a cast. In general, fractures of the long bones of the arm and leg require approximately 6 weeks of casting, and the smaller bones in the hands and feet may require as little as 3 weeks of either casting or splinting. In some instances, immobilization may not be required for healing. For example, breaks of the four small toes are difficult to splint or cast. Of course, complications such as infections may lengthen the time required for both casting and rehabilitation.

**osteoblasts (os** tee oh blasts**)**
Bone-forming cells.

**closed fracture**
Fracture does not penetrate superficial tissue.

**open fracture**
Overlying skin is lacerated by protruding bone fragments.

Long bones can be stressed by tension, compression, bending, torsion, and shear.

| MECHANISM | PATTERN | APPEARANCE |
|---|---|---|
| Bending | Transverse | |
| Torsion | Spiral | |
| Compression plus bending | Oblique-transverse | |
| Compression plus bending plus torsion | Oblique | |
| Variable | Comminuted | |
| Compression | Metaphyseal compression | |

**Figure 13-2**

Mechanisms, patterns, and
appearance of bone fractures

**callus**
New bone formation over a
fracture.

**osteoclasts (os** tee oh
klasts**)**
Cells that absorb and re-
move osseous tissue.

**stress fracture**
Spot of irritation on the
bone.

For a fracture to heal, osteoblasts must lay down extra bone formation, called a **callus,** over the fracture site during the immobilization period. Once the cast is removed, the bone must be subjected to normal
stresses and strains so that tensile strength may be regained before the
healing process is complete. Cells called **osteoclasts** function to reshape
the bone in response to normally applied stresses and strains.[9]

Stress Fractures

Perhaps the most common fracture that results from physical activity is a
**stress fracture.** Unlike the other types of fractures that have been discussed, the stress fracture results from overuse rather than acute
trauma.[2] Common sites for stress fractures include the weight-bearing
bones of the leg or foot. In either case, repetitive forces transmitted
through the bones produce irritations at specific spots on the bone. The
pain usually begins as a dull ache, which becomes progressively painful
day after day. Initially, pain is most severe during activity. However,
when a stress fracture develops, pain becomes worse after the activity is
stopped.

The biggest problem with a stress fracture is that often it does not
show up on an x ray until the osteoblasts begin laying down bone. At
that point, a small white line appears on the x ray. If a stress fracture is

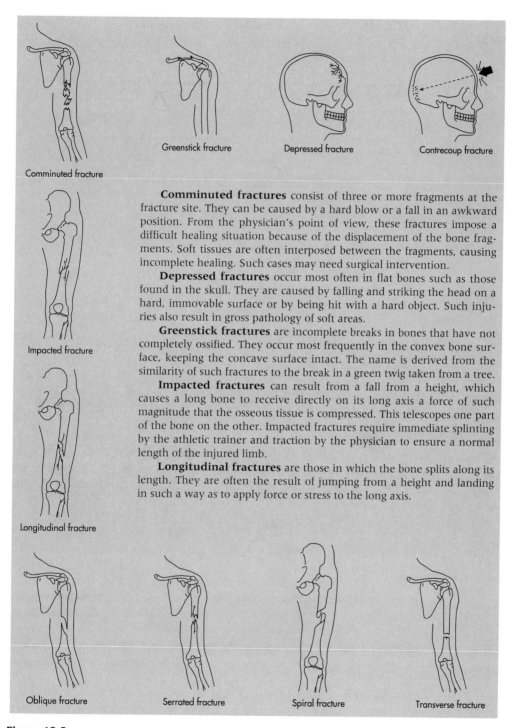

Comminuted fracture

Greenstick fracture

Depressed fracture

Contrecoup fracture

Impacted fracture

Longitudinal fracture

Oblique fracture

Serrated fracture

Spiral fracture

Transverse fracture

**Comminuted fractures** consist of three or more fragments at the fracture site. They can be caused by a hard blow or a fall in an awkward position. From the physician's point of view, these fractures impose a difficult healing situation because of the displacement of the bone fragments. Soft tissues are often interposed between the fragments, causing incomplete healing. Such cases may need surgical intervention.

**Depressed fractures** occur most often in flat bones such as those found in the skull. They are caused by falling and striking the head on a hard, immovable surface or by being hit with a hard object. Such injuries also result in gross pathology of soft areas.

**Greenstick fractures** are incomplete breaks in bones that have not completely ossified. They occur most frequently in the convex bone surface, keeping the concave surface intact. The name is derived from the similarity of such fractures to the break in a green twig taken from a tree.

**Impacted fractures** can result from a fall from a height, which causes a long bone to receive directly on its long axis a force of such magnitude that the osseous tissue is compressed. This telescopes one part of the bone on the other. Impacted fractures require immediate splinting by the athletic trainer and traction by the physician to ensure a normal length of the injured limb.

**Longitudinal fractures** are those in which the bone splits along its length. They are often the result of jumping from a height and landing in such a way as to apply force or stress to the long axis.

**Figure 13-3**

Various types of fractures

**Oblique fractures** are similar to spiral fractures. They occur when one end receives sudden torsion or twisting and the other end is fixed or stabilized.

**Serrated fractures** are sawtooth, sharp-edged fracture lines of the two bony fragments. They are usually caused by a direct blow. Because of the sharp and jagged edges, extensive internal damage such as the severance of vital blood vessels and nerves often occurs.

**Spiral fractures** have an S-shaped separation. They are fairly common in football and skiing, in which the foot is firmly planted and the body is suddenly rotated.

**Transverse fractures** occur in a straight line, more or less at right angles to the bone shaft. A direct outside blow usually causes this injury.

**Contrecoup fractures** occur on the side opposite to the part where trauma was initiated. Fracture of the skull is at times an example of the contrecoup. An athlete may be hit on one side of the head with such force that the brain and internal structures compress against the opposite side of the skull, causing a fracture.

**Avulsion fractures** are the separation of a bone fragment from its cortex at an attachment of a ligament or tendon. This fracture usually occurs as a result of a sudden, powerful twist or stretch of a body part. An example of a ligamentous episode is the sudden eversion of the foot that causes the deltoid ligament to avulse bone from the medial malleolus. An example of a tendinous avulsion is one that causes a patellar fracture, which occurs when an athlete falls forward while suddenly bending a knee. The stretch of the patellar tendon pulls a portion of the inferior patellar pole apart.

**Blow-out fractures** occur to the wall of the eye orbit as the result of a blow to the eye.

**Figure 13-3—cont'd**

13-1

**Critical Thinking** Exercise

A track athlete training for a marathon complains of pain in the lower leg. She consults with her physician, who determines that she has a stress fracture. When she returns to practice, she is confused about how a stress fracture is different from a real fracture.

? How should the coach explain the difference between the two, and what is the course of management?

suspected, it is best to stop the activity for a period of at least 14 days. Stress fractures do not usually require casting; however, if they are not handled correctly, they may become true fractures that must be immobilized (Focus Box 13-1).

## Dislocations and Subluxations

A **dislocation** occurs when at least one bone in an articulation is forced out of its normal and proper alignment and stays out until it is either manually or surgically put back into place or reduced. Dislocations most commonly occur in the shoulder joint, elbow, and fingers, but they can occur wherever two bones articulate (Figure 13-4A). A **subluxation** is like a dislocation except that in this situation a bone pops out of its normal articulation but then goes right back into place.[4] Subluxations most commonly occur in the shoulder joint and, in females, in the knee cap (Figure 13-4B).

In dislocations, deformity is almost always apparent; however, it may be obscured by heavy musculature, making it important for the examiner to routinely palpate, or feel, the injured site to determine the loss of normal contour. Comparison of the injured side with the uninjured side often reveals asymmetry.

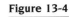

**13-1** ⟩ *Focus Box*

**Differentiating between Injuries to a Muscle or Joint**

Here is a simple procedure to help the coach determine whether an injury is to the muscle or joint:

1. To rule out the possibility of fracture, the coach has the athlete move the part through a full range of motion. Pain may indicate muscle injury.
2. The coach passively moves the relaxed part through a range of motion. Pain may indicate a joint condition.
3. The coach applies a resistance against the moving extremity. Pain may suggest a muscle injury.

Dislocations or subluxations may result in a rupture of the stabilizing ligaments and tendons surrounding the joint. Occasionally an avulsion fracture occurs in which an attached tendon or ligament pulls a small piece of bone away from the rest of the bone. In other cases, the force may separate growth plates or cause a complete fracture of a long bone. These possibilities indicate the importance of administering complete and thorough medical attention to first-time dislocations. It has often been said, "Once a dislocation, always a dislocation." In most cases this statement is true, because once a joint has been either subluxated or completely dislocated, the connective tissues that bind and hold it in its correct alignment are stretched to such an extent that the joint is extremely vulnerable to subsequent dislocations.

A first-time dislocation should always be considered and treated as a possible fracture. Once it has been ascertained that the injury is a dislocation, a physician should be consulted for further evaluation. However, before the athlete is taken to the physician, the injury should be properly splinted and supported to prevent any further damage.

*Dislocations should never be reduced immediately, regardless of where they occur.* The coach should take the athlete to an x-ray facility and rule out fractures or other problems before reduction. Inappropriate techniques of

**dislocation**
A bone is forced out of alignment and stays out until surgically or manually replaced or reduced.

**subluxation** (sub **lucks** ashun)
A bone is forced out of alignment but goes back into place.

**Figure 13-4**

A joint that is forced beyond its anatomical limits can be A, dislocated or B, subluxated.

A          B

reduction may only exacerbate the problem. Return to activity after dislocation or subluxation is largely dependent on the degree of soft tissue damage.

### Ligament Sprains

> **sprain**
> Injury to a ligament that connects bone to bone.

A **sprain** involves damage to a ligament that provides support to a joint.[5] A ligament is a tough, relatively inelastic band of tissue that connects one bone to another. Before discussing injuries to ligaments, a review of joint structure is necessary (Figure 13-5). All *synovial* joints are composed of two or more bones that articulate with one another to allow motion in one or more planes. The articulating surfaces of the bone are lined with a very thin, smooth, cartilaginous covering called an articular, or *hyaline, cartilage.* All joints are entirely surrounded by a thick, ligamentous *joint capsule.* The inner surface of this joint capsule is lined by a very thin *synovial membrane* that is highly vascularized and innervated. The synovial membrane produces *synovial fluid,* the functions of which include lubrication, shock absorption, and nutrition of the joint.[9]

> **mechanoreceptors**
> Located in muscles, tendons, ligaments, and joints; provide information on position of a joint.

The articular capsule, ligaments, outer aspects of the synovial membrane, and fat pads of the synovial joint are well supplied with nerves. The inner aspect of the synovial membrane, cartilage, and articular disks, if present, have nerves as well. These nerves, called **mechanoreceptors,** provide information about the relative position of the joint and are found in the fibrous capsule and ligaments.[9]

**Figure 13-5**

Structure of a synovial joint

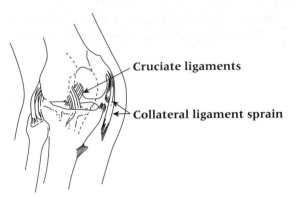

Cruciate ligaments

Collateral ligament sprain

**Figure 13-6**

A ligament sprain in the
knee joint

Some joints contain a thick fibrocartilage called a *meniscus*. The knee
joint, for example, contains two wedge-shaped menisci that deepen the
articulation and provide shock absorption in that joint. Finally, the main
structural support and joint stability is provided by the ligaments, which
may be either thickened portions of a joint capsule or totally separate
bands. The anatomical position of the ligaments partly determines what
motions a joint is capable of making.[9]

If a joint is forced to move beyond normal limits or planes of movement, injury to the ligaments is likely to occur (Figure 13-6). The severity of the damage is subject to many different classifications; however, the
most commonly used system involves three grades of sprain.

- *Grade 1 sprain.* There is some stretching and separation of the
  ligamentous fibers, with minimal instability of the joint. Mild to
  moderate pain, localized swelling, and joint stiffness should be
  expected.
- *Grade 2 sprain.* There is some tearing and separation of the ligament
  fibers, with moderate instability of the joint. Moderate to severe pain,
  swelling, and joint stiffness should be expected.
- *Grade 3 sprain.* There is total tearing of the ligament, which leads to
  major instability of the joint. Initially, severe pain may be present,
  followed by little or no pain as a result of total disruption of nerve
  fibers. Swelling may be great, and the joint tends to become very stiff
  some hours after the injury. In some cases, a grade 3 sprain with
  marked instability requires surgical repair. Frequently, the force
  producing the ligament injury is so great that other ligaments or
  structures surrounding the joint may also be injured. Rehabilitation
  of grade 3 sprains involving surgery is a long-term process.

The greatest problem in the rehabilitation of grade 1 and grade 2
sprains is restoring stability to the joint.[9] Once a ligament has been
stretched or partially torn, inelastic scar tissue forms, preventing the ligament from regaining its original tension. To restore stability to the joint,
the other structures surrounding that joint, primarily muscles and their

13–2

**Critical Thinking** Exercise

A volleyball player has
sprained her ankle just 2 days
before the beginning of the
conference tournament. The
athlete, her parents, and her
coach are extremely concerned
that she is going to miss the
tournament and want to know if
anything can be done to make
her get well more quickly.

? What can this athlete be
told about the process of
healing?

tendons, must be strengthened. The increased muscle tension provided by strength training can improve stability of the injured joint.

## Contusions

A contusion is another word for a bruise. The mechanism that produces a bruise is familiar. A blow from some external object causes soft tissues (i.e., skin, fat, and muscle) to be compressed against hard bone underneath[2] (Figure 13-7). If the blow is hard enough, capillaries are torn, which allows bleeding into the tissues. Minor bleeding often causes a bluish-purple discoloration of the skin that persists for several days. The contusion may be very sore to the touch, and if damage has occurred to muscle, pain may be experienced on active movement. In most cases the pain ceases within a few days and discoloration disappears usually in a few weeks.[6]

The major problem with contusions occurs in an area that is subjected to repeated blows. If the same area, or more specifically, a muscle, is bruised over and over again, small calcium deposits may begin to accumulate in the injured area. These pieces of calcium may be found between several fibers in the muscle belly, or calcium may build up to form a spur, which projects from the underlying bone. These calcium formations may significantly impair movement and are referred to as **myositis ossificans.**[4]

The key to preventing the occurrence of myositis ossificans from repeated contusions is to protect the injured area with padding. If the area is properly protected after the first contusion, myositis may never develop. Protection and rest may allow the calcium to be reabsorbed, eliminating any need for surgery.

The two areas that seem to be the most vulnerable to repeated contusions during physical activity are the quadriceps muscle group on the front of the thigh and the biceps muscle on the front of the upper arm. The formation of myositis ossificans in these or any other areas may be detected by x rays.

## Muscle Strains

The muscle is composed of separate fibers that are capable of simultaneous contraction when stimulated by the central nervous system. Each muscle is attached to bone at both ends by strong, relatively inelastic tendons that cross over joints.

If a muscle is overstretched or forced to contract against too much resistance, separation or tearing of the muscle fibers occurs. This damage is referred to as a **strain** (Figure 13-8).[4] Muscle strains, like ligament sprains, are subject to various classification systems. The following is a simple system of strain classification:

- *Grade 1 strain.* Some muscle fibers have been stretched or actually torn. There is some tenderness and pain on active motion. Movement is painful, but full range of motion is usually possible.

**Figure 13-7**

A contusion occurs when soft tissues are compressed between bone and some external force.

---

**myositis ossificans** (my oh **sigh** tis ah **sif** ah cans) Calcium deposits that result from repeated trauma.

---

**strain**
A stretch, tear, or rip in the muscle or its tendon.

Strained hamstring
muscles

**Figure 13-8**

A muscle strain results in
separation or tearing of
fibers.

- *Grade 2 strain.* A number of muscle fibers have been torn, and active contraction of the muscle is extremely painful. Usually a depression or divot can be felt somewhere in the muscle belly at the place at which the muscle fibers have been torn. Some swelling may occur because of capillary bleeding; therefore, some discoloration is possible.
- *Grade 3 strain.* A complete rupture of a muscle has occurred in the area of the muscle belly at the point at which muscle becomes tendon or at the tendinous attachment to the bone. There is significant impairment to or perhaps total loss of movement. Initially, pain is intense but quickly diminishes because of complete nerve fiber separation.

Muscle strains can occur in any muscle and usually result from some uncoordinated activity between muscle groups. Grade 3 strains are most common in the biceps tendon of the upper arm or in the Achilles heel cord in the back of the calf. When either of these tendons tears, the muscle tends to bunch toward its attachment at the bone site. Grade 3 strains involving large tendons that produce great amounts of force must be surgically repaired. Smaller musculotendinous ruptures such as those that occur in the fingers may heal by immobilization with a splint.

Regardless of the severity of the strain, the time required for rehabilitation is lengthy.[9] In many instances muscle strains are incapacitating, making rehabilitation time for a muscle strain even longer than for a ligament sprain. Incapacitating muscle strains occur most frequently in the large, force-producing hamstring and quadriceps muscles of the lower extremity. The treatment of hamstring strains requires a healing period of 6 to 8 weeks and a considerable amount of patience. Trying to return to activity too soon often causes reinjury to the area of the muscle that has been strained, and the healing process must begin again.

## Muscle Cramps

**Muscle cramps** are extremely painful involuntary muscle contractions that occur most commonly in the calf, abdomen, or hamstrings, although

 13-3

*Critical Thinking* Exercise

A football player sustains repeated contusions to the left quadriceps muscle.

? What should he be most concerned about?

**muscle cramps**
Involuntary muscle
contraction.

any muscle can be involved.[3] The occurrence of heat cramps is related to excessive loss of water and, to some extent, several electrolytes or ions (sodium, chloride, potassium, magnesium, and calcium) that are essential elements in muscle contraction (see Chapter 10).

## Muscle Guarding

Following injury, the muscles that surround the injured area contract to, in effect, splint that area, thus minimizing pain by limiting movement. Quite often this "splinting" is incorrectly referred to as a muscle spasm. The terms *spasm* and *spasticity* are more correctly associated with increased tone or contractions of muscle that occur because of some upper motor neuron lesion in the brain. Thus **muscle guarding** is a more appropriate term for the involuntary muscle contractions that occur in response to pain following musculoskeletal injury.[9]

**muscle guarding**
Muscle contraction in response to pain.

## Muscle Soreness

Overexertion in strenuous muscular exercise often results in muscular pain. All active people at one time or another have experienced muscle soreness, usually resulting from some physical activity to which they are unaccustomed. The older a person gets, the more easily muscle soreness seems to develop.

There are two types of muscle soreness. The first type of muscle pain is *acute-onset muscle soreness,* which accompanies fatigue. It is transient and occurs during and immediately after exercise. The second type of soreness involves delayed muscle pain that appears approximately 12 hours after injury. This *delayed-onset muscle soreness (DOMS)* becomes most intense after 24 to 48 hours and then gradually subsides so that the muscle becomes symptom-free after 3 or 4 days. DOMS is described as a syndrome of delayed muscle pain leading to increased muscle tension, swelling, and stiffness and to resistance to stretching.[3]

DOMS is thought to result from several possible causes. It may occur from very small tears in the muscle tissue, which seems to be more likely with eccentric or isometric contractions. It may also occur because of disruption of the connective tissue that holds muscle tendon fibers together.

Muscle soreness may be prevented by beginning exercise at a moderate level and gradually progressing the intensity of the exercise over time. Treatment of muscle soreness usually also involves static or PNF stretching activity. Another important treatment for muscle soreness, as for other conditions discussed in this chapter, is ice applied within the first 48 to 72 hours.[9]

## Nerve Injuries

In athletics, nerve injuries usually involve either compression or tension. Nerve injuries, as with injuries to other tissues in the body, can be acute or chronic. Trauma directly affecting nerves can produce a variety of sensory responses, including hypoesthesia (diminished sense of feeling), hyperesthesia (increased sense of feelings such as pain or touch), or paresthesia (numbness, prickling, or tingling, which may occur from a direct blow or stretch to an area). For example, a sudden nerve stretch or pinch can produce both a sharp burning pain that radiates down a limb and muscle weakness. **Neuritis,** a chronic nerve problem, can be caused by a variety of forces that usually have been repeated or continued for a long time. Symptoms of neuritis can range from minor nerve problems to paralysis. More serious injuries involve the crushing of a nerve or complete division (severing). This type of injury may produce a lifelong physical disability, such as paraplegia or quadriplegia, and should therefore not be overlooked in any circumstance.

Specialized tissue, such as nerve cells, cannot regenerate once the nerve cell dies. In an injured peripheral nerve, however, the nerve fiber can regenerate significantly if the injury does not affect the cell body. For regeneration to occur, an optimal environment for healing must exist.

Regeneration is slow, at a rate of only 3 to 4 mm per day. Damaged nerves within the central nervous system regenerate very poorly compared to nerves in the peripheral nervous system.[9]

> **neuritis**
> Chronic nerve irritation.

## CHRONIC OVERUSE INJURIES

### The Importance of Inflammation in Healing

For most people, the word *inflammation* has negative connotations. However, inflammation is an essential part of the healing process. Once a structure is damaged or irritated, inflammation must occur to initiate the healing process. Signs and symptoms of inflammation include pain, swelling, warmth, loss of function, and perhaps redness.[6] Inflammation is supposed to be an acute process that ends when its role in the healing process has been accomplished. However, if the source of irritation (e.g., the repetitive movements that cause stress to the tendon) is not removed, then the inflammatory process becomes chronic rather than acute. When this situation occurs, an acute condition may become a chronic disabling problem.

### Tendinitis

Of all the overuse problems associated with sport activity, **tendinitis** is probably the most common. Any term ending in the suffix-*itis* means inflammation is present. Tendinitis means inflammation of a **tendon.** During muscle activity, a tendon must move or slide on other structures around it whenever the muscle contracts. If a particular movement is performed repeatedly, the tendon becomes irritated and inflamed.[5] This inflammation is manifested by pain on movement, swelling, possibly some warmth, and usually crepitus. **Crepitus** is a crackling sound. It is usually caused by the tendon's tendency to stick to the surrounding structure while it slides back and forth. This sticking is caused primarily by the chemical products of inflammation that accumulate on the irritated tendon.

The key to the treatment of tendinitis is rest.[9] If the repetitive motion causing irritation to the tendon is eliminated, the inflammatory process

> **tendinitis**
> Inflammation of a tendon.

The suffix -*itis* means "inflammation of."

> **tendon**
> Tough band of connective tissue that attaches muscle to bone.

> **crepitus**
> A crackling feel or sound.

will allow the tendon to heal. Unfortunately, athletes find it difficult to totally stop activity and rest for 2 or more weeks while the tendinitis subsides. The athlete should substitute some form of activity, such as bicycling or swimming, to maintain present fitness levels while avoiding continued irritation of the inflamed tendon. In runners, tendinitis most commonly occurs in the Achilles tendon in the back of the lower leg; in swimmers, it often occurs in the muscle tendons of the shoulder joint. However, tendinitis can flare up in any activity in which overuse and repetitive movements occur.

### Tenosynovitis

> **tenosynovitis** (ten oh sin oh **vie** tis)
> Inflammation of a tendon and its synovial sheath.

**Tenosynovitis** is very similar to tendinitis in that the muscle tendons are involved in inflammation. However, many tendons are subject to an increased amount of friction because of the tightness of the space through which they must move. In these areas of high friction, tendons are usually surrounded by synovial sheaths that reduce friction on movement. If the tendon sliding through a synovial sheath is subjected to overuse, inflammation is likely to occur (Figure 13-9).[4] As with tendinitis, the inflammatory process produces by-products that are "sticky" and tend to cause the sliding tendon to adhere to the synovial sheath surrounding it.

Tenosynovitis occurs most commonly in the long flexor tendons of the fingers as they cross over the wrist joint and in the biceps tendon around the shoulder joint. Treatment for tenosynovitis is the same as for tendinitis. Because both conditions involve inflammation, antiinflammatory drugs may be helpful in chronic cases.

### Bursitis

Bursitis occurs around joints, where there is friction between tendon and bone, skin and bone, or muscle and other muscles. Without some mechanism of protection in these high-friction areas, chronic irritation would exist.

**Figure 13-9**

Tenosynovitis is an inflammation of the sheath covering a tendon. A, Normal. B, Inflamed.

A        B

**Bursae** are pieces of synovial membrane that contain a small amount of fluid (synovial fluid). Just as oil lubricates a hinge, these small pieces of synovium permit motion of these structures without friction.

If excessive movement or perhaps some acute trauma occurs around the bursae, they become irritated and inflamed and begin producing large amounts of synovial fluid.[8] The longer the irritation continues or the more severe the acute trauma, the more fluid is produced. As fluid continues to accumulate in the limited space available, pressure increases, causing pain in the area. Bursitis can be an extremely painful condition that may severely restrict movement, especially if it occurs around a joint. Synovial fluid continues to be produced until the movement or trauma producing the irritation is eliminated.

Occasionally, a bursa or synovial sheath completely surrounds a tendon, allowing more freedom of movement in a tight area. Irritation of this synovial sheath may restrict tendon motion. All joints have many bursae surrounding them. The three bursae that are most commonly irritated as a result of various types of physical activity are the subacromial bursa in the shoulder joint under the distal clavicle and acromion process; the olecranon bursa on the tip of the elbow; and the prepatellar bursa on the front surface of the patella. All three of these bursae produce large amounts of synovial fluid, affecting motion at their respective joints.

> **bursae**
> Pieces of synovial membrane that contain a small amount of fluid.

13–4

*Critical Thinking* Exercise

A wrestler complains of pain, swelling, and warmth around the knee that always seems to be worse after practice.

? What should the coach suspect is wrong with the knee and how should it be treated?

## Osteoarthritis

Any mechanical system wears out with time. The joints in the body are mechanical systems, and wear and tear, even from normal activity, is inevitable. The most common result of this wear and tear, a degeneration of the articular or hyaline cartilage, is referred to as **osteoarthritis**.[10] The cartilage may be worn away to the point of exposing, eroding, and polishing the underlying bone.

Any process that changes the mechanics of the joint eventually leads to degeneration of that joint. Degeneration is a result of repeated trauma to the joint and to tendons, ligaments, and fasciae surrounding the joint. Such injuries may be caused by a direct blow or fall, by pressure of carrying or lifting heavy loads, or by repeated trauma to the joint as in running or cycling.

Osteoarthritis most often affects the weight-bearing joints: the knees, hips, and lumbar spine. Also affected are the shoulders and cervical spine. Although many other joints may show pathological degenerative change, clinically the disease only occasionally produces symptoms in them. Any joint that is subjected to acute or chronic trauma may develop osteoarthritis.[9]

The symptoms of osteoarthritis are relatively local. Osteoarthritis may be localized to one side of the joint or may be generalized about the joint. One of the most distinctive symptoms is pain, which is brought about by friction that occurs with use and which is relieved by rest. Stiffness is a common complaint that occurs with rest and is quickly loosened with activity. This symptom is prominent upon rising in the morning.

> **osteoarthritis**
> A wearing down of hyaline cartilage.

Joints may also show localized tenderness, or grating that may be heard and felt.[6]

### Myofascial Trigger Points

trigger point
Area of tenderness in a
tight band of muscle.

A **trigger point** is an area of tenderness in a tight band of muscle. In the athlete, painful or active trigger points most often develop because of some mechanical stress to the muscle.[9] This stress could involve either an acute muscle strain or static postural positions that produce constant tension in the muscle. Trigger points occur most typically in the neck, upper back, and lower back. Palpation of the trigger point produces pain in a predictable distribution of referred pain. The pain may also cause some restricted range of motion. Pressure on the trigger point produces a twitch or a jump response from the pain. Pain can be increased by passive or active stretching of the involved muscle.

## THE IMPORTANCE OF THE HEALING PROCESS FOLLOWING INJURY

Phases of the healing process:
Inflammatory response phase
Fibroblastic repair phase
Maturation-remodeling phase

The coach must possess some understanding of both the sequence and time frames for the various phases of healing, realizing that certain physiological events occur during each of the phases. Any interference with the healing process during a rehabilitation program will likely slow return to full activity. The healing process must have an opportunity to accomplish what it is supposed to. At best, the coach can only try to create an environment that is conducive to the healing process. Little can be done to speed up the process physiologically, but many things may be done during rehabilitation to impede healing.

The healing process consists of three phases: the inflammatory response phase, the fibroblastic repair phase, and the maturation-remodeling phase.[1] Although the phases of healing are often discussed as three separate entities, the healing process is a continuum. Phases of the healing process overlap one another and have no definitive beginning or end points (Figure 13-10).[9]

### Inflammatory Response Phase

The inflammatory response phase begins immediately following injury. The inflammatory response phase is perhaps the most critical phase of the healing process. Without the physiological changes that take place during the inflammatory process, the later stages of healing cannot occur. The destruction of tissue produces direct injury to the cells of the various soft tissues. During this phase, phagocytic cells clean up the mess created by the injury. Injured cells release chemicals that facilitate the healing process. This phase is characterized symptomatically by redness, swelling, tenderness, increased temperature, and loss of function. This initial inflammatory response lasts for approximately 2 to 4 days following initial injury.

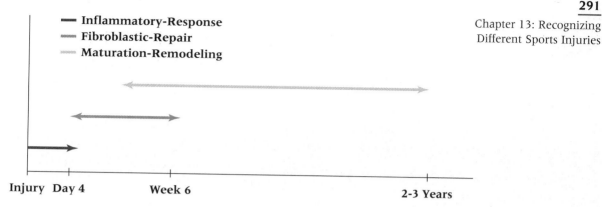

- Inflammatory-Response
- Fibroblastic-Repair
- Maturation-Remodeling

Injury  Day 4          Week 6                                    2-3 Years

**Figure 13-10**

The healing process is a
continuum in which the
three phases of healing
overlap one another.

## Fibroblastic Repair Phase

During the fibroblastic phase of healing, proliferative and regenerative
activity leading to scar formation and repair of the injured tissue occurs.
The period of scar formation, referred to as *fibroplasia,* begins within the
first few hours following injury and may last for as long as 4 to 6 weeks.
During this period many of the signs and symptoms associated with the
inflammatory response subside. The athlete may still indicate some tenderness to touch and usually complains of pain when particular movements stress the injured structure. As scar formation progresses, complaints of tenderness or pain gradually disappear.

## Maturation-Remodeling Phase

The maturation-remodeling phase of healing is a long-term process. This
phase features a realignment or remodeling of the scar tissue according
to the tensile forces to which that scar is subjected. With increased stress
and strain, the collagen fibers that make up the scar realign in a position
of maximum efficiency parallel to the lines of tension. The tissue gradually assumes normal appearance and function, although a scar is rarely as
strong as the normal uninjured tissue. Usually after about 3 weeks, a
firm, strong, contracted, nonvascular scar exists. The maturation phase of
healing may require several years to be totally complete.

## SUMMARY

- Fractures may be classified as either greenstick, transverse, oblique,
  spiral, comminuted, impacted, avulsive, or stress.
- Dislocations and subluxations are disruptions of the joint capsule and
  ligamentous structures surrounding the joint.
- Ligament sprains involve stretching or tearing the fibers that provide
  stability at the joint.
- Repeated contusions may lead to the development of myositis ossificans.

- Muscle strains involve a stretching or tearing of muscle fibers and their tendons and cause impairment to active movement.
- Muscle soreness may be caused by spasm, connective tissue damage, muscle tissue damage, or some combination of these factors.
- Tendinitis, an inflammation of a muscle tendon that causes pain on movement, usually occurs because of overuse.
- Tenosynovitis is an inflammation of the synovial sheath through which a tendon must slide during motion.
- Bursitis is an inflammation of the synovial membranes located in areas in which friction occurs between various anatomical structures.
- Osteoarthritis involves degeneration of the articular cartilage or subchondral bone.
- A trigger point is an area of tenderness in a tight band of muscle that develops from some mechanical stress to the muscle.
- The three phases of the healing process, the inflammatory response phase, the fibroblastic repair phase, and the maturation-remodeling phase, occur in sequence but overlap one another in a continuum.

---

### Solutions to Critical Thinking Exercises

**13-1** A stress fracture is not an actual break of the bone, it is simply an irritation of the bone. Treatment of a stress fracture requires about 14 days of rest. However, the coach should point out that a stress fracture can become a true fracture if it is not rested; if that happens, 4 to 6 weeks of immobilization in a cast is necessary. Thus, it is critical that this athlete rest for the required amount of time.

**13-2** Little can be done to speed up the healing process physiologically. This athlete must realize that certain physiological events must occur during each phase of the healing process. Any interference with this healing process during a rehabilitation program will likely slow

return to full activity. The healing process must have an opportunity to accomplish what it is supposed to.

**13-3** Repeated contusion of any muscle may lead to the development of myositis ossificans. The key to treating myositis ossificans is prevention. An initial contusion to any muscle should be immediately protected with padding to prevent reinjury.

**13-4** The coach should suspect that the wrestler has developed bursitis from constantly kneeling on the mat. Inflammation may best be treated by rest, ice, antiinflammatory medication, and protective padding of the knee.

## REVIEW QUESTIONS AND CLASS ACTIVITIES

1. What is the difference between an acute injury and a chronic injury? Give examples of each.
2. Describe various types of fractures and the mechanisms that cause fractures to occur.
3. How does a stress fracture differ from a regular fracture?

4. Differentiate between a subluxation and a dislocation.
5. What structures are found at a joint? What are their functions?
6. How do the three grades of ligament sprains differ?
7. What is myositis ossificans and how can it be prevented?
8. Differentiate between muscle strains, muscle cramps, muscle guarding, and muscle soreness.
9. How does a damaged nerve heal?
10. How are tendinitis, tenosynovitis, and bursitis related to one another?
11. Explain how osteoarthritis develops.
12. What are myofascial trigger points, where are they most likely to occur, and what are the signs and symptoms?
13. Discuss the physiological events that occur during each of the different phases of the healing process.
14. Invite an orthopedist to class to discuss common injuries to the musculoskeletal system.

## REFERENCES

1. American Orthopaedic Society for Sports Medicine: *Sports-induced inflammation*, Park Ridge, Ill, 1990, American Academy of Orthopaedic Surgeons.
2. Armstrong R, Warren G, Warren J: Mechanisms of exercise induced muscle fiber injury, *Sports Med* 12:184, 1991.
3. Arnheim D, Prentice WE: *Principles of athletic training*, Boston, 2000, McGraw-Hill.
4. Blauvelt CT, Nelson FRT: *A manual of orthopaedic terminology*, ed 4, St Louis, 1990, Mosby–Year Book.
5. Cailliet R: *Soft tissue pain and disability*, Philadelphia, 1988, FA Davis.

6. Gallaspie J, May D: *Signs and symptoms of athletic injuries*, St Louis, 1996, Mosby.
7. Malone T, McPhoil T, Nitz A: *Orthopedic and sports physical therapy*, St Louis, 1997, Mosby.
8. Morris A: *Sports medicine: prevention of athletic injuries*, Dubuque, Iowa, 1992, WC Brown.
9. Prentice W: *Rehabilitation techniques in sports medicine*, Dubuque, Iowa, 1999, WC Brown/McGraw-Hill.
10. Strauss R: *Sports medicine*, Philadelphia, 1996, WB Saunders.

## ANNOTATED BIBLIOGRAPHY

Booher JM, Thibodeau GA: *Athletic injury assessment*, Boston, 1999, McGraw-Hill.

*An excellent guide to the recognition, assessment, classification, and evaluation of athletic injuries.*

Garrick JG, Webb DR: *Sports injuries: diagnosis and management.* Philadelphia, 1999, WB Saunders.

*An overview of musculoskeletal injuries that are unique to sports and exercise.*

Griffith HW, Pederson M: *Complete guide to sports injuries: how to treat fractures, bruises, sprains, dislocations, and head injuries*, New York, 1997, Perigee.

*Tells readers how to treat, avoid, and rehabilitate nearly 200 of the most common sports injuries, including fractures, bruises, sprains, strains, dislocations, and head injuries.*

Micheli L: *The sports medicine bible*, New York, 1995, Harper Perennial.

*A clearly written basic text that explains how to recognize and prevent injuries from occurring. Also discusses principles and management of injuries that do occur.*

Peacinn M, Bojanic I: *Overuse injuries of musculoskeletal system*, Boca Raton, Fla, 1993, CRC Press.

*A comprehensive text describing overuse injuries of the tendon, tendon sheath, bursae, muscle, muscle-tendon function, cartilage, and nerve.*

Williams JGP: *Color atlas of injury in sport*, Chicago, 1990, Mosby–Year Book.

*An excellent visual guide to the area of sports injuries, covering the nature and incidence of sport injury, types of tissue damage, and regional injuries caused by a variety of sports activities.*

## WEBSITES

Cramer First Aider: http://www.ccsd.k12.wy.us/CCHS_web/sptmed/fstaider.htm

American Red Cross: http://www.arc.org

National Institute of Health: http://www.nih.gov

Wheeless' Textbook of Orthopedics: http://www.medmedia.com/med.htm

v

# The Foot

*When you finish this chapter you will be able to:*

- Briefly describe the anatomy of the foot.
- Explain the process of injury assessment for the foot.
- Identify steps that can be taken to minimize foot injuries.
- Explain the causes of various foot injuries commonly seen in athletes.
- Describe the appropriate care for injuries incurred in the foot.

# FOOT ANATOMY

## Bones

The human foot must function both to absorb forces and to provide a stable base of support during walking, running, and jumping. It contains twenty-six bones, (seven tarsal, five metatarsal, and fourteen phalangeal) that are held together by an intricate network of ligaments and fascia and moved by a complicated group of muscles (Figure 14-1). The tarsal bones that form the ankle include the talus and calcaneous. The navicular, cuboid, and three cuneiform bones form the instep of the foot.

## Ligaments

### Arches of the Foot

The foot is structured, by means of ligamentous and bony arrangements, to form several arches. The arches assist the foot in supporting the body weight and in absorbing the shock of weight bearing. There are four arches: the medial longitudinal, the lateral longitudinal, the metatarsal, and the transverse (Figure 14-2).

The *metatarsal arch* is shaped by the distal heads of the metatarsals. The arch stretches from the first to the fifth metatarsal. The *transverse arch* extends across the transverse tarsal bones and forms a half dome. The *medial longitudinal arch* originates along the medial border of the calcaneus

**Figure 14-1**

Bones of the foot: A, Medial.
B, Lateral.

and extends forward to the distal head of the first metatarsal. The main supporting ligament of the longitudinal arch is the plantar calcaneonavicular ligament, which acts as a spring by returning the arch to its normal position after it has been stretched. The *lateral longitudinal arch* is on the lateral aspect of the foot and follows the same pattern as the medial longitudinal arch. It is formed by the calcaneus, cuboic, and fifth metatarsal bones.

### Plantar Fascia (Plantar Aponeurosis)

The plantar fascia is a thick white band of fibrous tissue originating from the medial aspect of the calcaneus and ending at the distal heads of the metatarsals. Along with ligaments, the plantar fascia supports the foot against downward forces (Figure 14-3).

## Muscles

**Figure 14-2**

Arches of the foot: A,
Metatarsal and transverse
arches. B, Medial
longitudinal arch. C, lateral
longitudinal arch.

The medial movements include adduction (medial movement of the forefoot), and supination (a combination of inversion and adduction).

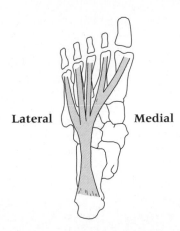

**Lateral**     **Medial**

**Figure 14-3**

Plantar fascia

Muscles that produce these movements pass behind and in front of the medial malleolus. Muscles passing behind are the tibialis posterior, flexor digitorum longus, and flexor hallucis longus. Muscles passing in front of the medial malleolus are the tibialis anterior and the extensor hallucis longus (Figure 14-4).

The lateral movements of the foot include abduction (lateral movement of the forefoot), and pronation (a combination of eversion and abduction). Muscles passing behind the lateral malleolus are the peroneus longus and the peroneus brevis. Muscles passing in front of the lateral malleolus are the peroneus tertius and extensor digitorum longus (Figure 14-5).

In general the small intrinsic muscles on the plantar surface of the foot cause toe flexion whereas those muscles on the dorsum of the foot cause toe extension.

**Figure 14-4**

Muscles and tendons of the
dorsum (top) of the foot

**Peroneus tertius**

**Extensor digitorum longus**

**Tibialis anterior**

**Extensor hallucis longus**

**Extensor hallucis brevis**

**Lateral**     **Medial**

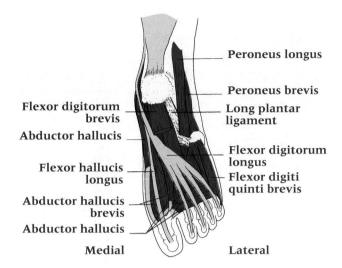

Peroneus longus

Peroneus brevis

Flexor digitorum
brevis

Long plantar
ligament

Abductor hallucis

Flexor digitorum
longus

Flexor hallucis
longus

Flexor digiti
quinti brevis

Abductor hallucis
brevis

Abductor hallucis

**Medial**                    **Lateral**

**Figure 14-5**

Muscles on the plantar
(bottom) surface of the foot

## PREVENTION OF FOOT INJURIES

Of major importance in preventing foot injuries is the understanding of
the foot's structure and mechanics, types of footwear, and surface concerns. Coaches must pay particular attention to athletes who may be predisposed to injuries caused by muscular or tendinous tightness or, conversely, weakness or hypermobility. Such situations, when recognized
early, can usually be remedied by exercise, by the use of appropriate shoe
inserts or *orthotics,* or by selecting appropriate shoes.[7] Strengthening,
stretching, and mobility exercises should be performed routinely by athletes in sports that place a great deal of stress and strain on the feet.

The foot must continually adapt to the contact surface. Training on surfaces that are irregular and variable in resilience can ultimately serve to
strengthen the foot over time. However, a nonyielding surface may in some
cases overstress joints and soft tissue, eventually leading to an acute or chronic
pathological condition in the foot or somewhere in the kinetic chain. In contrast, a surface that is too resilient and absorbs too much of the impact energy
may lead to early fatigue in sports such as basketball and indoor tennis.

The majority of foot skin conditions are preventable. The athlete
should be instructed on proper foot hygiene, which includes proper
washing and drying of the feet following activity and changing to clean
socks daily. The coach should emphasize wearing properly fitting shoes
and socks. Athletes who have abnormal foot stresses caused by faulty mechanics may find the use of custom orthotics to be helpful.

Nearly all blisters, calluses,
corns, and ingrown toenails
are preventable.

## FOOT ASSESSMENT

### History

A coach who is deciding how to manage a foot injury must make an assessment to determine the type of injury and its history. The following
questions should be asked:

- How did the injury occur?
- Did it occur suddenly or come on slowly?
- Was the mechanism a sudden strain, twist, or blow to the foot?
- What type of pain is there? Is there muscle weakness? Are there noises such as crepitation during movement? Is there any alteration in sensation?
- Can the athlete point to the exact site of pain? When is the pain or other symptoms more or less severe?
- On what type of surface has the athlete been training? What type of footwear was being used during training? Is it appropriate for the type of training? Is discomfort increased when footwear is worn?
- Is this the first time this condition has occurred, or has it happened before? If so, when, how often, and under what circumstances?

## Observation

The athlete should be observed to determine the following:

- Whether he or she is favoring the foot, is walking with a limp, or is unable to bear weight.
- Whether the injured part is deformed, swollen, or discolored.
- Whether the foot changes color when bearing weight and not bearing weight (changing rapidly from a darker to a lighter pink when not bearing weight).
- Whether the foot is well aligned and whether it maintains its shape when bearing weight.
- What do the wear patterns look like on the sole of the shoe? Is there symmetry between the two shoes?

## Palpation

Palpation of the bony structures should be done first for deformities or areas of point tenderness. Palpation of the muscles and their tendons in the foot is essential to detect **point tenderness,** abnormal swelling or lumps, muscle spasm, or muscle guarding.[3]

| **point tenderness** |
| --- |
| Pain is produced when the site of injury is palpated. |

| **exostoses** (ek **sosto** ses) |
| --- |
| A bony outgrowth. |

**Figure 14-6**

A pump bump that develops from retrocalcaneal bursitis can be protected using a doughnut-type pad.

## RECOGNITION AND MANAGEMENT OF FOOT INJURIES

### Retrocalcaneal Bursitis (Pump Bump)

**Cause of injury** The retrocalcaneal bursa lies between the calcaneous and the Achilles tendon on the back of the heel. This bursa can become chronically irritated and inflamed by constant rubbing or pressure from the heel counter of a shoe.[6] If inflammation continues for many months, a bone callus, or **exostoses,** is likely to form on the back of the heel (Figure 14-6). This exostoses has been referred to as a *pump bump.* (A pump is a type of woman's shoe with a heel counter that tends to cross right over the retrocalcaneal bursa).

**Signs of injury**  All the signs of bursitis—tenderness, swelling, warmth, and redness—will be present and will progress eventually to a palpable and tender bony bump on the back of the calcaneous.

**Care**  A doughnut-type pad should be constructed and placed around the area of tenderness to disperse pressure created by the heel counter. Also, a heel lift can help to change the site of pressure. The athlete may also want to choose a shoe with a heel counter that is either a little higher or lower than the one presently being worn.

### Heel Bruise

**Cause of injury**  Of the many contusions and bruises that an athlete may receive, none is more disabling than the heel bruise on the bottom of the calcaneous.[14] Sport activities that demand a sudden stop-and-go response or a sudden change from a horizontal to a vertical movement, such as basketball jumping, high jumping, and long horse vaulting, are particularly likely to cause heel bruises.[6] The heel has a thick, cornified skin layer and a heavy fat pad covering, but even this thick padding cannot protect against a sudden abnormal force directed to this area.

> The athlete who is prone to heel bruises should routinely wear a padded heel cup.

**Signs of injury**  When injury occurs, the athlete complains of severe pain in the heel and is unable to tolerate the stress of weight bearing. An acute bruise of the heel may progress to chronic inflammation of the bone covering (periosteum).

**Care**  Initially, cold is applied to the heel bruise, and if possible, the athlete should not step on the heel for at least 24 hours. If pain when walking has subsided by the third day, the athlete may resume moderate activity—with the protection of a heel cup or protective doughnut (Figure 14-7). The coach should be aware that an athlete who is prone to or who needs protection from a heel bruise should routinely wear a heel cup with a foam rubber pad as a preventive aid. Surrounding the heel with a firm heel cup diffuses traumatic forces.[12]

### Plantar Fasciitis

**Cause of condition**  Heel pain is a very common problem in both the athletic and nonathletic populations. The plantar fascia runs the

**Figure 14-7**

Protection of a heel bruise using, A and B, A heel cup. C, A doughnut pad.

A          B          C

14-1

*Critical Thinking* Exercise

A distance runner is
complaining of pain that started
on the bottom of her heel and
now seems to also be bothering
the long arch. She states that
pain seems to be the worst in
the morning when she first gets
out of bed.

? What condition usually
results in these complaints and
how should this problem be
managed?

length of the sole of the foot (refer to Figure 14-3). It assists in maintaining the stability of the foot and in supporting the longitudinal arch.[4] A number of conditions have been studied as possible causes of plantar fasciitis. They include leg length discrepancy, inflexibility of the longitudinal arch, tightness of the gastrocnemius-soleus unit, wearing shoes without sufficient arch support, a lengthened stride during running, and running on soft surfaces.[4]

**Signs of condition** The athlete complains of pain in the anterior medial heel, usually at the attachment of the plantar fascia to the calcaneus that eventually moves more centrally into the middle of the plantar fascia. This pain is particularly troublesome when the athlete rises in the morning or bears weight on the foot after sitting for a long period. However, the pain lessens after a few steps. Pain also is intensified when the toes and forefoot are forcibly dorsiflexed.

**Care** Management of plantar fasciitis generally requires an extended period of treatment. It is not uncommon for symptoms to persist for as long as 8 to 12 weeks. Vigorous heel cord stretching should be done, along with an exercise to stretch the plantar fascia in the arch. Use of a heel cup compresses the fat pad under the calcaneous and provides a cushion under the area of irritation (refer to Figure 14-7). A simple arch taping often allows pain-free ambulation. Orthotic therapy is very useful in the treatment of this problem. In some cases, particularly during a competitive season, the athlete may continue to train and compete if symptoms and associated pain are not prohibitive.

## Fractures of the Metatarsals

**Cause of injury** Fractures of the metatarsals can be caused by direct force, such as having the foot stepped on by another player, by being kicked or kicking another object, or by twisting or torsional stresses.[6] The most common acute fracture is to the neck of the fifth metatarsal (Jones fracture).

**Signs of injury** It is very difficult to differentiate a fracture from a sprain of the metatarsal ligaments. Fractures of the metatarsals are characterized by swelling and pain. A fracture may be more point tender and occasionally it may be possible to palpate a deformity. The most definitive way to distinguish a fracture from a sprain is to get an x ray.

**Care** Treatment is usually symptomatic, with RICE used to control swelling. Once swelling has subsided, a short leg walking cast is applied for 3 to 6 weeks. Ambulation is usually possible by the second week. A shoe with a large toe box should be worn.

### Jones Fracture

**Cause of injury** A Jones fracture involves a fracture at the neck of the fifth metatarsal that can occur from overuse, acute inversion, or high-velocity rotational forces (Figure 14-8). A Jones fracture occurs most often as a sequela of a stress fracture.

**Signs of injury** The athlete complains of a sharp pain on the lateral border of the foot and usually reports hearing a "pop." Because of a his-

**Medial**          **Lateral**

**Jones fracture of fifth metatarsal**

**Figure 14-8**

A Jones fracture occurs at the neck of the fifth metatarsal.

tory of poor blood supply and delayed healing, a Jones fracture may result in nonunion, requiring an extended period of rehabilitation.[5]

**Care**    A Jones fracture of the fifth metatarsal usually requires a non-weight-bearing short leg cast for 6 to 8 weeks for nondisplaced fractures. With cases of delayed union, nonunion, or especially displaced fractures, the Jones fracture requires internal fixation, with or without bone grafting. In the highly competitive athlete, immediate surgical internal fixation should be recommended.

### Second Metatarsal Stress Fractures

**Cause of injury**    Second metatarsal stress fractures, also referred to as *march fractures*, occur most often in running and jumping sports. As with other overuse injuries in the foot, the most common causes include structural deformities in the foot, training errors, changes in training surfaces, and wearing inappropriate shoes.[5]

*Morton's toe* is a condition in which the first metatarsal is abnormally short, making the second toe appear longer than the great toe (Figure 14-9). In a normal walking gait, the first metatarsal bears most of

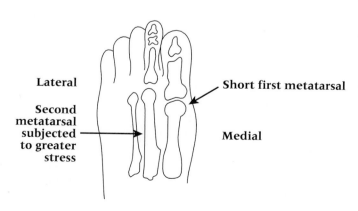

**Lateral**

**Second metatarsal subjected to greater stress**

**Short first metatarsal**

**Medial**

**Figure 14-9**

In a Morton's toe, the first metatarsal is abnormally short.

the weight. However, because the first metatarsal in a Morton's toe is short, the second metatarsal must bear a greater percentage of the forces during walking and even greater forces in a running gait. Thus a Morton's toe increases the chance of a stress fracture of the second metatarsal.[6]

**Signs of injury** The athlete usually complains of pain and point tenderness along the second metatarsal. Commonly the athlete indicates the presence of pain during running and perhaps also during walking. The athlete may also feel ongoing pain and aching during non-weight-bearing movements.

**Care** Treatment for stress fractures should focus on determining the precipitating cause or causes and alleviating those that created the problem. Athletes with second metatarsal stress fractures tend to do well with modified rest and non-weight-bearing exercises such as pool running or using an upper body ergometer or stationary bike to maintain cardiorespiratory fitness for 2 to 4 weeks. These exercises are followed by the athlete's progressive return to running and jumping sports over a 2- to 3-week period using appropriate shoes.

### Metatarsal Arch Strain

**Cause of injury** Athletes with hypermobility of the metatarsals caused by laxity in the ligaments are prone to sprain of the metatarsal arch.[5] Hypermobility allows the metatarsals in the foot to spread apart (splayed foot), giving the appearance of a fallen metatarsal arch (Figure 14-10).[11]

**Signs of injury** The athlete has pain or cramping in the metatarsal region. There is point tenderness, with signs of inflammation and weakness in the area. Pain in this region is called **metatarsalgia**.[11] Although meta-

Fatigue, poor posture, overuse, excessive weight, or improperly fitting shoes may damage the supporting tissue of the arch.

**Figure 14-10**

In hypermobility the metatarsals splay apart.

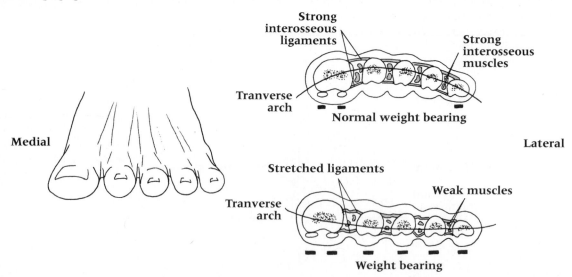

tarsalgia is a general term to describe pain or cramping in the ball of the foot, it is more commonly associated with pain under the second and sometimes the third metatarsal head. A heavy callus often forms in the area of pain.

**Care**   Treatment of acute metatarsalgia usually consists of applying a pad to elevate the depressed metatarsal heads. The pad is placed in the center and just behind the ball of the foot (metatarsal heads) (Figure 14-11). A daily regimen of exercise should concentrate on strengthening foot muscles and stretching the heel cord.

## Longitudinal Arch Strain

**Cause of injury**   Longitudinal arch strain is usually caused by subjecting the musculature on the plantar surface of the foot to unaccustomed stresses and forces when coming in contact with hard playing surfaces. In this condition, there is a flattening or depression of the longitudinal arch **(pes planus)** while the foot is in the midsupport phase, resulting in a strain to the arch.[13] Such a strain may appear suddenly, or it may develop slowly over a considerable length of time.

**Signs of injury**   As a rule, pain is experienced only when running is attempted and usually appears just below the medial malleolus and the posterior tibial tendon, accompanied by swelling and tenderness along the medial aspects of the foot. Prolonged strain will also involve the calcaneonavicular ligament and first cuneiform with the navicular. The flexor muscle of the great toe (flexor hallucis longus) often develops tenderness as a result of overuse in compensating for the stress on the ligaments.

Many people have what appears to be a flat foot or a fallen longitudinal arch with no associated symptoms or pain whatsoever. In these cases the rule that should always be followed is "If it's not broken, don't try to fix it" (Figure 14-12).

**Care**   The management of a longitudinal arch strain involves immediate care consisting of RICE followed by appropriate therapy and reduction of weight bearing. Weight bearing must be performed painfree. Arch taping might be used to allow earlier pain-free weight bearing.

**metatarsalgia** (metah tar **sal** gee ah)
Pain on the bottom of the foot.

**pes planus (pees** plan is)
Flat feet.

As long as an existing condition in the foot is *not* causing pain, don't try to fix it.

**Figure 14-11**

A metatarsal bar placed just behind the metatarsal heads is used to reduce metatarsalgia.

**Figure 14-12**

The approach to take with athletes who appear to have a flat foot or a fallen longitudinal arch but have no associated symptoms: "If it's not broken, don't try to fix it."

**Figure 14-13**

Hammer toes

Fractures and dislocations of
the toes can be caused by
kicking an object or stubbing
a toe.

 14-2

***Critical Thinking*** Exercise

A field hockey player complains
to the athletic trainer of
swelling, tenderness, and
aching in the head of the first
metatarsophalangeal joint of
her left foot. On inspection, the
athletic trainer observes that
the great toe is deviated
laterally.

**?** What is this condition
commonly called, and why
does it occur?

 14-3

***Critical Thinking*** Exercise

A soccer player complains of
intermittent pain in the region
between the third and fourth
toes of the left foot. Pain along
with tingling and numbness
seems to radiate from the base
to the tip of the toes during
weight bearing.

**?** What condition usually
causes these symptoms and
how can it be managed?

## Hammer Toes

**Cause of condition**    Hammer, or clawed, toes may be congenital, but more often the condition is caused by long-term wearing of shoes that are too short and that cramp the toes (Figure 14-13).[9] Hammer toe usually involves the second or third toe, whereas clawed toes involve more than one toe. In both conditions the toe joints become malaligned, and the foot develops overly contracted flexor tendons and overly stretched extensor tendons. This deformity eventually results in the formation of hard corns or calluses on the exposed joints.

**Care**    Quite often surgery is the only cure. However, wearing properly fitting shoes and protective taping can help prevent irritation.

## Fractures and Dislocations of the Toes (Phalanges)

**Cause of injury**    Fractures of the phalanges may be incurred by kicking an object or stubbing a toe or dropping a heavy object on the toes.

**Signs of injury**    Generally fractures and dislocations of the phalanges are accompanied by swelling and discoloration. If the fracture is to the proximal phalanx of the great toe or to the distal phalanx and also involves the interphalangeal joint, the injury should be referred to a physician.

**Care**    If the break is in the bone shaft, adhesive tape is applied. However, if more than one toe is involved, a cast may be applied for a few days. As a rule, 3 or 4 weeks of inactivity permit healing, although tenderness may persist for some time. A shoe with a wide toe box should be worn; in cases of great toe fracture, a stiff sole should be worn.

Dislocations of the phalanges are less common than fractures. If one occurs, it is usually a dislocation of the proximal joint of the middle phalanx. The mechanism of injury is the same as for fractures. Reduction is usually performed easily without anesthesia by a physician.

## Bunions (Hallux Valgus Deformity)

**Cause of injury**    A bunion, also referred to as an exostoses, is a painful deformity of the head of the first metatarsal. A bunion involves bony enlargement of the head of the first metatarsal that progresses to the point at which the great toe becomes malaligned and moves laterally toward the second toe, sometimes to such an extent that it eventually overlaps the second toe, creating what is called a hallux valgus deformity (Figure 14-14).[8] This type of bunion may also be associated with a depressed or flattened transverse arch. Often the bunion occurs from wearing shoes that are pointed, too narrow, too short, or have high heels.

**Signs of injury**    A bunion is one of the most frequent painful deformities of the great toe. As the bunion is developing, there is tenderness, swelling, and enlargement with calcification of the head of the first metatarsal. Poorly fitting shoes increase the irritation and pain.

**Care**    Shoe selection plays an important role in the treatment of bunions. Shoes of the proper width cause less irritation to the bunion. Protective devices such as some type of doughnut pad over the bunion

Hallux ← valgus

**Figure 14-14**

A bunion with a hallux valgus deformity

help disperse pressure, and tape can also be used. If the condition progresses, a special orthotic device may help normalize foot mechanics and significantly reduce the symptoms and progression of a bunion. Surgery to correct the hallux valgus deformity is very common during the later stages of this condition.

## Morton's Neuroma

**Cause of condition**   A **neuroma** is a mass occurring in the common plantar nerve. It occurs most commonly between the third and fourth metatarsal heads, where the nerve is the thickest because it is receiving both branches from the medial and lateral plantar nerves (Figure 14-15).[8]

**Signs of condition**   The athlete complains of severe intermittent pain radiating from the distal metatarsal heads to the tips of the toes; the pain is often relieved when the foot is not bearing weight. The athlete complains of a burning numbness in the forefoot that is often localized to the third web space and radiating to the toes. Hyperextension of the toes on weight bearing, as in squatting, stair climbing, or running, can increase the symptoms. Wearing shoes with a narrow toe box or high heel can increase the symptoms.

**Care**   Either a metatarsal bar is placed just proximal to the metatarsal heads or a teardrop-shaped pad is placed between the heads of the third and fourth metatarsals in an attempt to have these toes splay apart with weight bearing (Figure 14-16). Shoe selection also plays an important role in treatment of neuromas. A shoe that is wide in the toe box area should be selected.

**Figure 14-15**

A Morton's neuroma usually occurs between the third and fourth metatarsal heads.

**neuroma**
Enlargement of a nerve.

## Turf Toe

**Cause of injury**   Turf toe is a hyperextension injury resulting in a sprain of the great toe, either from repetitive overuse or trauma.[10] Typically, these injuries occur on unyielding synthetic turf, although they can occur on grass also. Many of these injuries occur because artificial turf shoes often are more flexible and allow more dorsiflexion of the great toe. Some shoe companies have addressed this problem by adding steel or other materials to the forefoot of their turf shoes to stiffen them. A sprain of the great toe can also occur from kicking some nonyielding object.

**Figure 14-16**

A teardrop-shaped pad will spread the metatarsal heads apart during weight bearing.

14–4

*Critical Thinking* Exercise

A football player who both
practices and plays on artificial
turf complains of pain in his
right great toe.

? What type of injury
frequently occurs to the great
toe when competing on
artificial turf?

**Care**   Flat insoles that have thin sheets of steel under the forefoot
are available. When commercially made products are not available, a
thin, flat piece of thermoplastic material may be placed under the shoe
insole or may be molded to the foot. Taping the toe to prevent dorsiflexion may be done separately or in addition to one of the shoe-stiffening
suggestions (refer to Figure 11-13). In less severe cases, the athlete can
continue to play with the addition of a rigid insole. With more severe
sprains, 3 to 4 weeks may be required for pain to subside to the point at
which the athlete can push off on the great toe.

### Calluses

**Cause of condition**   Foot calluses may be caused by shoes that are
too narrow or too short. Calluses that develop from friction can be
painful because the fatty layer loses its elasticity and cushioning effect.
The excess callus moves as a gross mass, becoming highly vulnerable to
tears, cracks, and ultimately, infections.[2]

**Care**   Athletes who are prone to excess calluses should be encouraged to use an emery callus file after each shower. Massaging small
amounts of lanolin into devitalized calluses once or twice a week after
practice may help maintain some tissue elasticity. The coach may have
the athlete decrease the calluses' thickness and increase their smoothness
by sanding or pumicing. NOTE: *Great care should be taken not to remove the callus totally and the protection it affords at a given pressure point.*

Athletes whose shoes are properly fitted but who still develop heavy
calluses commonly have faulty foot mechanics that may require special
orthotics. Special cushioning devices such as wedges, doughnuts, and
arch supports may help to distribute the weight on the feet more evenly
and thus reduce skin stress. Excessive callus accumulation can be prevented by (1) wearing at least one layer of socks; (2) wearing shoes that
are the correct size and in good condition; and (3) routinely applying materials such as petroleum jelly to reduce friction.

### Blisters

**Cause of injury**   As a result of shearing forces acting on the skin,
blisters develop in which fluid accumulates below the outer skin layer.
This fluid may be clear, bloody, or infected. Soft feet coupled with this
shearing skin stress can produce severe blisters. The application of petroleum jelly can protect the skin against abnormal friction. Wearing socks
with no folds or wrinkles can protect the athlete with sensitive skin or the
one who perspires excessively.[2] Wearing the correct-size shoe is essential.
Shoes should be broken in before being used for long periods.

**Care**   If a blister or hot spot arises, the athlete has several options:
(1) cover the irritated skin with a friction-proofing material, such as petroleum jelly, (2) cover the blister with an adhesive bandage, or (3) apply a doughnut pad that surrounds the blister.

When caring for a blister, the coach must be aware at all times of
the possibility of infection from contamination. Any blister that appears

**BIOHAZARD**

**14-1** *Focus Box*

**Caring for a Torn Blister**

1. Cleanse the blister and surrounding tissue with soap and water; rinse with an antiseptic.
2. Using sterile scissors, make a small cut along the perimeter of the blister.
3. Drain the fluid using a sterile gauze pad.
4. Apply antibiotic ointment under and around the loose skin; cover the area with a sterile dressing.
5. Apply a doughnut pad around blister.
6. Change dressing daily and check for signs of infection.
7. Within 2 or 3 days, or when the underlying tissue has hardened sufficiently, remove the dead skin by trimming the skin on a bevel and as close as possible to the perimeter of the blister.

**Figure 14-17**

In some cases a blister should be opened and padded to allow the athlete to continue to play.

to be infected requires medical attention. In sports, two approaches are generally used to care for blisters. The conservative approach is that a blister should not be contaminated by cutting or puncturing but should be protected from further insult by a small doughnut until the initial irritation has subsided (Figure 14-17). However, the pressure of the fluid inside the blister can often be extremely painful and in some cases debilitating. Puncturing may be necessary to allow the athlete to continue to play or practice. Focus Box 14-1 details the technique for opening a blister. Conservative care of blisters is preferred when there is little danger of tearing or aggravation through activity. A product called Second Skin by Spenco is widely used on blisters to provide a protective coating.

### Corns

**Cause of condition**  The hard corn is the most serious type of corn. It is caused by the pressure of improperly fitting shoes, the same mechanism that causes calluses. Hammer toes and hard corns are usually associated; the hard corns form on the tops of the deformed toes. The soft corn is the result of a combination of wearing narrow shoes and excessive foot perspiration (Figure 14-18).[2]

**Signs of condition**  The corn usually forms between the fourth and fifth toes. A circular area of thickened, white, macerated skin appears between and at the base of the toes. There also appears to be a black dot in the center of the corn. Both pain and inflammation are likely to be present. Symptoms are local pain and disability, with inflammation and thickening of soft tissue.

**Care**  When caring for a soft corn, the best procedure is to have the athlete wear properly fitting shoes, keep the skin between the toes clean and dry, and decrease pressure by keeping the toes separated with cotton

**Figure 14-18**

A, Hard corns appear on the
top of a toe and are usually
associated with hammer toes.
B, Soft corns usually appear
between the fourth and fifth
toes.

or lamb's wool. The athlete should soak feet daily in warm, soapy water
to soften the corn. To alleviate further irritation, the corn should be protected by a small felt or sponge rubber doughnut.

Ingrown Toenails

**Cause of condition**   An ingrown toenail is a condition in which the
leading side edge of the toenail has grown into the soft tissue nearby,
usually resulting in severe inflammation and infection.[1]

**Care**   It is important that the athlete's shoes be of the proper length
and width, because continued pressure on a toenail can lead to serious
irritation or cause it to become ingrown. In most cases ingrown toenails can be prevented by trimming the nails correctly. The nail must
be trimmed so that its margins do not penetrate the tissue on the sides.
Also, the nail should be left sufficiently long that it is clear of the underlying tissue but should be cut short enough that it is not irritated by
either shoes or socks. Focus Box 14-2 details the care for an ingrown
toenail.

---

14-2   *Focus Box*

---

**Managing the Ingrown Toenail**

1. Soak the toe in hot water (110° to 120° F) [43.3° to 48.8° C]) for
   approximately 20 minutes, two or three times daily.
2. When the nail is soft and pliable, use forceps to insert a wisp of cotton
   under the edge of the nail and lift it from the soft tissue.
3. Continue this procedure until the nail has grown out sufficiently to be
   trimmed straight across.

An ingrown toenail can easily become infected. If this occurs, the athlete
should be immediately referred to a physician for treatment.

## Toenail Hematoma

**Cause of injury**    Blood can accumulate under a toenail as a result of the toe being stepped on, of dropping an object on the toe, or of kicking another object. Repetitive shearing forces on toenails, as may occur in the shoe of a long-distance runner, may also cause bleeding into the nail bed. In any case, blood that accumulates in a confined space underneath the nail is likely to produce extreme pain and can ultimately cause loss of the nail.[1]

**Signs of injury**    Bleeding into the nail bed may be either immediate or slow, producing considerable pain. The area under the toenail assumes a bluish-purple color and gentle pressure on the nail greatly exacerbates pain.

**Care**    An ice pack should be applied immediately, and the foot should be elevated to decrease bleeding. Within the next 12 to 24 hours, the pressure of the blood under the nail should be released by drilling a small hole though the nail into the nail bed. This drilling must be done under sterile conditions and is best done by either a physician or an athletic trainer. It is not uncommon to have to drill the nail a second time because more blood is likely to accumulate.

BIOHAZARD

## SUMMARY

- The human foot must function both to absorb forces and to provide a stable base of support during walking, running, and jumping.

- The twenty-six bones in the foot are held together by an intricate network of ligaments and fascia and are moved by a complicated group of muscles.

- Foot injuries may be prevented by selecting appropriate footwear and using various orthotic devices inserted into the shoe to protect the foot from abnormal forces, stresses, and strains.

- A pump bump develops from chronic retrocalcaneal bursitis on the back of the heel.

- Plantar fasciitis is pain in the anterior medial heel, usually at the attachment of the plantar fascia to the calcaneus. Orthotics in combination with stretching exercises can significantly reduce pain.

- A Jones fracture is a fracture of the neck of the fifth metatarsal that often results in delayed healing.

- The most common stress fracture in the foot involves the second metatarsal (march fracture).

- Metatarsal and longitudinal arch sprains are best treated by inserting appropriate support pads into the shoes.

- A bunion is a deformity of the head of the first metatarsal in which the large toe assumes a hallux valgus position.

- To treat a Morton's neuroma, a metatarsal bar is placed just proximal to the metatarsal heads or a teardrop-shaped pad is placed between the heads of the third and fourth metatarsals in an attempt to have these toes splay apart with weight bearing.

- Turf toe is a hyperextension injury resulting in a sprain of the great toe.

- The foot within the shoe can sustain forces that produce calluses, blisters, corns, or ingrown toenails.

---

*Solutions to Critical Thinking* Exercises

**14-1** These complaints are most typically associated with plantar fasciitis, which can be treated with a combination of vigorous heel cord stretching, stretching the plantar fascia in the arch, using a heel cup, arch taping, and using an orthotic with increased arch support.

**14-2** This condition is a bunion or hallux valgus deformity. It is associated with wearing shoes that are too pointed, narrow, or short. It may begin with an inflamed bursa over the metatarsophalangeal joint. It can be as-

sociated with a depressed transverse arch or a pronated foot.

**14-3** Most likely the athlete has a Morton's neuroma. A metatarsal bar or a teardrop-shaped pad applied in the correct position on the sole of the foot can help to spread the metatarsal heads apart and take pressure off the neuroma, reducing the symptoms.

**14-4** A sprain of the great toe is often referred to as turf toe. It results from a hyperextension of the great toe and usually occurs in athletes playing on artificial turf.

## REVIEW QUESTIONS AND CLASS ACTIVITIES

1. Briefly describe the anatomy of the foot.
2. In evaluating an acute condition in the foot region, what general observations can be made?
3. What measures can be taken to prevent foot injuries?
4. What is the relationship between a pump bump and retrocalcaneal bursitis?
5. What is a Jones fracture, and why does it take so long to heal?
6. How is it possible for a heel bruise to lead to plantar fasciitis?
7. How are stress fractures of the second metatarsal managed?
8. Discuss how various arch sprains can be treated.
9. What injuries may potentially result from wearing shoes that are too tight?
10. How does a Morton's toe differ from a Morton's neuroma?
11. How would you care for a chronic case of turf toe?
12. What is the recommended procedure in caring for a blister on the foot?

 **Dynamic Human CD**

For more information on skeletal anatomy of the foot click on:

- Skeletal
- Anatomy
- Gross anatomy
- Lower limbs

- Tibia/fibula
- Then, Foot

To take a closer look at the muscles that are involved in foot movement click on:

- Muscular
- Anatomy
- Body regions
- Lower leg
- Then, Foot

## REFERENCES

1. Adams BB: Running-related toenail abnormality, *Physician Sportsmed* 27(13):85, 1999.
2. Burkhart CG: Skin disorders of the foot in active patients, *Physician Sportsmed* 27(2):88, 1999.
3. Cornwall MW: Common pathomechanics of the foot, *Ath Ther Today* 5(1):10, 2000.
4. Cornwall MW, McPoil TG: Plantar fasciitis: etiology and treatment, *JOSPT* 29(12):756, 1999.
5. Coughlin MJ: Forefoot disorders. In Baxter DE, editor: *The foot and ankle in sports,* St Louis, 1995, Mosby.
6. Crosby LA, McMullen ST: Heel pain in an active adolescent? *Physician Sportsmed* 21:125, 1993.
7. Dolan MG: The use of foot orthotic devices in clinical practice, *Ath Ther Today* 5(1):17, 2000.
8. Hunter S, Prentice WE: Rehabilitation of ankle and foot injuries. In Prentice WE, editor: *Rehabilitation techniques in sports medicine,* ed 3, Boston, 1999, WCB/McGraw-Hill.
9. Jaivin JS: Foot injuries and arthroscopy in sport, *Sports Med* 29(1):65, 2000.
10. Mann RA: Great toe disorders. In Baxter DE, editor: *The foot and ankle in sports,* St Louis, 1995, Mosby.
11. Myerson M: Tarsometatarsal joint injury, *Physician Sportsmed* 21:97, 1993.
12. Pfeffer GB: Plantar heel pain. In Baxter DE, editor: *The foot and ankle in sport,* St Louis, 1995, Mosby.
13. Sherman KP: The foot in sport, *Br J Sports Med* 33(1):6, 1999.
14. Stephens MM: Heel pain, *Physician Sportsmed* 20:87, 1992.

## ANNOTATED BIBLIOGRAPHY

Alexander I: *The foot: examination and diagnosis,* New York, 1997, Churchill-Livingston.

*Practical guide to clinical care of the foot and ankle. Presents anatomy, biomechanics, and a systematic approach to evaluation. Discusses common complaints.*

Baxter DE: *The foot and ankle in sport,* St Louis, 1995, Mosby.

*A complete medical text on all aspects of the foot and ankle. It covers common sports syndromes, anatomical disorders in sports, unique problems, shoes, orthoses, and rehabilitation.*

Tremaine MD, Elias M: *The foot and ankle source book: everything you need to know,* 1998, Lowell House.

*Discusses common problems affecting feet and ankles; from bunions and corns to flat feet and sports injuries. Surveys the range of problems, preventive treatments, orthopedic inserts, and other health solutions to foot ailments, providing an uncommon range of disorders and treatments ranging from self-help to surgery.*

**WEBSITES**

Foot and Ankle Web Index: http://
www.footandankle.com
*The foot and ankle link library at this
site is very helpful.*

Premiere Medical Search Engine:
http://www.medsite.com
*Type in any medical condition at this
site and it will search the Net to find relevant articles.*

Dr. Pribut's Running Injuries Page:
http://www.clarknet/pub/pribut/
spsport.html

Wheeless' Textbook of Orthopaedics:
http://www.medmedia.com/
med.htm
*An excellent page for injuries, anat-
omy, and x rays.*

North Shore Podiatry Foot Care Center: http://www.BUNIONBUSTERS.
com

# The Ankle and Lower Leg

*When you finish this chapter you will be able to:*

- Describe the bony, ligamentous, and muscular anatomy of the ankle and lower leg.
- List considerations for preventing injuries to the ankle and lower leg.
- Explain how to assess common ankle and lower leg injuries.
- Identify the possible causes and signs of various injuries that can occur in the ankle and lower leg.
- Explain the procedures that can be used in caring for ankle and lower leg injuries.

The ankle joint is composed of:
- Tibia
- Fibula
- Talus

The talocrural joint allows two motions:
- plantarflexion
- dorsiflexion

The subtalar joint allows two motions:
- inversion
- eversion

Medial ligament includes:
- Deltoid

## ANKLE AND LOWER LEG ANATOMY

### Bones

The portion of the anatomy below the knee and above the ankle is the lower leg. It is composed of the thicker tibia, which is more medial, and the thinner fibula, which is more lateral. The ankle joint or *talocrural joint* (sometimes called the ankle mortise) is formed by the thickened distal portion of the fibula, called the lateral malleolus; the thickened distal portion of the tibia, called the medial malleolus; and the more-or-less cube-shaped tarsal bone, called the talus, that fits between the two malleoli. The ankle joint allows two motions: plantarflexion and dorsiflexion. The joint between the talus and the calcaneous is called the *subtalar joint.* Inversion and eversion take place at the *subtalar joint* (Figure 15-1).

### Ligaments

The tibia and fibula are held together by the interosseous membrane, which extends the entire length of the two bones. The anterior and posterior tibiofibular ligaments bridge the tibia and fibula and form the distal portion of the interosseous membrane. The medial aspect of the ankle is relatively stable because of the thick deltoid ligament. The presence of this strong deltoid ligament combined with the fact that the lateral malleolus of the fibula extends further distally than the medial malleolus lim-

**Figure 15-1**

The ankle joint is formed by
the tibia, fibula, and talus.
The subtalar joint is formed
by the talus and calcaneus.

its the ability of the ankle to evert. Thus eversion ankle sprains are considerably less common than inversion sprains. The three lateral ligaments include the anterior talofibular, the posterior talofibular, and the calcaneofibular. The lateral ligaments collectively limit inversion and are much more susceptible to injury (Figure 15-2).

## Muscles

Contraction of the muscles in the lower leg produces movement at the ankle joint. The muscles of the lower leg are divided into four distinct groups. Each of the four muscle groups is contained separately within a compartment by thick sheets of fascia (connective tissue) that surround them. The muscles in the anterior compartment dorsiflex the ankle, the muscles in the superficial posterior compartment plantarflex the ankle, the muscles in the lateral compartment evert the ankle, and the muscles in the deep posterior compartment invert the ankle (Figure 15-3).

## PREVENTION OF LOWER LEG AND ANKLE INJURIES

Many lower leg and ankle injuries, especially sprains, can be reduced by heel cord (Achilles tendon) stretching, strengthening of key muscles,

Lateral ligaments include:
• Anterior talofibular
• Posterior talofibular
• Calcaneofibular

Muscle actions by
compartment:
• Anterior compartment—
  dorsiflex the ankle
• Superficial posterior
  compartment—plantarflex
  the ankle
• Lateral compartment—
  evert the ankle
• Deep posterior
  compartment—invert the
  ankle

**Figure 15-2**

Major ligaments of the ankle:
A, Lateral aspect. B, Medial
aspect.

**Figure 15-3**

The muscles of the lower leg are divided into four distinct groups contained separately within individual compartments: the anterior compartment, superficial posterior compartment, lateral compartment, and deep posterior compartment.

Preventing lower leg and ankle injuries:
• Heel cord stretching
• Strength training
• Neuromuscular control
• Appropriate footwear
• Ankle taping and bracing

improving neuromuscular control, choosing appropriate footwear, and when necessary, proper taping or bracing.[10,11]

## Heel Cord Stretching

The athlete with a tight heel cord should routinely stretch before and after practice.[21] To properly stretch the heel cord, the ankle should be dorsiflexed and the knee fully extended to stretch the gastrocnemius muscle, and then the knee should be flexed to about 30 degrees to stretch the soleus muscle (Figure 15-4). There should be at least 10 degrees of dorsiflexion for normal ankle motion to occur.

## Strength Training

Achieving both static and dynamic joint stability through strength training is critical in preventing ankle injury (Figure 15-5). A balance in strength throughout the full range of motion must be developed and maintained in each of the four muscle groups that surround the ankle joint.[17] Strengthening exercises should be done in eversion and inversion, which can be done by rocking the ankle back and forth on a wobble board, and also in plantarflexion and dorsiflexion, which can be done using surgical tubing.

## Neuromuscular Control

As is the case with strength training, maintaining neuromuscular control is critical to prevention of injury to the ankle joint. Neuromuscular control relies on the central nervous system to interpret and integrate proprioceptive and kinesthetic information and then to control individual muscles and joints to produce coordinated movements that collectively protect the joint from injury. Thus, the foot and ankle must respond quickly to any uneven surface condition. Ankle joint position sense can be enhanced by training on uneven surfaces or by spending time each day on a balance board, or wobble board (Figure 15-6).

### Footwear

As discussed in Chapters 6 and 14, proper footwear can be an important factor in reducing injuries to both the foot and the ankle. Shoes should not be used in activities for which they were not intended—for example, running shoes, which are designed for straight-ahead activity, should not be worn to play basketball, a sport demanding a great deal of lateral movement.

**Figure 15-4**

Stretching techniques for the heel cord complex: A, Stretching position for the gastrocnemius muscle. B, Stretching position for the soleus muscle.

**Figure 15-5**

Strengthening exercises are important in prevention of ankle sprains and may be done using. A, surgical tubing resistance or B, a wobble board.

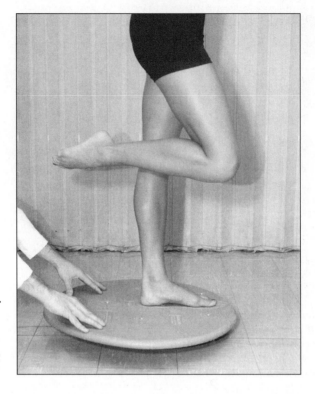

**Figure 15-6**

The BAPS board is an
excellent device both for
strengthening and for
reestablishing neuromuscular
control.

## Preventive Ankle Wrapping, Taping, and Bracing

There is some doubt about whether it is beneficial to routinely tape ankles that have no history of sprain. Tape, properly applied, can provide some prophylactic protection. Poorly applied tape does more harm than good. Tape that constricts soft tissue and blood circulation or disrupts normal biomechanical function can, in time, create unnecessary problems.

Ankle bracing can also offer protection to the ankle joint (Figure 15-7).[4] Braces may prevent lateral and inversion movement of the foot without inhibiting plantar flexion (see Chapter 6).

## ASSESSING THE LOWER LEG

### History

An athlete who complains of discomfort in the lower leg region should be asked the following questions:

- How long has it been hurting?
- Where is the pain or discomfort?
- Has the feeling changed or is there numbness?
- Is there a feeling of warmth?
- Is there any sense of muscle weakness or difficulty in walking?
- How did the problem occur?

**Figure 15-7**

Ankle braces may be used to
support weakened ankles.

## Observation

The athlete is generally observed for the following:

- Any postural deviations, such as toeing in, should be noted.
- Any walking difficulty should be noted, along with leg deformities or swelling.

## Palpation

Palpation should be done over the musculature in each of the four compartments. When fracture is suspected, a gentle percussive blow can be given to the tibia or fibula below or above the suspected site. Percussion can also be applied upward on the bottom of the heel. Such blows set up a vibratory force that resonates at the fracture, causing pain.

## ASSESSING THE ANKLE JOINT

The injured or painful ankle should be carefully evaluated to determine the possibility of fracture and whether medical referral is necessary.

## History

The athlete's history may vary, depending on whether the problem is the result of sudden trauma or is chronic. The athlete with an acute sudden trauma to the ankle should be asked the following questions:

- What trauma or mechanism occurred?
- What was heard when the injury occurred—a crack, snap, or pop?

- What were the duration and intensity of pain?
- How disabling was the occurrence? Could the athlete walk right away, or was he or she unable to bear weight for a time?
- Has a similar injury occurred before?
- Was there immediate swelling, or did the swelling occur later (or at all)? Where did the swelling occur?
- What past ankle injuries have occurred?

### Observation

In an initial look at the ankle, the athletic trainer determines the following:

- Is there an obvious deformity?
- Are the bony contours of the ankle normal and symmetrical, or is there a deviation such as a bony deformity?
- Is there any discoloration?
- Is there crepitus or abnormal sound in the ankle joint?
- Is heat, swelling, or redness present?
- Is the athlete in obvious pain?
- Does the athlete have a normal ankle range of motion?
- If the athlete is able to walk, is there a normal walking pattern?

### Palpation

Palpation in the ankle region should start with key bony landmarks and ligaments and progress to the musculature, especially the major ligaments that surround the ankle. The purpose of palpation in this region is to detect obvious structural deformities, swelling, and localized tenderness.

### Functional Examination

Muscle function is important in evaluating the ankle injury. If the athlete cannot execute or has difficulty performing the following functional activities, the athlete is not ready to return to activity.

- Walk on toes
- Walk on heels
- Hop on affected foot without heel touching surface
- Start or stop the running motion
- Change direction rapidly
- Run figure eights

## RECOGNITION AND MANAGEMENT OF INJURIES TO THE ANKLE

### Ankle Sprains

**Cause of injury**  Ankle sprains are among the more common injuries seen in athletics (Figure 15-8).[5] Injuries to the ligaments of the ankle may be classified by the mechanism of injury.

**Critical Thinking** Exercise

A basketball player sustains a grade I inversion sprain of her left ankle during a game. There is immediate pain and swelling, and she is unable to bear weight.

**?**  What is the most important first-aid goal immediately following injury, and how may that first-aid goal best be accomplished?

Ankle sprain classifications:
Inversion
Eversion
Dorsiflexion

**Figure 15-8**

Ankle sprains are very
common in athletics.

*Inversion sprains*    An inversion ankle sprain is most common and often
results in injury to the lateral ligaments. The anterior talofibular ligament
is the weakest of the three lateral ligaments. It is injured in an
inverted and plantarflexed position. The calcaneofibular and posterior
talofibular ligaments are also likely to be injured in inversion sprains as
the force of inversion is increased. Increased inversion force is needed to
tear the calcaneofibular ligament (Figure 15-9).[11]

*Eversion sprains*    Eversion ankle sprains are less common than inversion ankle sprains largely because of the bony and ligamentous anatomy.
Eversion injuries may involve an avulsion fracture of the tibia before the
deltoid ligament tears. The deltoid ligament may also be contused in inversion sprains because of impingement between the medial malleolus and
the calcaneous. Although eversion sprains are less common, these sprains
may take longer to heal than do inversion sprains (Figure 15-10).[11]

*Dorsiflexion sprains*    The anterior and posterior tibiofibular ligaments
are torn with forced dorsiflexion and are often injured in conjunction
with a severe sprain of the medial and lateral ligament complexes.
Sprains of these ligaments are extremely hard to treat and often take
months to heal. Return to sport may be delayed for a longer time than
for inversion or eversion sprains (Figure 15-11).[11]

**Signs of injury**    In a grade 1 sprain, there is some stretching or perhaps tearing of the ligamentous fibers with little or no joint instability.
Mild pain, little swelling, and joint stiffness may be apparent.

With a grade 2 sprain, there is some tearing and separation of the ligamentous fibers and moderate instability of the joint. Moderate-to-severe
pain, swelling, and joint stiffness should be expected.

The most important factor in
rehabilitation of an ankle
sprain is controlling initial
swelling with RICE.

**Figure 15-9**

Mechanism of an inversion
ankle sprain

Lateral          Medial

**Figure 15-10**

Mechanism of an eversion
ankle sprain

Grade 3 sprains involve total rupture of the ligament, manifested primarily by gross instability of the joint. Severe pain may be present initially, followed by little or no pain because of total disruption of nerve fibers. Swelling may be profuse, and thus the joint tends to become very stiff some hours after the injury. A grade 3 sprain with marked instability usually requires some form of immobilization lasting several weeks. Surgical repair or reconstruction may be necessary to correct an instability.

**Care**   For ankle sprains, as for all acute musculoskeletal injuries, initial treatment efforts should be directed toward limiting the amount of swelling. This treatment is more essential for ankle sprains than for any other injury. Controlling initial swelling is the single most important treatment measure that can be taken during the entire rehabilitation process. Limiting the amount of acute swelling can significantly reduce the time required for rehabilitation. Initial management includes ice, compression, elevation, rest, and protection.[11]

Coaches should follow exactly the technique described here to be maximally effective in controlling swelling following ankle sprain:

- As soon as possible following the injury, cut out a horseshoe-shaped pad made of felt or foam and fit it around the malleolus on the side of injury (Figure 15-12).[19]
- Apply a wet compression wrap over this pad. Wetting the elastic wrap helps facilitate the passage of cold from ice packs. Wrapping should begin covering the toes and progress proximally, completely

**Figure 15-11**

Mechanism of dorsiflexion
ankle sprain

**Figure 15-12**

A horseshoe-shaped pad
provides an excellent
compression when held in
place by an elastic wrap.

compressing the ankle joint and ending just below the level of the
gastrocnemius muscle (Figure 15-13A).

- Surround the ankle joint entirely with ice bags and secure them in
  place with a second, dry, elastic wrap. Ice bags should be left on for
  45 minutes initially and then 1 hour off and 30 minutes on as much
  as possible over the next 24 hours. During the following 48-hour
  period, ice should be applied as often as possible (Figure 15-13B).
- The foot and ankle should be elevated to a minimum of 45 degrees
  while icing. The ankle should be elevated as much as possible during
  the 72-hour period after injury. Keeping the injured part elevated
  while sleeping is particularly important (Figure 15-13C).
- The athlete should be placed on crutches to avoid weight bearing for
  a minimum of 24 hours following injury to allow the healing process
  to accomplish what it needs to. After 24 hours the athlete should be
  encouraged to begin weight bearing as soon as tolerated.

In the past, athletes were simply returned to sports once the pain was
low enough to tolerate the activity. Returning to full activity should include a gradual progression of functional activities (i.e., walking, jogging,
running, cutting, etc.) that slowly increase the stress on the ligament. The
specific demands of each individual sport dictate the individual drills of
this progression.

Ideally, the athlete should return to sport without the aid of ankle
support. However, it is common practice to wear some type of ankle support initially. Ankle taping has a stabilizing effect on unstable ankles
without interfering with motor performance. Taping the ankle and also
taping the shoe onto the foot to make the shoe and ankle function as one
unit has been recommended. High-topped footwear may further stabilize
the ankle. If cleated shoes are worn, cleats should be outset along the periphery of the shoe to provide stability. A protective ankle brace can also
be worn for support as a substitute for taping.[11]

## Ankle Fractures

**Cause of injury**  When assessing an ankle injury, the coach must
always be cautious about suspecting an ankle sprain when a fracture

A

B

C

**Figure 15-13**

RICE technique: A, A wet
compression wrap should be
applied over the horseshoe
pad; B, Ice bags should be
secured in place by a dry
compression wrap; and C,
The leg should be elevated
during the initial treatment
period.

**Lateral**                    **Medial**

**Figure 15-14**

The mechanism that
produces an ankle sprain can
also cause an avulsion
fracture.

actually exists. Ankle fractures can occur from several mechanisms that are similar to those that cause ankle sprains. In an inversion injury, medial malleolus fractures often occur along with a sprain of the lateral ligaments of the ankle (Figure 15-14). A fracture of the lateral malleolus is often more likely to occur than a sprain if an eversion force is applied to the ankle. With a fracture of the lateral malleolus, however, there may also be a sprain of the deltoid ligament. With avulsion injuries it is often the injured ligaments rather than the fracture that prolong the rehabilitation period.

**Signs of injury**    A fracture of the malleoli generally results in immediate swelling. There is point tenderness over the bone and apprehensiveness by the athlete when asked to bear weight.

**Care**    If the possibility of a fracture exists, the coach should splint the ankle and refer the athlete to the physician for x-ray examination and immobilization. Usually a physician treats fractures by casting the leg in a short walking cast for 6 weeks with early weight bearing. The course of rehabilitation following this period of immobilization is generally the same as for ankle sprains. Once near-normal levels of strength, flexibility, and neuromuscular control have been regained and the injured athlete can perform functional activities, full activity may be resumed.[11]

## Tendinitis

**Cause of injury**    Inflammation of the tendons surrounding the ankle joint is a common problem in athletes. The tendons most often involved are the posterior tibialis tendon behind the medial malleolus, the anterior tibialis on the dorsal surface of the ankle, and the peroneal tendons behind the lateral malleolus (Figure 15-15). Tendinitis in these tendons may result from one specific cause or from a collection of mechanisms including faulty foot mechanics, inappropriate or poor footwear that can create faulty foot mechanics, acute trauma to the tendon, tightness in the heel cord complex, or training errors.[9]

**Signs of injury**    Athletes who develop tendinitis are likely to complain of pain with both active movement and passive stretching; swelling

Common sites for tendinitis:
Anterior tibialis
Posterior tibialis
Peroneals

**Figure 15-15**

Common sites of tendinitis
around the ankle

**Critical Thinking** Exercise

A jogger, after running downhill
for an extended period,
experiences pain in the anterior
medial aspect of the left foot.
The condition is diagnosed as
anterior tibialis tendinitis.

**?** How should this condition
be managed?

around the area of the tendon caused by inflammation of the tendon;
crepitus on movement; and stiffness and pain following periods of inactivity but particularly in the morning.[9]

**Care** Techniques that reduce or eliminate inflammation, including
rest, therapeutic modalities (ice), and antiinflammatory medications,
should be used. The use of an orthotic device to correct the biomechanics
or taping the foot may also be helpful in reducing stress on the tendons.

In many instances, if the mechanism that is causing the irritation and
inflammation of the tendon is removed and the inflammatory process is
allowed to run its normal course, the tendinitis will resolve within 10
days to 2 weeks. It is best to allow the athlete to rest for a sufficient time
for tendon healing to take place.

## RECOGNITION AND MANAGEMENT
## OF INJURIES TO THE LOWER LEG

### Tibial and Fibular Fractures

The tibia is more commonly
fractured than the fibula.

**Cause of injury** The tibia and fibula constitute the bony components of the lower leg and are primarily responsible for weight bearing
and muscle attachment. The tibia is the most commonly fractured long
bone in the body; this injury is usually the result either of direct trauma
to the area or of indirect trauma, such as a combination rotatory/
compressive force. Fractures of the fibula are usually seen in combination
with a tibial fracture or as a result of direct trauma to the area (Figure 15-16).

**Signs of injury** Tibial fractures present with immediate pain, swelling, and possible deformity and may be open or closed. Fibular fractures
alone are usually closed and present with pain and point tenderness on
palpation and with ambulation.

**Care** Treatment of these fractures is immediate medical referral and
most likely a period of immobilization and restricted weight bearing for
weeks to possibly months, depending on the severity and involvement of
the injury.

**Figure 15-16**

Fractures of the lower leg can
be serious injuries.

## Tibial and Fibular Stress Fractures

**Cause of injury**   Stress fractures of the tibia and fibula are common in
sports. Studies indicate that tibial stress fractures occur at a higher rate than
those of the fibula. Stress fractures in the lower leg are usually the result of
repetitive loading during training and conditioning (Figure 15-17). Tibial
stress fractures are prevalent in athletes involved with jumping.[2]

**Signs of injury**   The athlete complains of pain with activity that
sometimes becomes worse when activity is stopped. Focal point tenderness on the bone helps differentiate a stress fracture from medial tibial
stress syndrome, which is located in the same area but is more diffuse.
Tibial stress fractures usually occur in the middle of the shaft whereas
fibular stress fractures are more likely to occur in the distal part of the
bone.[15]

**Care**   An athlete with a suspected stress fracture should be referred
to a physician for diagnosis. The physician will most likely do a bone
scan, looking for signs of inflammation. Immediate elimination of the of-
fending activity is most important. Generally recuperation requires about
a 2-week period during which the athlete can continue to be weight
bearing but must not engage in the activity that caused the problem in
the first place. The athlete must be educated on the importance of adhering to this advice to prevent further damage to the bone. Progressively
increasing stresses and strains can be placed on the bone so the athlete
can gradually return to normal training.[2,15]

## Shin Splints (Medial Tibial Stress Syndrome)

**Cause of injury**   The term **shin splints** is a catchall that has traditionally referred to any type of pain in the anterior aspect of the lower
leg. Medial tibial stress syndrome, as it is more correctly called, is a condition that involves increasing pain specifically at the distal two-thirds of
the posterior medial aspect of the tibia. A strain of the posterior tibialis

> **shin splints**
> Medial tibial stress syn-
> drome; anterior lower leg
> pain.

**Figure 15-17**

X ray film of a stress fracture
in the tibia

muscle and its fascial sheath at its attachment to the periosteum of the
distal tibia during running activities is the most likely mechanism for this
injury.[5] Pain can arise secondary to a combination of faulty foot mechanics, tightness of the heel cord, muscle weakness, improper footwear,
and training errors usually involving running on changing surfaces.[10]

**Signs of injury**   Pain is usually diffuse about the distal medial tibia
and the surrounding soft tissues. Initially, the area may only hurt after an
intense workout. As the condition worsens, daily ambulation may be
painful and morning pain and stiffness may be present. Medial tibial stress
syndrome can progress to a stress fracture if not treated appropriately.[13]

**Care**   Management of this condition should include physician referral to rule out the possibility of stress fracture via the use of bone scan
and plain films. Activity modification along with measures to maintain
cardiovascular fitness are set in place immediately. Correction of abnormal foot mechanics during walking and running must also be addressed
with shoes and, if needed, custom foot orthotics. Ice massage to the
area may be helpful in the reduction of localized pain and inflammation. A stretching program for the heel cord should be initiated (refer to
Figure 15-4). Occasionally, supportive taping to the longitudinal arch
might be helpful[10] (refer to Figure 11-12).

## Compartment Syndromes

**Cause of injury**   Compartment syndromes are conditions in which
increased pressure within one of the four compartments of the lower leg

Compartment syndrome
classifications:
• Acute compartment
  syndrome
• Acute exertional
  compartment syndrome
• Chronic compartment
  syndrome

causes compression of muscular and neurovascular structures within that compartment (refer to Figure 15-3). The anterior and deep posterior compartments are usually involved.[18]

Compartment syndromes can be divided into three categories: acute compartment syndrome, acute exertional compartment syndrome, and chronic compartment syndrome.[3] *Acute compartment syndrome* occurs secondary to direct trauma to the area, such as being kicked in the anterior aspect of the lower leg. Acute compartment syndrome is considered to be a medical emergency. *Acute exertional compartment syndrome* occurs without any precipitating trauma and can evolve with minimal to moderate activity. *Chronic compartment syndrome* is activity related in that the symptoms arise rather consistently at a certain point in the activity. Chronic compartment syndrome usually occurs during running and jumping activities, and symptoms cease when activity stops.[6,20]

**Signs of injury**  Because of increased intracompartmental pressure associated with compartment syndromes, the athlete complains of a deep aching pain, tightness and swelling of the involved compartment, and pain with passive stretching of the involved muscles. Reduced circulation and sensory changes can be detected in the foot. Intracompartmental pressure measurements further define the severity of the condition. A compartment syndrome that is not recognized, diagnosed, and treated properly can lead to a poor functional outcome for the athlete.[16]

**Care**  Immediate first aid for acute compartment syndrome should include the application of ice and elevation. However, in this situation a compression wrap should not be used to control swelling because there is already a problem with increased pressure in the compartment. Using a compression wrap only acts to increase the pressure.

In the case of both acute compartment syndrome and acute exertional compartment syndrome, measurement of intracompartmental pressures by a physician confirms the diagnosis with emergency fasciotomy to release the pressure within that compartment being the definitive treatment. Athletes undergoing anterior or deep posterior compartment fasciotomy may not return to full activity for 2 to 4 months post surgery.[12]

Management of chronic compartment syndrome is initially conservative, with activity modification, icing, and stretching of the anterior compartment musculature and heel cord complex. If conservative measures fail, fasciotomy of the affected compartments has shown favorable results in an athlete's return to higher levels of activity.

### Achilles Tendon Rupture

**Cause of injury**  The Achilles tendon is the largest tendon in the human body. It serves as a common tendon for the gastrocnemius and soleus muscles and inserts on the calcaneus. This heel cord complex produces plantarflexion of the ankle. Injury may range from a grade 1 strain of the muscle to complete rupture of the tendon. A tight heel cord is prone to strain, particularly of the gastrocnemius muscle, which is sometimes referred to as a **tennis leg**[8] (Figure 15-18). Achilles tendon rupture is usually caused by a sudden, forceful plantarflexion of the ankle. A

*Critical Thinking* Exercise

A soccer player who is not wearing shin guards is kicked on the outside shin of his right leg. After several minutes the pain begins to increase and he feels some tingling and numbness in his foot.

**?**  What is the primary concern with this injury, and what steps should be taken to manage this situation?

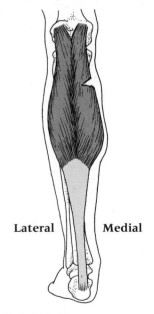

**Lateral**　　　**Medial**

**Figure 15-18**

Strain of the gastrocnemius muscle

---

**tennis leg**
Strain of gastrocnemius muscle.

**Medial** ◄ **Lateral**

**Figure 15-19**

Achilles tendon rupture

rupture of the Achilles tendon is more common in athletes above the age of 30 years and occurs in activities requiring ballistic movement, such as tennis and basketball[14] (Figure 15-19).

**Signs of injury**   Athletes may feel or hear a pop and feel as if they have been kicked in the back of the leg. Plantarflexing the ankle will be painful and limited but still possible with the assistance of the tibialis posterior and the peroneals. A palpable defect will be noted along the length of the tendon. The athlete will require the use of crutches to continue ambulation without an obvious limp.[14]

**Care**   After an Achilles tendon rupture, the question of surgical repair versus cast immobilization arises. Surgical repair of the tendon is recommended to allow the athlete to return to previous levels of activity. Surgical repair of the Achilles tendon may require a period of immobilization for 6 to 8 weeks to allow for proper tendon healing. It is important that the athlete not only regain full range of motion without harming the repair, but also regain normal muscle function through controlled progressive strengthening exercises.[10]

## Achilles Tendinitis

**Cause of injury**   Achilles tendinitis is an inflammatory condition that occurs because of repetitive stresses and strains placed on the tendon such as with running or jumping activities.[7] Repetitive weight-bearing activities such as running or early season conditioning in which the duration and intensity are increased too quickly with insufficient recovery time worsen the condition. Uphill running or hill workouts usually aggravate the condition. The athlete may experience reduced gastrocnemius and soleus muscle flexibility in general that may worsen as the condition progresses and adaptive shortening occurs.

**Signs of injury**   The athlete often complains of generalized pain and stiffness about the Achilles tendon just proximal to the calcaneal insertion. Achilles tendinitis often begins with a gradual onset over time. Symptoms may progress to morning stiffness and discomfort with walking after periods of prolonged sitting. The tendon may be warm and painful to palpation, and if the inflammation persists, the tendon may thicken[1] (Figure 15-20).

**Care**   Achilles tendinitis generally takes a long time to resolve. It is important to create a proper healing environment by limiting or restricting the activity that caused the inflammation. Aggressive stretching of the heel cord complex (refer to Figure 15-4), inserting a heel lift under the calcaneus, using taping techniques to provide support to the Achilles tendon (refer to Figure 11-16), and using antiinflammatory medication have all been recommended as treatments.[10] Chronic Achilles tendinitis may eventually predispose the athlete to rupture of the Achilles tendon.

## Shin Contusions

**Cause of injury**   The shin (tibia), lying just under the skin, is exceedingly vulnerable and sensitive to blows or bumps. Because of the absence of muscular or adipose padding, force is not dissipated and the pe-

**Figure 15-20**

Diffuse swelling and tendon
thickening in Achilles
tendinitis

riosteum receives the impact delivered to the shin. Shin contusions occur
frequently in soccer, and the incidence can be minimized by wearing appropriate shin guards (refer to Figure 6-23).

**Signs of injury**   The athlete complains of intense pain, swelling, and
increased warmth. A bulging hematoma with a jellylike consistency develops rapidly. In some instances the hematoma may increase to the size
of a golf ball (Figure 15-21).

**Care**   A compressive wrap along with ice and elevation should be
applied immediately to minimize swelling. Occasionally a physician may

Achilles tendinitis generally
takes a long time to resolve.

A ruptured Achilles tendon
can occur following chronic
inflammation.

Severe blows to an
unprotected shin can lead to
a chronic inflammation.

**Figure 15-21**

A serious shin bruise can
destroy bony tissue.

decide to aspirate the hematoma. A protective doughnut pad constructed to disperse pressure away from the contusion should be worn to protect the area from additional injury.

## SUMMARY

- The movements that take place at the talocrural joint are ankle plantarflexion and dorsiflexion. Inversion and eversion occur at the subtalar joint.

- Many lower leg and ankle injuries, especially sprains, can be reduced by heel cord (Achilles tendon) stretching, strengthening of key muscles, improving neuromuscular control, choosing appropriate footwear, and when necessary, proper taping or bracing.

- Ankle sprains are very common. Inversion sprains usually involve the lateral ligaments of the ankle, and eversion sprains frequently involve the medial ligaments of the ankle. Dorsiflexion injuries often involve the tibiofibular ligaments and may be very severe.

- The early phase of treatment following ankle sprain uses ice, compression, elevation, rest, and protection, all of which are critical components in preventing swelling.

- Tendinitis in the posterior tibialis, anterior tibialis, and the peroneal tendons may result from one specific cause or from a collection of mechanisms. Techniques that act to reduce or eliminate inflammation, including rest, ice, and antiinflammatory medications, should be incorporated into rehabilitation.

- Although some injuries that occur in the region of the lower leg are acute, the majority of injuries seen in an athletic population result from overuse, most often from running.

- Tibial fractures can create long-term problems for the athlete if inappropriately managed, whereas fibular fractures generally require much shorter periods for immobilization. Treatment of these fractures is immediate medical referral and most likely a period of immobilization and restricted weight bearing.

- Stress fractures in the lower leg are usually the result of the bone's inability to adapt to the repetitive loading response during training and conditioning of the athlete and are more likely to occur in the tibia.

- Care for medial tibial stress syndrome must be comprehensive and must address several factors, including musculoskeletal training and conditioning as well as proper footwear and orthotics intervention.

- Compartment syndromes can occur from acute trauma or from repetitive trauma or overuse. They can occur in any of the four compartments but are most likely to occur in the anterior compartment or deep posterior compartment.

- Perhaps the greatest question after an Achilles tendon rupture is whether surgical repair or cast immobilization is the best method of treatment. Regardless, the time required for rehabilitation is significant.

- Achilles tendinitis often presents with a gradual onset over time and may be resistant to a quick resolution.

---

**Solutions to Critical Thinking** Exercises

---

**15-1** The most important care that can be given immediately following ankle sprain is to control or minimize the swelling. This goal is accomplished by using a combination of ice, compression, elevation, and rest beginning immediately and continuing for at least the next 72 hours.

**15-2** The athlete is instructed to rest or reduce the stress of running. Application of ice packs followed by stretching is carried out before and after activity. A strengthening program is carried out along with treatment by oral antiinflammatory medications as needed.

**15-3** This athlete may be developing an acute compartment syndrome in the anterior compartment. If so, this condition should be handled as an emergency. The coach should immediately elevate the leg and apply ice but no compression wrap, and the athlete should be given medical attention as soon as possible.

**15-4** This scenario is a classic description of a ruptured Achilles tendon. In cases of a complete rupture, surgery is necessary to repair the tendon, followed by a reasonably long period of rehabilitation.

## REVIEW QUESTIONS AND CLASS ACTIVITIES

1. Describe the anatomy of the ankle and lower leg.
2. How can ankle and lower leg injuries be prevented?
3. What questions should be asked when assessing injuries to the lower leg or ankle?
4. Describe the common mechanisms of injury for acute ankle sprains. What structures are damaged?
5. How can the coach rule out fractures in the lower leg and ankle?
6. What is the appropriate care for stress fractures of the tibia and fibula?
7. Which of the tendons surrounding the ankle joint can potentially develop tendinitis?
8. What are some indications of a heel cord rupture? How is a heel cord rupture cared for?
9. How does Achilles tendinitis develop? How should it be cared for?
10. Contrast acute compartment syndrome with chronic compartment syndrome.
11. What exactly are shin splints and what measures can be taken to eliminate this problem?
12. What is the most important thing that can be done in caring for a shin contusion?

### Dynamic Human CD

For more information on skeletal anatomy of the ankle and lower leg click on:

- Skeletal
- Anatomy
- Gross anatomy
- Lower limbs
- Tibia/fibula
- Then, Ankle

To take a closer look at the muscles that are involved in ankle movement click on:

- Muscular
- Anatomy
- Body regions
- Lower leg
- Then, Ankle

### REFERENCES

1. Alfredson H, Lorentzon R: Chronic Achilles tendinosis: recommendations for treatment and prevention, *Sports Med* 29(2):135, 2000.
2. Bennell K et al: Risk factors for stress fractures in track and field athletes: a twelve-month prospective study, *Am J Sports Med* 24(6): 810, 1996.
3. Blackman PG: A review of chronic exertional compartment syndrome in the lower leg, *Med Sci Sports Exerc* 32(3 suppl):S4, 2000.
4. Bot SDM, van Mechelen W: The effect of ankle bracing on athletic performance, *Sports Med* 27(3): 171, 1999.
5. Case W: Relieving the pain of shin splints, *Physician Sportsmed* 22(4): 31, 1994.
6. Fehlandt A, Micheli L: Acute exertional anterior compartment syndrome in an adolescent female, *Med Sci Sports Exerc* 27(1):3, 1995.
7. Galloway M, Jokl P, Dayton W: Achilles tendon overuse injuries, *Clin Sports Med* 11(4):771, 1992.
8. Garrick J, Couzens G: Tennis leg: how I manage gastrocnemius strains, *Physician Sportsmed* 20(5): 203, 1992.
9. Gross M: Chronic tendinitis: pathomechanics of injury factors affecting the healing response, and treatment, *J Ortho Sports Phys Ther* 16(6):248, 1992.
10. Hirth C: Rehabilitation of lower leg injuries. In Prentice WE, editor: *Rehabilitation techniques in sports medicine*, ed 3, Boston, 1999, WCB/McGraw-Hill.
11. Hunter S, Prentice W: Rehabilitation of foot and ankle injuries. In Prentice WE, editor: *Rehabilitation techniques in sports medicine*, ed 3, Boston, 1999, WCB/McGraw-Hill.
12. Kohn H: Shin pain and compartment syndromes in running, In Guten G, editor: *Running injuries*, Philadelphia, 1997, WB Saunders.
13. Kortebein PM et al: Medial tibial stress syndrome, *Med Sci Sports Exerc* 32(3 suppl):S27, 2000.
14. Leppilahti J, Orava S: Total achilles tendon rupture: a review, *Sports Med* 25(2):79, 1998.
15. Reeder M et al: Stress fractures: current concepts of diagnosis and treatment, *Sports Med* 22(3):198, 1996.
16. Stuart M, Karaharju T: Acute compartment syndrome: recognizing the progressive signs and symp-

toms, *Physician Sportsmed,* 22(3):
91, 1994.

17. Thacker SB et al: The prevention
of ankle sprains in sports: a systematic review of the literature,
*Am J Sports Med* 27(6):753, 1999.

18. Vincent N: Compartment syndromes. In Harries M et al, editors:
*Oxford textbook of sports medicine,*
New York, 1994, Oxford University Press.

19. Wilkerson GB: Treatment of the
inversion ankle sprain through

20. synchronous application of focal
compression and cold, *Ath Rain*
26(3):220, 1991.

20. Willy C, Becker B, Evers H: Unusual development of acute exertional compartment syndrome
due to delayed diagnosis: a case
report, *Int J Sports Med,* 17(6):458,
1996.

21. Wright IC et al: The effects of ankle compliance and flexibility on
ankle sprains, *Med Sci Sports Exerc*
32(2):260, 2000.

## ANNOTATED BIBLIOGRAPHY

Baxter D: *The Foot and Ankle in Sport,* St
Louis, 1995, Mosby.

*Discusses all aspects of dealing with
foot and ankle injuries as they occur in
an athletic population.*

Brown DE, Neumann RD, editors: *Orthopedic secrets,* Philadelphia, 1995,
Hanley & Belfus.

*Presents an overview of orthopedics in*
*a question-and-answer format. The an-
kle and lower leg are well presented.*

Pfeffer, R: *Athletic injuries to the foot
and ankle,* Park Ridge, IL American
Academy of Orthopedic Surgeons,
2000.

*This book goes into great detail on a
wide variety of injuries that occur in the
ankle joint.*

**WEBSITES**

Cramer First Aider: http://www.ccsd.
k12.wy.us/CCHS_web/sptmed/
fstaider.htm

Ankle and lower leg anatomy cross
section: http://rpiwww.mdacc.tmc.
edu/cgibin/ankle_engine

The University of Texas Anatomy of
The Human Body: http://rpiwww.
mdacc.tmc.edu/mmlearn/anatomy.
html

American Othopaedic Foot and Ankle
Society: http://aofas.org

World Ortho: http://www.worldortho.
com

*Use the search engine in this site to lo-
cate relevant information.*

# The Knee and Related Structures

*When you finish this chapter you will be able to:*

- Describe the anatomical relationships of the bones, ligaments, and muscles that surround the knee joint.
- Explain how to prevent knee injuries.
- Briefly describe how to assess an injury of the knee joint.
- Describe injuries to the stabilizing structures of the knee.
- Identify injuries to the knee that can occur either from acute trauma or from overuse.
- Identify injuries that can occur to the patella.
- Describe injuries that can occur to the extensor mechanism.

T he knee is considered one of the most complex joints in the human body. Because so many sports place extreme stress on the knee, it is also one of the most frequently injured joints. The knee is commonly considered a hinge joint because its two principal movements are flexion and extension. However, because rotation of the tibia is an essential component of knee movement, the knee is not a true hinge joint. The stability of the knee joint depends primarily on the ligaments, the joint capsule, and the muscles that surround the joint. The knee functions to provide stability in weight bearing and mobility in locomotion.

## KNEE ANATOMY

### Bones

Muscles and ligaments provide the main source of stability in the knee.

The knee joint consists of four bones: the femur, the tibia, the fibula, and the patella (Figure 16-1). These four bones form several articulations between the femur and the tibia; the femur and the patella; the femur and the fibula; and the tibia and fibula. The articular surfaces of the knee joint are completely enveloped by the largest joint capsule in the body. Synovial membrane lines the inner surface of the joint capsule.

The distal end of the femur expands into the lateral and medial femoral condyles, which are designed to articulate with the tibia and the patella. The patella, or kneecap, is located in the tendon of the quadriceps muscle group on the front of the knee and moves up and down in a

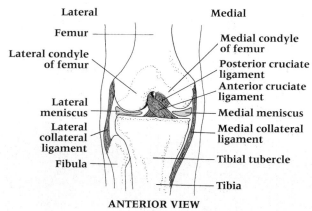

Lateral — Medial

Femur

Lateral condyle of femur

Lateral meniscus

Lateral collateral ligament

Fibula

Medial condyle of femur

Posterior cruciate ligament

Anterior cruciate ligament

Medial meniscus

Medial collateral ligament

Tibial tubercle

Tibia

**ANTERIOR VIEW**

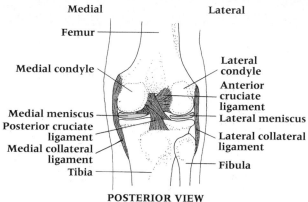

Medial — Lateral

Femur

Medial condyle

Medial meniscus
Posterior cruciate ligament
Medial collateral ligament
Tibia

Lateral condyle

Anterior cruciate ligament

Lateral meniscus

Lateral collateral ligament

Fibula

**POSTERIOR VIEW**

**Figure 16-1**

The bony and ligamentous arrangement of the knee

groove between the two femoral condyles as the quadriceps muscle group contracts and relaxes. The proximal end of the tibia, or the tibial plateau, is very flat and must articulate with the round condyles of the femur.

The medial meniscus and lateral meniscus are fibrocartilage disks that are shaped like bowls, thicker on the outside border and thinner on the inside (Figure 16-2). They lie on top of the flat tibial plateau and function to make the rounded femoral condyles fit better on the flat tibial plateau, thus increasing the stability of the joint. They also help cushion any stresses placed on the knee joint by keeping the bony surface of the femur separated from the tibial plateau.

Generally the meniscus has a poor blood supply.

## Ligaments

The major stabilizing ligaments of the knee include the cruciate ligaments and the collateral ligaments (refer to Figure 16-1).

The anterior and posterior cruciate ligaments account for a considerable amount of stability in the knee. In general, the anterior cruciate ligament (ACL) prevents the femur from moving posteriorly during weight bearing. It also stabilizes the tibia against excessive internal rotation and serves as a secondary stabilizer when there is injury to the collateral

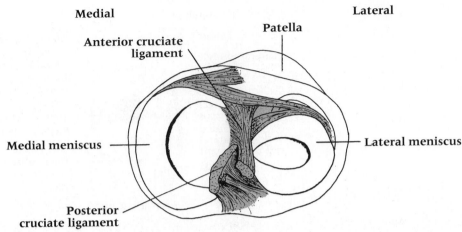

**Figure 16-2**

Menisci of the knee

Major movements of the
knee:
• Flexion
• Extension
• Rotation

ligaments. The posterior cruciate ligament (PCL) prevents the femur from sliding forward during weight bearing.

The medial and lateral collateral ligaments function to stabilize the knee against the side to side (valgus/varus) forces at the knee joint. The medial collateral ligament (MCL) attaches above the joint line on the medial condyle of the femur and inserts well below the joint line on the tibia. Its major purpose is to protect the knee from valgus forces that are applied to the lateral surface of the joint and to resist external tibial rotation. There are two parts of the MCL: the superficial portion and the deep portion, which is actually a thickened part of the medial joint capsule. The medial meniscus is attached to the deep portion of the medial collateral ligament.

The lateral collateral ligament (LCL) is attached to the lateral condyle of the femur and to the head of the fibula. The lateral collateral ligament resists varus forces that are applied to the medial surface of the knee. Both the medial and lateral collateral ligaments are tightest during knee extension but relaxed during flexion.

## Muscles

For the knee to function properly, a number of muscles must work together in a highly complex fashion (Figure 16-3). In general, contraction of the quadriceps muscle group (the rectus femoris, and the vastus medialis, intermedialis, and lateralis) on the front of the thigh causes knee extension. Contraction of the hamstring muscle group (the biceps femoris, semitendinosus, and semimembranosus) on the back of the thigh, along with the gracilis, sartorius, popliteus, gastrocnemius, and plantaris causes knee flexion. The hamstrings, popliteus, sartorius, and gracilis contribute to knee rotation. Table 16-1 summarizes all of the muscles that produce various movements at the knee joint.

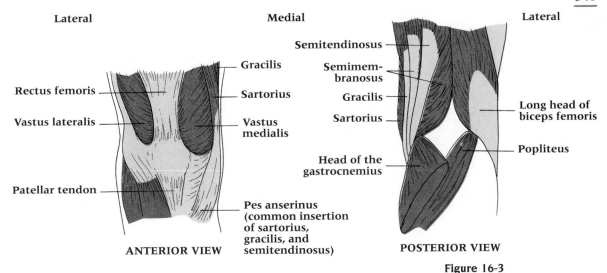

Lateral     Medial     Lateral

Rectus femoris

Vastus lateralis

Patellar tendon

Gracilis

Sartorius

Vastus medialis

Pes anserinus (common insertion of sartorius, gracilis, and semitendinosus)

**ANTERIOR VIEW**

Semitendinosus

Semimem- branosus

Gracilis

Sartorius

Head of the gastrocnemius

Long head of biceps femoris

Popliteus

**POSTERIOR VIEW**

**Figure 16-3**

Musculature of the knee

## PREVENTION OF KNEE INJURIES

Preventing knee injuries in sports is a complex problem. Of major importance are effective physical conditioning, rehabilitation, and skill development, as well as shoe type. The routine use of protective bracing may be a questionable practice.

**TABLE 16-1** Muscles of the knee joint

| | |
|---|---|
| Knee flexion | Hamstring group |
| |    Biceps femoris |
| |    Semitendinosus |
| |    Semimembranosus |
| | Gracilis |
| | Sartorius |
| | Gastrocnemius |
| | Popliteus |
| | Plantaris |
| Knee extension | Quadriceps muscle group |
| |    Vastus medialis |
| |    Vastus lateralis |
| |    Vastus intermedius |
| |    Rectus femoris |
| External tibial rotation | Biceps femoris |
| Internal tibial rotation | Popliteus |
| | Semitendinosus |
| | Semimembranosus |
| | Sartorius |
| | Gracilis |

## Physical Conditioning and Rehabilitation

To avoid knee injuries, the athlete must be as highly conditioned as possible, meaning total body conditioning that includes strength, flexibility, cardiovascular and muscle endurance, agility, speed, and balance.[11] Specifically, the muscles surrounding the knee joint must be as strong as possible. Depending on the requirements of a sport, some balance in strength should exist between the quadriceps and hamstring muscle groups. For example, in football players the hamstring muscles should have about 60 percent of the strength of the quadriceps muscles.[7] The gastrocnemius muscle should also be strengthened to help stabilize the knee. Although maximizing muscle strength may prevent some injuries, it fails to prevent rotational injuries.

Knees that have been injured must be properly rehabilitated. Once the ligaments that stabilize the knee have been injured, the knee relies to a great extent on the strength of all the muscles that surround the joint to provide the inherent stability that was lost with the injury. Thus strengthening exercises are essential in preventing reinjury. Repeated minor injuries to a knee make it susceptible to a major injury.

## Shoe Type

During recent years, collision sports such as football have been using soccer-style shoes. The change from a few long conical cleats to a large number of cleats that are short and broad has significantly reduced knee injuries in football. The more numerous and shorter cleats are better because the foot does not become fixed to the surface and the shoe still allows controlled running and cutting.

## Functional and Prophylactic Knee Braces

Functional and prophylactic knee braces were discussed in Chapter 6. These braces have been designed to prevent or reduce the severity of knee injuries.[13] Prophylactic knee braces are worn on the lateral surface of the knee to protect the medial collateral ligament (Figure 16-4A).[11] Their usefulness, however, is questionable and some studies have even shown that they increase the chance of injury.

Functional knee braces are worn to provide some degree of support to the unstable knee once an athlete returns to activity following injury.[13] All functional braces are custom fitted to some degree and use hinges and posts for support. Some braces use custom-molded thigh and calf enclosures to hold the brace in place, whereas others rely on straps for suspension (Figure 16-4B). These braces are designed to control excessive rotational stress or tibial translation. The effectiveness of protective knee braces is at best controversial.[13] However, if combined with an appropriate rehabilitation program, these braces have been shown to restrict anterior/posterior translation of the tibia at low loads.[10]

A                                    B

**Figure 16-4**

A, Prophylactic knee brace
B, Functional knee brace

## ASSESSING THE KNEE JOINT

The coach is usually the first person to observe the injury and thus assumes responsibility for initial evaluation and immediate care. Unquestionably, the most important aspect of understanding what pathological process has taken place is to become familiar with the traumatic sequence and mechanisms of injury, either through having seen the injury occur or through learning its history. If an athletic trainer is not present when the injury occurs, the coach must relate the pertinent information and then provide the appropriate first aid measures as discussed in Chapter 7.

### History

To determine the history and major complaints involved in a knee injury, the following questions should be asked.

#### Current Injury

- What were you doing when the knee was hurt?
- What position was your body in?
- Did the knee collapse?
- Did you hear a noise or feel any sensation at the time of injury, such as a pop or crunch? (A pop could indicate an anterior cruciate tear, a crunch could be a sign of a torn meniscus, and a tearing sensation might indicate a capsule tear.)

- Could you move the knee immediately after the injury? If not, was it locked in a bent or extended position? (Locking could mean a meniscal tear.) After being locked, how did it become unlocked?
- Did swelling occur? If yes, was it immediate, or did it occur later? (Immediate swelling could indicate a cruciate or tibial fracture, whereas later swelling could indicate a capsular, synovial, or meniscal tear.)
- Where was the pain? Was it local, all over, or did it move from one side of the knee to the other?
- Have you hurt the knee before?

When first assessing the injury, the athletic trainer or coach should observe whether the athlete is able to support body weight flat-footed on the injured leg or whether the athlete finds it necessary to stand and walk on the toes. Toe walking is an indication that the athlete is holding the knee in a splinted position to avoid pain or that the knee is being held in a flexed position by a wedge of dislocated meniscus.

In first-time acute knee sprains, fluid and blood effusion is not usually apparent until after a 24-hour period. However, in an anterior cruciate ligament sprain, blood may accumulate in the joint (hemarthrosis) during the first hour after injury. Swelling and discoloration (ecchymosis) will occur unless the swelling is controlled through the use of compression, elevation, and ice.

### Recurrent or Chronic Injury

- What is your major complaint?
- When did you first notice the condition?
- Is there recurrent swelling?
- Does the knee ever lock or catch? (If yes, it may be a torn meniscus or a loose body in the knee joint.)
- Is there severe pain? Is it constant, or does it come and go?
- Do you feel any grinding or grating sensations? (If yes, it could indicate chondromalacia or traumatic arthritis.)
- Does your knee ever feel like it is going to give way or has it actually done so? (If yes and often, it may be a capsular, cruciate, or meniscal tear, a loose body, or a subluxating patella.)
- What does it feel like to go up and down stairs? (Pain may indicate a patellar irritation or meniscal tear.)
- What past treatment, if any, have you received for this condition?

### Observation

If possible, the athlete with an injured knee should be observed in the following actions:
- Walking
- Half-squatting
- Going up and down stairs

A visual examination should be performed after the major complaints have been determined. The athlete should be observed in a number of situations: walking, half-squatting, and going up and down stairs. The leg also should be observed for asymmetry. The coach must establish whether both the athlete's knees look the same:

- Do the knees appear symmetrical?
- Is one knee obviously swollen?
- Is muscle atrophy apparent?

### Walking

- Does the athlete walk with a limp, or is the walk free and easy? Is the athlete able to fully extend the knee during heel strike?
- Can the athlete fully bear weight on the affected leg?
- Is the athlete able to perform a half-squat to extension?
- Can the athlete go up and down stairs with ease? (If stairs are unavailable, stepping up on a box or stool will suffice.)

## Palpation

For palpation to yield any valuable information about the nature of the injury, the coach must know at least a little about the anatomy of the bones, ligaments, and the muscles. The athlete should either be lying on the back (supine) or sitting on the edge of the training table or a bench with the knee flexed to 90 degrees.

The bone structures of the knee are palpated for areas of tenderness or pain or for deformities, which might indicate a fracture or dislocation.

After palpation of the bony structures, the lateral collateral ligament and medial collateral ligament should be palpated for areas of tenderness. Because the anterior and posterior cruciate ligaments are inside the joint capsule they cannot be palpated. However the *joint line*, which is the articulation between the femoral condyles and the flat tibial plateau, should be palpated all around the knee joint. Tenderness at the joint line may indicate injury to either the medial or lateral menisci or the joint capsule.

## Special Tests

Both acute and chronic injury to the knee can produce ligamentous instability.[11] It is critical that the injured knee's stability be evaluated as soon after injury as possible. To be able to correctly conduct a series of stability tests and then determine the exact nature of the injury takes a considerable amount of training. However, because the coach is almost always on the field when the athlete is injured, a quick initial assessment of knee stability may give important information about the extent of the injury.

Perhaps the simplest test is to compare the injured knee with the uninjured knee to determine any differences in stability. Determination of the degree of instability is made by the endpoint feel during stability testing. As stress is applied to a joint, some motion is limited by an intact ligament. In a normal joint, the endpoint is abrupt with little or no give and no reported pain. With a grade 1 sprain, the endpoint is still firm with little or no instability and some pain is present. With a grade 2 sprain, the endpoint is soft with some instability present and a moderate amount of

**Figure 16-5**

Valgus knee stress test

pain. In a grade 3 complete rupture, the endpoint is very soft with
marked instability, and pain is severe initially, then mild.

There are many different tests that should be performed by a trained
individual to accurately assess ligament stability. However, the valgus/
varus stress test, the drawer test, and the McMurray test may be easily
done to determine the degree of instability in the knee caused by ligament or meniscal injury. These tests are not definitive but rather are possible indicators of injury. If they appear to be positive the athlete should
be referred to a physician.

### Valgus/Varus Stress Tests

Valgus and varus stress tests are intended to reveal laxity of the medial
and lateral collateral ligaments. The athlete lies supine with the leg
extended. To test the medial collateral ligament, valgus stress is applied
with the knee fully extended and at 30 degrees of flexion (Figure 16-5).

To test the lateral collateral ligament, the examiner holds the ankle
firmly with one hand while placing the other over the medial joint line.
The examiner then places a varus force laterally in an attempt to open the
lateral side of the knee (Figure 16-6).

**Figure 16-6**

Varus knee stress test

**Figure 16-7**

Anterior and posterior
drawer tests for cruciate
laxity

### Drawer Test

The drawer test is used to test the stability of the anterior and posterior cruciate ligaments. To perform this test, the athlete lies on the back with the injured knee flexed to 90 degrees. The examiner faces the anterior aspect of the athlete's leg and encircles the tibia immediately below the knee joint with both hands. The fingers of the examiners' hands are positioned on the back of the knee with the thumbs on the medial and lateral joint lines (Figure 16-7).

An anterior drawer test assesses the stability of the anterior cruciate ligament. The examiner's hands pull the tibia forward. If a positive anterior drawer sign occurs, the test should be repeated with the athlete's leg rotated internally 30 degrees and externally 15 degrees to see if the degree of instability changes.

A posterior drawer test is performed to assess the stability of the posterior cruciate ligament. Force is exerted in a posterior direction at the proximal tibial plateau. A tibia that slides backward excessively from under the femur is considered a positive posterior drawer sign (refer to Figure 16-7).

### McMurray's Test

The McMurray test (Figure 16-8) is used to determine the presence of a meniscus tear within the knee. The athlete is positioned supine on the table with the injured leg fully flexed. The examiner places one hand on the foot and one hand over the top of the knee, fingers touching the joint line. The hand on the foot scribes a small circle and pulls the leg into extension. As this movement occurs, the hand on the knee feels for a clicking response. Medial meniscal tears can be detected at the medial joint line when the tibia is externally rotated, whereas lateral meniscal tears can be detected at the lateral joint line when the tibia is internally rotated.

### Functional Tests

It is important that the athlete's knee also be tested for function. The athlete should begin with walking (forward, backward, straight line, curve)

**Figure 16-8**

The McMurray meniscal test

and progress to jogging (straight, curve, uphill, downhill), running (forward, backward), and then sprinting (straight, curve, large figure eight, small figure eight, zig-zag, carioca).

## RECOGNITION AND MANAGEMENT OF INJURIES TO THE KNEE

### Ligament Injuries

The major ligaments of the knee can be torn in isolation or in combination.[3] Depending on the application of forces, injury can occur from a direct straight-line or single-plane force, from a rotary force, or from a combination of the two.

### Medial Collateral Ligament Sprain

**Cause of injury**  Injury to the MCL most often occurs either as a result of a medially directed valgus force from the lateral side or from external rotation of the tibia (Figure 16-9). MCL tears resulting from rotation combined with valgus stress with the foot fixed frequently result in ACL and occasionally PCL tears.[11]

**Figure 16-9**

A valgus force with the tibia in external rotation injures the medial collateral and capsular ligaments, the medial meniscus, and sometimes the anterior cruciate ligaments.

Lateral          Medial

**Figure 16-10**

A, Grade 1 MCL sprain. B,
Grade 2 MCL sprain. C,
Grade 3 MCL sprain

16-1

***Critical Thinking*** Exercise

A football running back is hit on
the lateral surface of his knee
by an opponent making a
tackle. He has significant pain
and some immediate swelling
on the medial surface of his
knee. The athletic trainer
suspects that the athlete has
sustained a sprain of the MCL.

**?** What are the most appropriate tests that the athletic
trainer should do to determine
the exact nature and extent of
the injury?

More significant injury usually occurs with medial sprains than
from lateral sprains because of the increased potential of injury to the
joint capsule and the medial meniscus. Many mild-to-moderate sprains
leave the knee unstable and thus vulnerable to additional internal
derangements.

**Signs of injury** The force and angle of the trauma usually determine
the extent of injury. Even after witnessing the occurrence of a knee injury, coaches have difficulty predicting the extent of tissue damage. The
most revealing time for testing joint stability is immediately after injury
before effusion masks the extent of derangement.

In a grade 1 MCL sprain, a few ligament fibers are torn or stretched;
the joint is stable during valgus stress tests; there is little or no joint effusion; there may be some joint stiffness and point tenderness just below
the medial joint line; even with minor stiffness, there is almost full passive and active range of motion (Figure 16-10A).

A                                    B

**Figure 16-11**

Knee immobilizers. A,
Universal knee immobilizer.
B, Adjustable angle
immobilizer. Both types
may be used depending on
whether full extension or
some other angle is desired.

A grade 2 MCL sprain involves moderate tearing or partial separation of ligament fibers; no gross instability, but minimum or slight laxity during full extension; slight or absent swelling unless the meniscus or ACL has been torn; moderate-to-severe joint tightness with an inability to fully actively extend the knee (the athlete is unable to place the heel flat on the ground); definite loss of passive range of motion; and pain in the medial aspect with general weakness and instability (Figure 16-10B).

A grade 3 MCL sprain means a complete tear of the ligament; complete loss of medial stability; minimum-to-moderate swelling; immediate severe pain followed by a dull ache; loss of motion because of effusion and hamstring guarding; a valgus stress test that reveals some joint opening in full extension and significant opening at 30 degrees of flexion (Figure 16-10C).

**Care** Immediate care consists of RICE for at least 24 hours. Crutches may be used if the athlete is unable to walk without a limp. Depending on the severity and possible complications, a postoperative knee immobilizer may be applied by the physician (Figure 16-11) for 2 to 5 days, after which range-of-motion exercises are begun. Isometric exercise emphasizing quadriceps strengthening (quad sets, straight leg lifts) should progress to active, resisted, full-range exercise as soon as possible. The athlete then graduates to stationary biking, stair climbing, and resisted flexion/extension exercises as soon as possible. Use of tape or perhaps a hinged brace when attempting to return to running activities is encouraged.

Conservative nonoperative treatment is recommended for isolated grade 2 and even grade 3 MCL sprains. Conservative treatment usually involves limited immobilization with range-of-motion and progressive weight bearing for 2 weeks followed by protection with a functional hinged brace for another 2 to 3 weeks.

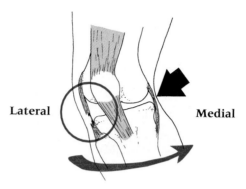

**Lateral**          **Medial**

**Figure 16-12**

A varus force with the tibia
internally rotated injures the
lateral collateral ligament; in
some cases both the cruciate
ligaments and the
attachments of the iliotibial
band and biceps muscle of
the thigh may be torn.

The athlete is allowed to return to full participation when the knee
has regained normal strength, power, flexibility, endurance, and coordination. Usually 1 to 3 weeks is necessary for recovery. When returning to
activity, the athlete may require tape support for a short period.

## Lateral Collateral Ligament Sprain

**Cause of injury**    Injury to the LCL most often occurs either as a result of a laterally directed varus force from the medial side or from internal rotation of the tibia (Figure 16-12). If the force is great enough, bony
fragments can be avulsed from the femur or tibia. Sprain of the LCL is
much less prevalent than sprain of the MCL.

**Signs of injury**    An LCL sprain causes pain and tenderness over the
ligament; swelling and effusion; some joint laxity with a varus stress test at
30 degrees (if laxity exists in full extension, ACL and possibly PCL injury
should be evaluated); and pain is greatest with grade 1 and grade 2 sprains.
In grade 3 sprains, pain is intense initially, then subsides to a dull ache.

**Care**    Management of the LCL injury should follow the same procedures as for MCL injuries.

## Anterior Cruciate Ligament Sprain

**Cause of injury**    The ACL is usually injured when the foot is on the
ground, the femur is externally rotated, and the knee is in a valgus position (Figure 16-13). In this position, the ACL becomes taut and vulnerable to sprain. Hyperextension from a force to the front of the knee with
the foot planted can tear the ACL (Figure 16-14) and, if severe enough,
can also sprain the MCL. Tears of the anterior cruciate are often associated
with injury to other supporting structures in the knee.

**Signs of injury**    The athlete with a torn ACL experiences a pop followed by immediate disability and will complain that the knee feels like
it is coming apart. ACL tears produce rapid swelling at the joint line. Usually the athlete experiences intense pain initially. However, within minutes the athlete begins to feel that the knee is not badly hurt and will pro-
fess an ability to get up and walk. The athlete with an isolated ACL tear
will exhibit a positive anterior drawer sign.

**Figure 16-13**

A major mechanism causing
an anterior cruciate tear
occurs when a running
athlete suddenly decelerates
and makes a sharp cutting
motion.

**Figure 16-14**

An anterior force with the
foot planted can tear the
anterior cruciate ligament.

Lateral          Medial

A lateral knee sprain can be
caused by a varus force when
the tibia is internally rotated.

**Care**  Even with application of proper first aid and immediate RICE, swelling begins within 1 to 2 hours and peaks within 4 to 6 hours.[3] The athlete typically cannot walk without help.

Anterior cruciate ligamentous injury can lead to serious knee instability; an intact ACL is necessary for a knee to function in high-performance situations. Controversy exists among physicians about how best to treat an acute ACL rupture and when surgery is warranted. Surgery may involve joint reconstruction to replace the lost anterior cruciate support. This type of surgery involves a brief hospital stay, 3 to 5 weeks in braces, and 4 to 6 months of rehabilitation.[8] Little scientific evidence exists to support the use of functional knee braces following ACL injury, yet many physicians feel that the braces can provide some protection during activity.[13]

### Posterior Cruciate Ligament Sprain

**Cause of injury**  The PCL is most likely to be injured when the knee is hyperflexed from falling with full weight on the anterior aspect of the bent knee with the foot in plantar flexion. A posteriorly directed force to the front of the bent knee can tear the PCL (Figure 16-15). In addition, it can be injured by a rotational force, which also affects the medial or lateral side of the knee.[6]

**Signs of injury**  The athlete will report feeling a pop in the back of the knee; tenderness and relatively little swelling will be evident in the popliteal fossa; laxity will be demonstrated in a posterior drawer test.

**Care**  RICE should be initiated immediately. Nonoperative rehabilitation of grade 1 and 2 injuries should focus on quadriceps strengthening. Controversy exists as to whether a grade 3 PCL tear should be treated nonoperatively or with surgical intervention. Unlike the situation faced by athletes with ACL tears, many high-level athletes can do very well without the PCL. Rehabilitation following surgery generally involves 6 weeks of immobilization in extension with full weight bearing on crutches. Range of motion exercises are begun at 6 weeks, progressing to the use of progressive resistance exercise at 4 months.[4]

**Figure 16-15**

A fall or a hit on the anterior
aspect of the bent knee can
tear the PCL.

### Meniscus Injuries

**Cause of injury**  A tear of the meniscus most often results from weight bearing combined with a rotational force while extending or

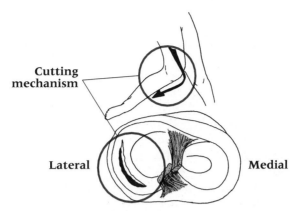

**Cutting mechanism**

**Lateral**

**Medial**

**Figure 16-16**

Common mechanisms of
injury to the meniscus.
Forced flexion produces a
peripheral tear, whereas
cutting with the foot fixed is
likely to produce a "bucket
handle" tear.

flexing the knee (Figure 16-16). The medial meniscus has a much
higher incidence of injury than does the lateral meniscus. Because of
its attachment to the deep portion of the MCL, the medial meniscus
is prone to disruption from valgus and rotational forces. The lateral
meniscus does not attach to the capsule and is more mobile during knee
movement.

A large number of medial meniscus lesions are the outcome of a sudden, strong, internal rotation of the femur with a partially flexed knee
while the foot is firmly planted.[2] As a result of the force of this action, the
meniscus is pulled out of its normal bed and pinched between the
femoral condyles. Tears within the cartilage fail to heal because of inadequate blood supply. However, some peripheral meniscus tears do heal
when an adequate supply of blood is available.

**Signs of injury**   An absolute diagnosis of meniscal injury is difficult. A meniscal tear may result in the following: effusion developing
gradually over 48 to 72 hours; joint-line pain and loss of motion; intermittent locking and giving way; and pain when squatting. Chronic
meniscal lesions may also display recurrent swelling and obvious muscle
atrophy around the knee. Often the athlete complains of an inability
to perform a full squat or to change direction quickly when running
without experiencing pain, a sense of the knee collapsing, or a popping
sensation.

**Care**   Immediate care involves RICE. Even if the knee is not locked
but shows indications of a tear, the athlete should be sent to a physician
for diagnosis. The knee that is locked by a displaced meniscus may require
unlocking with the athlete under anesthesia so that a detailed examination can be conducted. Management of the nonlocking acute meniscus
tear should follow a course similar to that for MCL injuries and does not
necessarily require surgery.

If discomfort, disability, and locking of the knee continue, arthroscopic surgery may be required to remove a portion of the meniscus. Surgical management of meniscal tears should make every effort to minimize loss of any portion of the meniscus.

16-2

*Critical Thinking* Exercise

A lacrosse player carrying the
ball attempts to avoid a
defender by planting his right
foot firmly on the ground and
cutting hard to his left. His
knee immediately gives way,
and he hears a loud pop. He
has intense pain immediately
but after a few minutes he feels
as if he can get up and walk.

**?**  What ligament has most
likely been injured? What
stability tests should be done
by the coach to determine the
extent of the injury to this
ligament?

## Joint Contusions (Bruises)

**Cause of injury**   A blow struck against the muscles crossing the knee joint can result in a handicapping condition. One of the muscles frequently involved is the vastus medialis of the quadriceps group, which is primarily involved in locking the knee in a position of full extension.

**Signs of injury**   Bruises of the vastus medialis produce all the appearances of a knee sprain, including severe pain, loss of movement, and signs of acute inflammation. Such bruising is often manifested by swelling and discoloration caused by the tearing of muscle tissue and blood vessels. If adequate first aid is given immediately, the knee usually returns to functional use 24 to 48 hours after the trauma.

**Care**   Care of a bruised knee depends on many factors. However, management principally depends on the location and severity of the contusion. The following procedures are suggested. Apply compression bandages and cold until resolution has occurred. Recommend inactivity and rest for 24 hours. If swelling occurs, continue cold application for 72 hours. If swelling and pain are intense, refer the athlete to the physician. Once the acute stage has ended and the swelling has diminished to little or none, cold application with active range-of-motion exercises should be conducted within a pain-free range. Allow the athlete to return to normal activity with protective padding when pain and the initial irritation have subsided. If swelling is not resolved within a week, a chronic condition of either synovitis or bursitis may exist, indicating the need for rest and medical attention.

## Bursitis

The knee has many bursae; the prepatellar and deep infrapatellar bursae are most often irritated.

**Cause of injury**   Bursitis in the knee can be acute, chronic, or recurrent. Although any one of the numerous knee bursae can become inflamed, the prepatellar and the deep infrapatellar bursae on the front of the knee have the highest incidence of irritation in sports (Figure 16-17).

**Figure 16-17**

Common bursae of the knee

Suprapatellar
bursa

Prepatellar
bursa

Medial
gastrocnemius
bursa

Infrapatellar
bursa

Pretibial bursa

The prepatellar bursa often becomes inflamed from continued kneeling or falling directly on the knee, whereas the deep infrapatellar becomes irritated from overuse of the patellar tendon.[11]

**Signs of injury** Prepatellar bursitis results in localized swelling above the knee that is similar to a balloon. Swelling occurs outside the joint, and there may be some redness and increased temperature. Swelling in the back of the knee does not necessarily indicate bursitis but could instead be a sign of Baker's cyst (Figure 16-18). A Baker's cyst is connected to the joint, which swells because of a problem in the joint and not because of bursitis. A Baker's cyst is commonly painless, causing no discomfort or disability. Some inflamed bursae may be painful and disabling because of the swelling and should be treated accordingly.

**Care** Management usually follows a pattern of eliminating the cause, prescribing rest, and reducing inflammation. Perhaps the two most important techniques for controlling bursitis are the use of elastic compression wraps and antiinflammatory medication. When the bursitis is chronic or recurrent and the synovial lining of the joint capsule has thickened, a physician may cautiously use aspiration and a steroid injection.

**Figure 16-18**

A Baker's cyst causes very little or no pain in the popliteal fossa.

### Loose Bodies within the Knee

**Cause of condition** Because of repeated trauma to the knee during sports activities, loose bodies, sometimes called *joint mice*, can develop within the joint cavity. Loose bodies can result from osteochondritis dissecans (fragments of bone and cartilage), fragments from the menisci, pieces of torn synovial tissue, or a torn cruciate ligament.

**Signs of condition** The loose bodies may move in the joint space and become lodged to cause locking and popping. The athlete complains of pain, instability, and a feeling that the knee is giving way.

**Care** When the loose body becomes wedged between articulating surfaces, irritation can occur. If not surgically removed, the loose body can create conditions that lead to joint degeneration.

A knee that locks and unlocks during activity may indicate a torn meniscus.

### Iliotibial Band Friction Syndrome (Runner's Knee)

**Cause of injury** **Iliotibial band friction syndrome** is an overuse condition commonly occurring in runners or cyclists that can be attributed to malalignment and structural asymmetries of the foot and lower leg. Irritation develops over the lateral femoral condyle or at the band's insertion on the lateral side of the knee where friction is created.[12]

**Signs of injury** There may be tenderness, some mild swelling, increased warmth, and possibly some redness over the lateral femoral condyle. Pain increases during running or cycling activities.

**Care** Treatment includes stretching the iliotibial band and performing techniques for reducing inflammation.[12] Management of runner's or cyclist's knee involves correction of foot and leg alignment problems. Therapy includes cold packs or ice massage before and after activity, proper warm-up and stretching, and avoiding activities that aggravate the

> **iliotibial band friction syndrome**
> (**eel** e oh **tib** ee ul) Runner's knee.

problem, such as running on inclines. Other procedures may include administering antiinflammatory medications. A transverse friction massage done over the site of irritation can also help eliminate chronic inflammation.

## RECOGNITION AND MANAGEMENT OF INJURIES AND CONDITIONS OF THE EXTENSOR MECHANISM

The extensor mechanism of the knee consists of the quadriceps muscle group, the patellar tendon, the patella located within that tendon, and the tibial tubercle, which is the site of attachment for the patellar tendon.[14]

### Fracture of the Patella

**Cause of injury**   Fractures of the patella can be caused by either direct or indirect trauma. Most patellar fractures are the result of indirect trauma in which a severe pull of the patellar tendon occurs against the femur when the knee is semiflexed. This position subjects the patella to maximum stress from the quadriceps tendon and the patellar ligament. Forcible muscle contraction may then fracture the patella at its lower half. Direct injury most often produces fragmentation with little displacement. Falls, jumping, or running may result in a fracture of the patella.

**Signs of injury**   The fracture causes hemorrhage, resulting in generalized swelling. An indirect fracture causes tearing of the joint capsule, separation of bone fragments, and possible tearing of the quadriceps tendon. Direct fracture involves little bone separation.

**Care**   Diagnosis usually requires x-ray confirmation. As soon as the examiner suspects a patellar fracture, a cold wrap should be applied, followed by an elastic compression wrap and splinting. The athlete should then be referred to the team physician. The athlete is normally immobilized for 2 to 3 months.

### Acute Patellar Subluxation or Dislocation

**Cause of injury**   When an athlete plants the foot, decelerates, and simultaneously cuts in an opposite direction from the weight-bearing foot, the thigh rotates internally while the lower leg rotates externally, causing a medially directed valgus force at the knee.[1] The quadriceps muscle attempts to pull in a straight line and as a result pulls the patella laterally—a force that may dislocate the patella. As a rule, displacement takes place outwardly, with the patella resting on the lateral condyle.

**Signs of injury**   The athlete experiences a complete loss of knee function along with pain and swelling; the patella rests in an abnormal position. A first-time patellar dislocation should always be suspected of being associated with a fracture.

**Care**   The knee should be immobilized in the position it is in (do not try to straighten the knee). Ice should be applied around the joint. The

Knees that give way or catch have a number of possible pathological conditions:
Subluxating patella
Meniscal tear
Anterior cruciate ligamentous tear

**16–3**

***Critical Thinking*** Exercise

A track athlete complains of pain in the anterior aspect of the knee while walking, running, ascending and descending stairs, or squatting. There is a grating sensation when flexing and extending the knee.

**?** What condition should the coach suspect and what should be the recommended treatment?

athlete should be taken to the physician, who will reduce the kneecap (put it back into place). After reduction, the knee is immobilized in extension for 4 weeks or longer, and the athlete is instructed to use crutches when walking. Muscle rehabilitation should involve strengthening all the muscles of the knee, thigh, and hip.

The athlete may find it helpful to wear a neoprene brace that has a horseshoe-shaped felt pad designed to push the patella medially; the brace is worn while running or performing in sports (Figure 16-19).

## Chondromalacia Patella

**Cause of condition**   Chondromalacia patella is a softening and deterioration of the articular cartilage on the back of the patella. The exact cause of chondromalacia is unknown but it is often related to either abnormal movement of the patella within the femoral groove or to overuse. Normally the patella moves up and down in the femoral groove between the femoral condyles as the knee flexes and extends. In some athletes the patella has a tendency to move or track in a lateral direction as the quadriceps group contracts (Figure 16-20).[7] This tracking most often occurs in athletes with weakness in the quadriceps muscle group or in female athletes who have a wider pelvis.

**Signs of condition**   The athlete may experience pain in the anterior aspect of the knee while walking, running, ascending and descending stairs, or squatting. There may be recurrent swelling around the kneecap and a grating sensation when flexing and extending the knee. The athlete may experience pain on the back of the patella or when the patella is compressed within the femoral groove while the knee is passively flexed and extended.

**Care**   Conservative treatment includes avoiding irritating activities such as stair climbing and squatting; doing pain-free isometric exercises that concentrate primarily on strengthening the quadriceps muscles; and wearing a neoprene knee sleeve (Figure 16-21). If conservative measures fail to help, surgery may be the only alternative.

## Jumper's Knee (Patellar Tendinitis)

**Cause of injury**   Jumping, kicking, or running may place extreme tension on the knee extensor muscle complex. As a result of either a single acute injury or, more commonly, repetitive injuries, **patellar tendinitis** occurs in the patellar or quadriceps tendon. On rare occasions, a patellar tendon may completely fail and rupture. Sudden or repetitive forceful extension of the knee may begin an inflammatory process that eventually leads to tendon degeneration.[9]

**Signs of injury**   The athlete indicates vague pain and tenderness generally around the bottom of the patella on the posterior aspect that worsens when engaging in jumping or running activities. Quite often athletes say that if they could take their finger and reach under the kneecap at the bottom, the pain would be there.[5]

**Figure 16-19**

A special pad for the dislocated patella

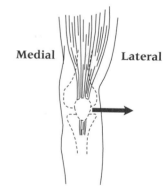

**Figure 16-20**

Lateral patellar tracking. There is a tendency for the patella to move laterally when the knee goes into full extension.

| patellar tendinitis (pa **teller**) |
| --- |
| Jumper's knee. |

**Care** Any pain in the patellar tendon must preclude sudden explosive movement such as that characterized by heavy plyometric-type exercising. Several approaches to treating athletes with inflammation associated with jumper's knee have been reported, including rest, the use of ice, and antiinflammatory medications. A patellar tendon tenodesis brace or strap may also be used (Figure 16-22). Transverse friction massage has also been demonstrated to be an effective technique for care of jumpers' knee.

### Osgood-Schlatter Disease

**Cause of condition** Osgood-Schlatter disease is a condition common to the immature adolescent's knee. The most commonly accepted cause is the repeated pull of the patellar tendon at the tibial tubercle on the front of the tibia. The tibial tubercle is an important bony landmark because it is the site of attachment for the tendon of the entire quadriceps muscle group. Osgood-Schlatter disease is characterized by ongoing pain at the attachment of the patellar tendon at the tibial tubercle. Over time, a bony callus forms and the tubercle enlarges. This condition usually resolves when the athlete reaches the age of eighteen or nineteen. The only remnant is an enlarged tibial tubercle.[11]

**Signs of condition** Repeated irritation causes swelling, hemorrhage, and gradual degeneration at the tibial tubercle. The athlete complains of severe pain when kneeling, jumping, and running. There is point tenderness over the anterior proximal tibial tubercle.

**Care** Treatment is usually conservative and includes the following: Stressful activities are decreased for approximately 6 months to 1 year; severe cases may require a cylindrical cast; ice is applied to the knee before and after activities; and isometric strengthening of quadriceps and hamstring muscles is performed.

**Figure 16-21**

Neoprene sleeve

**Figure 16-22**

The tenodesis strap or
brace for patellar tendinitis

# SUMMARY

- The knee is one of the most complex joints in the human body. Stability of the knee depends primarily on the bony articulations, ligaments, joint capsule, and muscles that surround the joint.

- Prevention of knee injuries involves maximizing muscle strength and wearing appropriate shoes. Use of protective knee bracing is questionable.

- Assessing an injury to the knee joint requires taking a history, observing both the appearance of the injured part and how the athlete moves, palpating the injured structures around the joint, and using special tests, including valgus/varus stress tests, drawer tests, and the McMurray test to determine the existing stability of the joint.

- The stabilizing structures most often injured are the medial and lateral collateral ligaments, the anterior and posterior cruciate ligaments, and the menisci.

- Other knee joint injuries that can occur either from acute trauma or from overuse are contusions, bursitis, joint mice, and iliotibial band friction syndrome.

- The patella and its surrounding area can develop a variety of injuries from sports activities, including fractures, subluxation and dislocation, and chondromalacia patella.

- The extensor mechanism of the knee consists of the quadriceps muscle group, the patellar tendon, the patella located within that tendon, and the tibial tubercle. Jumper's knee and Osgood-Schlatter disease are conditions associated with the extensor mechanism.

## *Solutions to Critical Thinking* Exercises

**16-1** A valgus stress test should be used to test the MCL. The examination in full extension tests the MCL, posteromedial capsule, and the cruciates. At 30 degrees of flexion the MCL is isolated. If there is some instability present with the knee in full extension, the athletic trainer should closely evaluate the integrity of the cruciate ligaments.

**16-2** This mechanism is typical for a sprain of the anterior cruciate ligament, although other ligamentous, capsular, and meniscal structures may be injured as well. An appropriate stability test for determining an injury to the ACL is the anterior drawer test.

**16-3** It is likely that this athlete has chondromalacia patella. The coach should recommend avoiding irritating activities such as stair climbing and squatting; isometric exercises that are pain free to strengthen the quadriceps and hamstring muscles; and wearing a neoprene knee sleeve. If conservative measures fail to help, surgery may be the only alternative.

**16-4** A conservative approach is to use normal techniques—reduce inflammation, rest, ice, ultrasound, anti-inflammatory medications, and so on. An alternative and more aggressive approach is to use a deep friction massage technique to increase the inflammatory response, which will ultimately facilitate healing. If successful, the more aggressive treatment may allow a quicker return to full activity.

## REVIEW QUESTIONS AND CLASS ACTIVITIES

1. What are the various structures that give the knee stability? What movements do these various structures prevent?
2. What motions can occur at the knee? Which muscles produce these movements?
3. Explain how a knee injury can best be prevented. What injuries are most difficult to prevent?
4. Demonstrate the steps that should be taken when assessing the knee.
5. Describe the mechanisms of injury for the collateral ligaments, the cruciate ligaments, and the menisci.
6. Contrast the signs and characteristics of grades 1, 2, and 3 medial collateral ligament sprains.
7. How might a contusion of the knee joint be related to bursitis of the knee?
8. How does a patellar subluxation or dislocation usually occur?
9. What factors can contribute to the development of chondromalacia?
10. What types of conditions can develop in the extensor mechanism? How are they cared for?
11. Invite an orthopedic physician to discuss the latest treatment and rehabilitation techniques for treating an injured knee.

 **Dynamic Human CD**

For more information on skeletal anatomy of the knee click on:

- Skeletal
- Anatomy
- Gross anatomy
- Lower limbs
- Then, Femur
- Then, Patella
- Then, Tibia/fibula

To take a closer look at the muscles that are involved in knee movement click on:

- Muscular
- Anatomy
- Body regions
- Thigh

To look at the effects of a torn lateral meniscus on joint range of motion click on:

- Skeletal
- Clinical Concepts
- Arthroscopy

## REFERENCES

1. Baker MM, Juhn MS: Patello-femoral pain syndrome in the female athlete, *Clin Sports Med* 19(2): 315, 2000.

2. Bernstein J: Meniscal tears of the knee: diagnosis and individualized treatment, *Physician Sportsmed* 28(3):83, 2000.

3. Boden BP, Griffin LY, Garrett WE: Etiology and prevention of non-contact ACL injury, *Physician Sportsmed* 28(4):53, 2000.

4. Edson CJ, Feldmann DD: Rehabilitation of posterior cruciate ligament injuries treated by operative methods, *Sports Med Arthroscop Rev* 7(4):303, 1999.

5. Fredberg U, Bolvig L: Jumper's knee: review of the literature, *Scand J Med Sci Sports* 9(2):66, 1999.

6. Janousek AT et al: Posterior cruciate ligament injuries of the knee joint, *Sports Med* 28(6):429, 1999.

7. Johnson RM, Poppe TR: Considering patellofemoral pain: exercise prescription, *Streng Condition J* 21(1):73, 1999.

8. Mullin MJ: Functional rehabilitation of the knee, *Ath Ther Today* 5(2):28, 2000.

9. Pellecchia G, Hame H, Behnke P: Treatment of infrapatellar tendinitis: a combination of modalities and transverse friction massage. *J Sport Rehab* 3(2):125, 1994.

10. Powers CM et al: Effect of bracing on patellar kinematics in patients with patellofemoral joint pain, *Med Sci Sports Exerc* 31(12):1714, 1999.

11. Prentice W, Davis M: Rehabilitation of the knee. In Prentice W: *Rehabilitation techniques in sports medicine*, Boston, 1999, WCB/McGraw-Hill.

12. Racioppi EA, Gulick DT: Iliotibial band friction syndrome, *Ath Ther Today* 4(5):9, 1999.

13. Styf J: The effects of functional knee bracing on muscle function and performance, *Sports Med* 28(2):77, 1999.

14. Thomee R, Augustsson J, Karlsson J: Patellofemoral pain syndrome: a review of current issues, *Sports Med* 28(4):245, 1999.

## ANNOTATED BIBLIOGRAPHY

Ellenbecker T: *Knee ligament rehabilitation*, Philadelphia, 2000, Churchill-Livingston.
   *Provides information to help diagnose and rehabilitate knee ligament injuries.*
Griffin L: *Rehabilitation of the knee*, St Louis, 1995, Mosby.
   *This text incorporates new advances in rehabilitation techniques and equipment and gives emphasis to sport-specific functional rehabilitation programs.*
Tria AJ, Klein K: *An illustrated guide to the knee*, New York, 1992, Churchill-Livingstone.
   *A basic, concise, easy-to-read guide to the knee.*

**WEBSITES**

World Ortho: http://www.worldortho.com
   *Use the search engine in this site to locate relevant information.*

Wheeless' Textbook of Orthopaedics: http://www.medmedia.com/med/htm
   *An excellent page for injuries, anatomy, and x rays.*

Anatomy of the Knee Tutorial: http://ncl.ac.uk/~nccc/tutorials/knee

Knee Surgery Information: http://www.arthroscopy.com/sp04000.htm

Knee I.com: http://www.kneel.com/
gotoindex.cfm

*A complete, free knee resource. Find
healing technology and rehabilitation for
knee pain, ACL injuries, osteoarthritis,
other diseases, knee replacements. Talk
online to surgeons and patients.*

Iliotibial Band Syndrome: http://www.
sover.net/~sstryker/itbs.html

*ITBS is a common running and cycling
injury around the knee. This site lists*
*causes, therapies, treatments, and per-
sonal experiences with this problem.*

What is Chondromalacia?: http://
healthlink.mcw.edu/article/
926052680.html

*Article on the causes and treatment
of the knee disorder chondromalacia
patella.*

# The Thigh, Hip, Groin, and Pelvis

*When you finish this chapter you will be able to:*

- Describe the major anatomical features of the thigh, hip, groin, and pelvis as they relate to sports injuries.
- Identify the major sports injuries to the thigh, hip, groin, and pelvis.
- Demonstrate appropriate emergency procedures for injuries to the thigh, groin, and pelvis.

Although the thigh, hip, groin, and pelvis have lower incidences of injury than do the knee and lower limb, they receive considerable trauma from a variety of sports activities. Of major concern are thigh strains and contusions and chronic and overuse stresses affecting the thigh and hip.

## ANATOMY OF THE THIGH REGION

### Bones

The thigh is generally considered that part of the leg between the hip and the knee. The *femur* is the longest and strongest bone in the body (Figure 17-1). It is designed for maximum support and mobility during weight-bearing activity. The proximal head of the femur articulates with the pelvis to form the hip joint and the distal femoral condyles articulate with the tibia at the knee joint.

### Muscles

The muscles located on the anterior thigh are the four quadriceps that function to extend the knee (Figure 17-2). One of the quadriceps, the rectus femoris muscle also acts to flex the hip. The sartorius muscle is also on the anterior thigh and acts to flex the hip and outwardly rotate the thigh (Figure 17-3). The three hamstring muscles on the back of the thigh are flexors of the knee and act to extend the hip (Figure 17-4). The five

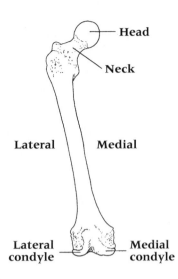

Head

Neck

Lateral    Medial

Lateral
condyle

Medial
condyle

**Figure 17-1**

Femur (or femoris)

medial muscles are known as the adductor group and collectively act as adductors of the hip. They include the gracilis, pectineus, and the adductor magnus, longus, and brevis (Figure 17-5).

## ASSESSING THIGH INJURIES

Thigh injury evaluation is concerned with the femur and the soft tissue that surrounds it.

### History

The coach should ask the following questions:

- Was the onset of injury fast or slow?
- Has this injury occurred before?
- How was the thigh injured?

**Figure 17-2**

Quadriceps femoris

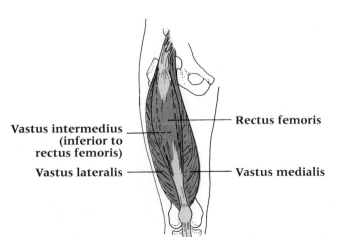

Vastus intermedius
(inferior to
rectus femoris)

Rectus femoris

Vastus lateralis

Vastus medialis

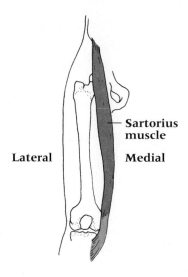

**Figure 17-3**

The sartorius flexes and
externally rotates the femur.

- Can you describe the intensity or duration of the pain?
- Is the pain constant? If not, when does it occur?
- Can you point to the pain site?

The coach should recognize that muscle pain is hard to localize, dull, and achy. Bone pain is described as deep, penetrating, and localized.

## Observation

The coach observes the thigh for:

- Symmetry with the noninjured thigh
- Swelling

**Figure 17-4**

Hamstring muscles

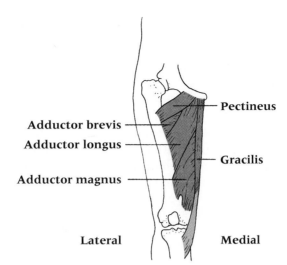

Pectineus

Adductor brevis

Adductor longus

Gracilis

Adductor magnus

Lateral          Medial

**Figure 17-5**

Hip adductors

- Normal skin coloration and texture
- The obvious presence of pain

Is the athlete willing to move the thigh?

## PREVENTION OF THIGH INJURIES

As with all muscles in sports, the thigh must have maximum strength, endurance, and extensibility to withstand strain. In collision sports such as football, the thigh must be protected against contusion by the wearing of thigh guards.

## RECOGNITION AND MANAGEMENT OF INJURIES TO THE THIGH

Injuries to the thigh muscles are among the most common in sports. Contusions and strains occur often to the thigh, with the former having the highest incidence.

### Quadriceps Contusions

**Cause of injury**   The quadriceps group is continually exposed to traumatic blows in a variety of sports. Contusions of the quadriceps display all the classic symptoms of most muscle bruises.

**Signs of injury**   Quadriceps contusions usually develop as the result of a severe impact on the relaxed thigh, compressing the muscle against the hard surface of the femur. At the instant of trauma, pain, a temporary loss of function, and the immediate bleeding of the affected muscles usually occur. The extent of the force and the degree of thigh relaxation determine the depth of the injury and the amount of structural and functional disruption that take place.[10]

Early detection and avoidance of profuse internal bleeding are vital, both in effecting a fast recovery by the athlete and in the prevention of

**Figure 17-6**

Quadriceps contusion: A, Grade 1 mild internal bleeding. B, Grade 1 mild pain and point tenderness. C, Grade 2 moderate pain and swelling. D, Grade 3 deep muscle bleeding.

widespread scarring of the muscle tissue. The athlete usually describes having been hit by a sharp blow to the thigh, which produced intense pain and weakness. The coach observes that the athlete is limping and holding the thigh. Palpation by the coach may reveal a swollen area that is painful to the touch. The seriousness or extent of injury is determined by the amount of weakness and decreased range of motion.

*Grade 1 (mild) contusions*   A Grade 1 quadriceps contusion can be either a very superficial intramuscular bruise or a slightly deeper one. The very superficial contusion (Figure 17-6A) creates a mild hemorrhage, little pain, no swelling, and a mild point tenderness with no restriction of the range of motion. In contrast, a deeper first-degree contusion (Figure 17-6B) produces pain, mild swelling, point tenderness, and a knee flexion of no more than 90 degrees.

*Grade 2 (moderate) contusions*   The Grade 2 quadriceps contusion is of moderate intensity, causing pain, swelling, and a range of knee flexion that is less than 90 degrees with an obvious limp present (Figure 17-6C).

*Grade 3 (severe) contusions*   The severe, or grade 3 quadriceps, contusion represents a major disability. A blow may have been so intense as to split the fasciae, allowing the muscle to protrude (muscle herniation) (Figure 17-6D). A characteristically deep intramuscular hematoma with an intermuscular spread is present. Pain is severe, and swelling may lead to hematoma. Movement of the knee is severely restricted, and the athlete has a decided limp.

**Care**   On-site action by the coach includes compression by elastic bandage; the application of a cold medium can help control superficial hemorrhage (Figure 17-7). The thigh contusion should be handled conservatively with RICE followed by a very gentle static stretch and crutch walking when a limp is present.

Once an athlete has sustained a grade 2 or 3 thigh contusion, great care must be taken to avoid the occurrence of another one. The athlete should routinely wear a protective pad held in place by an elastic wrap while engaged in sports activity.

Note: With grade 3, there is between 45 and 90 degrees of restriction flexion. With grade 4, there is a restriction of less than 45 degrees of flexion.

## Muscle Ossification (Myositis Ossificans)

**Cause of injury**   A severe blow or repeated blows to the thigh, usually the quadriceps muscle, can cause ectopic bone formation within the muscle, known as **myositis ossificans traumatica.**

**Signs of injury**   Myositis ossificans commonly develops following bleeding into the quadriceps muscle and formation of a blood tumorous formation. The contusion causes a disruption of muscle fibers, blood vessels, connective tissue, and periosteum of the femur. Acute inflammation follows resolution of hemorrhage. The irritated tissue may produce tissue formations resembling cartilage or bone. In 2 to 4 weeks, formation of bone may be noted under x-ray examination. If the injury is to a muscle

**Figure 17-7**

Immediate care of the thigh
contusion: Applying a cold
pack and pressure bandage
along with a mild stretch
may provide some relief.

belly, complete absorption or a decrease in size of the formation may occur. This absorption is less likely if calcification is at a muscle origin or insertion. Some formations are completely free of the femur, whereas another may be stalklike and yet another broadly attached (Figure 17-8).

Improper care of a thigh contusion can lead to ossification in muscle.
The following can cause the condition or, once present, aggravate it,
causing it to become more pronounced:

- Attempting to run off a quadriceps contusion
- Too vigorous treatment of a contusion—for example, massage directly
  over the contusion or superficial heat to the thigh.

**Care**  Once myositis ossificans traumatica is apparent, treatment
should be extremely conservative. If the condition is painful and restricts
motion, the formation may be surgically removed after 1 year with much
less likelihood of its return. Too early removal of the formation may cause
it to return. Recurrent myositis ossificans may indicate a problem with
blood clotting.[4]

## Quadriceps Muscle Strain

**Cause of injury**  The rectus femoris muscle of the quadriceps muscle
group occasionally becomes strained by a sudden stretch (e.g., falling on
a bent knee) or a sudden contraction (e.g., jumping in volleyball or kicking in soccer). Usually this muscle strain is associated with a muscle that
is weakened or overly constricted.[9]

A tear in the region of the rectus femoris may cause partial or
complete disruption of muscle fibers (Figure 17-9). The incomplete tear
may be located centrally within the muscle or more peripheral to the
muscle.

**Signs of injury**  A peripheral quadriceps rectus femoris tear causes
fewer symptoms than the deeper tear. In general, there is less point tenderness and little bleeding. A more centered partial muscle tear causes

17–1

*Critical Thinking* Exercise

A basketball player performing
a layup shot receives a sharp
blow to his right quadriceps
muscle.

**?**  How may the grade of this
contusion be determined?

---

**myositis ossificans
traumatica**
Bone formation occurring
in an abnormal place.

**Figure 17-8**

Myositis ossificans

**Figure 17-9**

Rupture of the rectus femoris

Myositis ossificans traumatica
can occur following:
• A single severe blow
• Many blows to a muscle
area
• Improper care of a contusion

In order of incidence of
sports injury to the thigh,
quadriceps contusions rank
first and hamstring strains
rank second.

**Figure 17-10**

A neoprene sleeve may be
worn for soft tissue support.

more pain and discomfort than does the peripheral tear. The deep tear
causes a great deal of pain, point tenderness, spasm, and loss of function,
but little discoloration from internal bleeding. In contrast, complete muscle tear of the rectus femoris may leave the athlete with little disability
and discomfort but with some deformity of the anterior thigh.

**Care**  On-site care of the quadriceps strain by the coach includes
rest, cold application, and pressure to control internal bleeding. The extent of the tear should be ascertained as soon as possible before swelling
masks the extent of injury (refer to Figure 17-9). To stabilize the muscle,
the coach might consider having the athlete wear a neoprene sleeve as
healing occurs (Figure 17-10).

## Hamstring Muscle Strains

Of all the thigh muscles subject to strain, the hamstring group has the
highest incidence of strain.

**Cause of injury**  The exact cause of hamstring strain is not known.
It is speculated that a quick change of the hamstring muscle from knee
stabilization to extension of the hip when running may be a major cause
of this strain (Figure 17-11). What leads to this muscle failure and deficiency in the complementary action of opposing muscles is not clearly
understood. Some possible reasons are muscle fatigue, sciatic nerve irritation, faulty posture, leg-length discrepancy, tight hamstrings, using improper form, and imbalance of strength between hamstring muscle
groups.

In most athletes, the hamstring muscle group should have at least 60
to 70 percent of the strength of the opposing quadriceps group. Stretching after exercise is imperative to avoid muscle tightness.

Hamstring strain can involve the muscle belly or bony attachment.
The extent of injury can vary from the pulling apart of a few muscle fibers
to a complete rupture or an avulsion fracture (Figure 17-12).

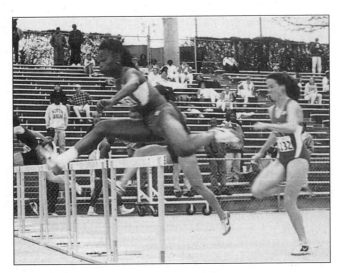

**Figure 17-11**

In many sports, stretching
of the hip region can cause
a hamstring strain.

**Signs of injury**   Internal bleeding, pain, and immediate loss of function vary according to the degree of trauma. Discoloration may occur 1 or 2 days after injury.

**Grade 1 hamstring strain**   A grade 1 hamstring strain is usually evidenced by muscle soreness on movement and is accompanied by point tenderness. These strains are often difficult to detect when they occur. Irritation and stiffness do not become apparent until the athlete has cooled down after activity. The soreness of the mild hamstring strain in most instances can be attributed to muscle spasm rather than to the tearing of tissue.[1]

 17-2

**Critical Thinking** Exercise

A sprinter competing in a 100-yard dash experiences a sudden snap, severe pain, and weakness in the left hamstring muscle.

**?**  What kind of injury can be expected by the coach?

**Figure 17-12**

Hamstring tear

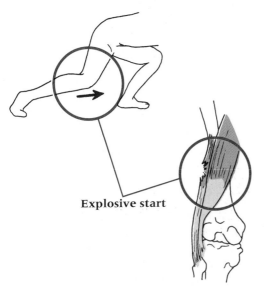

**Explosive start**

*Grade 2 hamstring strain*    A grade 2 muscle strain represents partial tearing of muscle fibers and can be identified by a sudden snap or tear of the muscle accompanied by severe pain and a loss of function of knee flexion. It is possible to palpate a defect in the muscle with a grade 2 strain.

*Grade 3 hamstring strain*    A grade 3 hamstring strain is the rupturing of tendinous or muscular tissue, involving major hemorrhage and disability.

**Care**    Initially an ice pack and compression by an elastic wrap should be employed. Activity should be restricted until soreness has been minimized. Ballistic stretching and explosive sprinting should be avoided initially.

Strains are always a problem to the athlete; they tend to recur because they sometimes heal with inelastic fibrous scar tissue. The higher the incidence of strains at a particular muscle site, the greater the amount of scar tissue and the greater the likelihood of further injury.

### Acute Femoral Fracture

**Cause of injury**    In sports, fractures of the femur occur most often in the shaft rather than at the bone ends and are almost always caused by a great force, such as falling from a height or being hit directly by another participant. A fracture of the shaft most often takes place in the middle third of the bone because of the anatomical curve at this point and because the majority of direct blows are sustained in this area.

**Signs of injury**    Shock generally accompanies a fracture of the femur as a result of the extreme amount of pathology and pain associated with this injury. Bone displacement is usually present as a result of the great strength of the quadriceps muscle, which causes overriding of the bone fragments. Direct impact produces extensive soft-tissue injury with muscle lacerations, major internal bleeding, and muscle spasms.

An acute fractured femur is recognized by these classic signs:

- Deformity, with the thigh rotated outward
- A shortened thigh, caused by bone displacement
- Loss of thigh function
- Pain and point tenderness
- Swelling of the soft tissues

To prevent a life-threatening situation, the coach must secure immediate emergency assistance and medical referral.[4]

### Stress Fracture of the Femur

**Cause of injury**    The popularity of jogging and the increased mileage covered by serious runners have increased the incidence of stress fractures to the femur bone.

**Signs of injury**    Stress fracture must be considered when the athlete complains of constant pain. It occurs most often at the neck of the femur. Rest and limited weight bearing is the treatment of choice.[7]

Femoral stress fractures are becoming more prevalent because of the increased popularity of repetitive, sustained activities such as distance running.

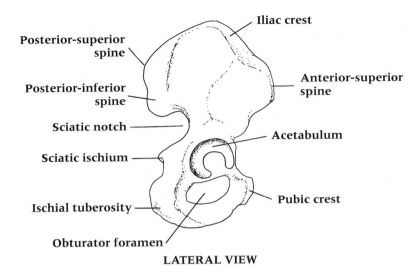

Posterior-superior spine

Posterior-inferior spine

Sciatic notch

Sciatic ischium

Ischial tuberosity

Obturator foramen

Iliac crest

Anterior-superior spine

Acetabulum

Pubic crest

**LATERAL VIEW**

**Figure 17-13**

The innominate bone of the pelvis

## ANATOMY OF THE HIP, GROIN, AND PELVIC REGION

### Bones

The pelvis is a bony ring formed by the two innominate bones, the sacrum, and the coccyx (Figure 17-13). The two innominate bones are each made up of an ilium, ischium, and pubis. The functions of the pelvis are to support the spine and trunk and tso transfer their weight to the lower limbs. In addition to providing skeletal support, the pelvis serves as a place of attachment for the trunk and thigh muscles and protection for the pelvic organs.

The hip and pelvis form the core for full body movement. The body's center of gravity is just in front of the upper part of the sacrum. Injuries to the hip or pelvis cause the athlete disability in the lower limb or trunk or both.[2]

### Ligaments

The hip joint is formed by articulation of the femur with the innominate. The head of the femur fits into a deep socket, the acetabulum, and is stabilized by strong ligaments and a joint capsule (Figure 17-14). The

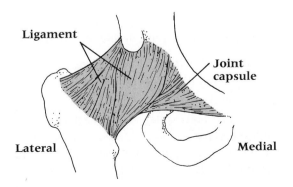

Ligament

Joint capsule

Lateral

Medial

**Figure 17-14**

The hip joint with surrounding ligament and joint capsule

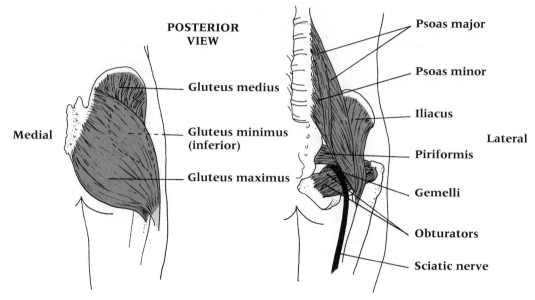

**POSTERIOR VIEW**

Medial

Gluteus medius

Gluteus minimus (inferior)

Gluteus maximus

Psoas major

Psoas minor

Iliacus

Piriformis

Lateral

Gemelli

Obturators

Sciatic nerve

**Figure 17-15**

Muscles of the hip

sacrum is joined to other parts of the pelvis by strong ligaments, forming the sacroiliac joint. A small backward-forward movement is present at the sacroiliac junction. The coccyx is composed of five small fused vertebral bodies that articulate with the sacrum. The sacroiliac joint is discussed in detail in Chapter 20.

## Muscles

Major movements of the hip and groin:
- Internal and external rotation
- Adduction
- Abduction
- Extension
- Flexion
- Internal and external circumduction

The muscles of the hip can be divided into anterior and posterior groups (Figure 17-15). The anterior group includes the iliacus and psoas muscles, which flex the thigh on the trunk. The posterior group includes the tensor fasciae latae and gluteus medius, which abduct the thigh, the gluteus maximus, which extends the thigh, the gluteus minimus, which internally rotates the thigh, and the six deep outward rotators—the piriformis, superior gemellus, inferior gemellus, obturator internus, obturator externus, and quadratus femoris.

## ASSESSING THE PELVIS AND HIP

### History

The coach should ask the following questions:

- What does the injury feel like (e.g., weakness, pain, etc.)?
- When did you first notice this problem with your hip or pelvis?
- Describe the type of pain you have (e.g., sharp, dull, pulsating, etc.)
- Does your pain radiate to the back or front of your thigh or to your buttocks area?
- When does the pain occur most intensely (e.g., during activity, at rest, or at night in bed)?

## Observation

- The athlete should be observed for postural asymmetry while standing on one leg and during ambulation.
- From the front view, do the hips look even?
- From the side view, is the pelvis abnormally tilted anteriorly or posteriorly?
- The patella should also be noted for relative position and alignment.
- Does standing on one leg produce pain in the hip?
- The athlete should be observed during walking and sitting. Pain in the hip and pelvic region is normally reflected in movement distortions.

## Palpation

Bony palpation should include the iliac crest, femur, sacrum, and coccyx. The soft-tissue sites of major concern are those lying in the groin region and major muscles.

## RECOGNITION AND MANAGEMENT OF HIP INJURIES

The hip joint, the strongest and best-protected joint in the human body, is seldom seriously injured during sports activities. The hip joint is substantially supported by the ligamentous tissues and muscles that surround it, so any unusual movement that exceeds the normal range of motion may result in tearing of tissue.

### Hip Sprain

**Cause of injury**  Hip sprains may occur as the result of a violent twist, either produced through an impact force delivered by another participant or by forceful contact with another object or sustained in a situation in which the foot is firmly planted and the trunk is forced in an opposing direction.

**Signs of injury**  A hip sprain displays all the signs of a major acute injury but is best revealed through the athlete's inability to circumduct the thigh. Symptoms are similar to a stress fracture. There is significant pain in the hip region.  Hip rotation increases pain.

**Care**  X rays should be taken to rule out fracture; RICE and analgesics are used as needed. Depending on the grade of sprain, weight bearing is restricted. Crutch walking is used for grade 2 and 3 sprains. Range-of-motion and progressive resistance exercises are delayed until the hip is pain free.

### Dislocated Hip Joint

**Cause of injury**  Dislocation of the hip joint rarely occurs in sports. The dislocated hip is caused by traumatic force along the long axis of the femur or by the athlete falling on his or her side. Such dislocations are produced when the knee is bent.

**atrophic necrosis** (ah **tro**
fick **necro** sis)
Death of an area caused by
lack of circulation.

**Signs of injury**  The incomplete dislocation or luxation presents a
picture of a flexed, adducted, and internally rotated thigh. Palpation reveals that the head of the femur has moved to a position posterior to the
acetabulum. A hip dislocation causes serious pathology by tearing capsular and ligamentous tissue. A fracture is often associated with this injury,
accompanied by possible damage to the sciatic nerve and the nutrient artery, causing **atrophic necrosis.**

**Care**  Medical attention must be secured immediately after displacement, or muscle contractures may complicate the initial treatment.
Immobilization usually consists of 2 weeks of bed rest and the use of a
crutch for walking for a month or longer.

**Complications**  Complication of the posterior hip dislocation is
likely. Such complications include muscle paralysis as a result of nerve injury in the area and later development of degeneration of the femoral
head.

### Groin Strain

The groin is the depression between the thigh and the abdomen. The
muscles in the groin region are responsible for adduction and internal rotation of the thigh.

**Cause of injury**  Any one of the muscles in the groin region can be
torn in sports activity and elicit a groin strain (Figure 17-16). In addition, overextension of the groin musculature may result in a strain.
Running, jumping, and twisting with external rotation can produce such
injuries.[5]

**Figure 17-16**

Contact and collision sports
can produce serious pelvic
injuries.

**Figure 17-17**

Commercial restraints such as the Sowa groin and thigh braces are increasingly being used in athletic training.

**Signs of injury**   The strain can appear as a sudden twinge or feeling of tearing during a movement, or it may not be noticed until after termination of activity. As is characteristic of most tears, the groin strain also produces pain, weakness, and internal bleeding.

**Care**   If it is detected immediately after it occurs, the strain should be treated by intermittent ice, pressure, and rest for 48 to 72 hours.[6]

Rest has been found to be the best treatment for groin strains. Until normal flexibility and strength return, a protective spica bandage should be applied. Commercial restraints are also available to protect the injured groin (Figure 17-17). Note that a pelvic stress fracture may produce groin pain. Any athlete complaining of severe groin pain should be referred for medical attention.

## Immature Hip Joint Problems

The coach working with a child or adolescent should understand two major problems stemming from the immature hip joint. They are coxa plana, or Legg-Perthes disease, which is caused by a death of the articular cartilage as a result of disruption of blood circulation; and a slipping of the femoral head's growth center, or epiphysis.[11]

### Coxa Plana or Legg-Perthes Disease

**Cause of condition**   Coxa plana is due to a loss of blood circulation to the articular head of the femur (Figure 17-18). It occurs in children ages three to twelve and in boys more often than in girls. The reason for this condition is not clearly understood. Because of a disruption of circulation to the head of the femur, the articular cartilage dies and becomes flattened.

**Figure 17-18**

Coxa plana (Legg-Perthes disease); arrow indicates the avascular necrosis of the femoral head.

Recognition and
Management of Specific
Injuries and Conditions

A young athlete who
complains of pain in the
groin, abdomen, or knee and
who walks with a limp may
display signs of coxa plana or
a slipped femoral epiphysis.

**Figure 17-19**

Slipped femoral epiphysis

*Critical Thinking* Exercise

A 15-year-old male football
player complains of pain in his
hip off and on during the season. There is increasing hip and
knee pain during movement.
The athlete has a restriction of
hip abduction, flexion, and
medial rotation. He is beginning to walk with a limp.

**?** What should the coach be
concerned about in this
15-year-old, and what steps
should be taken?

**Signs of condition**   The young athlete commonly complains of pain
in the groin that sometimes is referred to the abdomen or knee. Limping
is also typical. The condition can have a rapid onset, but more often it
comes on slowly over a number of months. Examination may show limited hip movement and pain.[3]

**Care**   This condition can warrant complete bed rest to reduce the
chances of a chronic hip condition. A special brace to avoid direct weight
bearing on the hip may have to be worn. If treated in time, the head of
the femur will revascularize and regain its original shape.

**Complications**   If the condition is not treated early enough, the
head of the femur will become ill shaped, producing osteoarthritis in later
life.

### Slipped Growth Site of the Femoral Head

The slipped femoral epiphysis (Figure 17-19) is found mostly in boys between the ages of ten and seventeen who are very tall and thin or are
obese.

**Cause of condition**   Although the cause is unknown, the slipped
femoral epiphysis may be related to the effects of a growth hormone. In
one-quarter of the cases, both hips are affected.[8]

**Signs of condition**   Symptoms of this condition are similar to those
for Legg-Perthes disease. The athlete has a pain in the groin that arises
suddenly as a result of trauma or over weeks or months as a result of prolonged stress. In the early stages of this condition, signs may be minimal;
however, in its most advanced stage there is hip and knee pain and major limitations on movement together with a limp.

**Care**   In cases of minor displacement, rest and no weight bearing
may prevent further slipping. Major displacement usually requires corrective surgery.

**Complications**   If the displacement goes undetected or if surgery
fails to restore normal hip mechanics, severe hip problems may occur in
later life.

## RECOGNITION AND MANAGEMENT OF INJURIES TO THE PELVIS

Athletes who perform activities involving violent jumping, running, and
collisions can sustain serious acute and overuse injuries to the pelvic region (Figure 17-20).

### Iliac Crest Contusion (Hip Pointer)

Iliac crest contusion, commonly known as a *hip pointer,* occurs most often
in contact sports.

**Cause of injury**   The hip pointer results from a blow to the inadequately protected iliac crest (Figure 17-21). The hip pointer is one of
the most handicapping injuries in sports. A direct impact to the unprotected iliac crest causes a severe pinching action to the soft tissue of that
region.

**Figure 17-20**

Athletes who perform
activities involving jumping,
running, and collisions can
sustain serious acute and
overuse injuries to the pelvic
region.

**Signs of injury**  The hip pointer produces immediate pain, spasms,
and transitory paralysis of the soft structures. As a result, the athlete is
unable to rotate the trunk or to flex the thigh without pain.[13]

**Care**  Cold and pressure should be applied immediately after injury
and should be maintained intermittently for at least 48 hours. In severe
cases bed rest for 1 to 2 days will speed recovery. Referral to a physician
must be made and an x-ray examination given.

**Figure 17-21**

A blow to the pelvic rim can
cause a bruise and hematoma
known as a hip pointer.

## Osteitis Pubis

**Course of injury**   Since the popularity of distance running has increased, a condition known as *osteitis pubis* has become more prevalent. It is also caused by soccer, football, and wrestling. Repetitive stress on the *pubic symphysis* and adjacent bony structures by the pull of muscles in the area creates a chronic inflammatory condition.

**Signs of injury**   The athlete has pain in the groin region and in the bony projection under the pubic hair called the symphysis pubis. There is point tenderness on the pubic tubercle and pain when movements such as running, sit-ups, and squats are performed.[12]

**Care**   Follow-up care usually consists of rest and an oral antiinflammatory agent. A return to activity should be gradual.

## Acute Fracture of the Pelvis

The pelvis is an extremely strong structure, and fractures stemming from sports are rare.

**Cause of injury**   The acute pelvic fracture usually occurs as the result of a direct trauma.

**Signs of injury**   The athlete responds to this injury with severe pain, loss of function, and shock.

**Care**   If a pelvic fracture is suspected, the athlete should be immediately treated for shock and referred to a physician. The seriousness of this injury depends on the extent of shock and the possibility of internal injury.

## Stress Fractures of the Pelvis

**Cause of injury**   As with other stress fractures, pelvic and femur stress fractures can be produced by repetitive abnormal overuse forces. Pelvic stress fractures tend to occur during intensive training or competitive racing.

**Signs of injury**   Commonly the athlete complains of groin pain along with an aching sensation in the thigh that increases with activity and decreases with rest.

**Care**   The coach must listen to the athlete who complains of pelvic pain following intense exercise. Referral to a physician for a detailed examination with an x ray is a must. Once this injury is verified, rest is the treatment of choice for 2 to 5 months.

## Avulsion Fractures

The pelvis has a number of sites at which major muscles attach. Pain at these sites can mean that a muscle has begun to pull away from its attachment.

**Cause of injury**   Avulsion fractures in the pelvic region occur during sudden acceleration or deceleration such as in football, soccer, and basketball.

**Signs of injury**   The athlete complains of a sudden localized pain with limited movement. On inspection the coach observes swelling and a point tenderness.

**Care**   Early conditions require rest, limited activity, and graduated exercise.

## SUMMARY

- The thigh is composed of the femoral shaft, musculature, nerves and blood vessels, and the fascia that envelops the soft tissue. It is the part of the leg between the hip and the knee.

- The quadriceps contusion and hamstring strain are the most common sports injuries to the thigh, with the quadriceps contusion having the highest incidence.

- Of major importance in acute thigh contusion is early detection and the avoidance of internal bleeding.

- One major complication to repeated contusions is myositis ossificans.

- It is not clearly known why hamstring muscles become strained. Strain occurs most often to the short head of the biceps femoris.

- The groin is the depression between the thigh and abdominal region. Groin strain can occur to any one of a number of muscles in this region. Running, jumping, or twisting can produce a groin strain.

- The hip joint, the strongest and best-protected joint in the human body, has a low incidence of acute sports injuries.

- Some young athletes develop conditions that stem from an immature hip joint. These conditions are coxa plana, or Legg-Perthes disease, and the slipped femoral epiphysis.

- A common problem in the pelvic region is the hip pointer, which results from a blow to the inadequately protected iliac crest. The contusion causes pain, spasm, and malfunction of the muscles in the area.

---

*Solutions to Critical Thinking* Exercises

---

**17-1**   One of the best ways to determine the grade of a contusion to the quadriceps muscle is through the degree of restriction of knee flexion. With grade 1 there is a knee flexion of no more than 90 degrees; with grade 2, less than 90 degrees; with grade 3, between 45 and 90 degrees; and with grade 4, less than 45 degrees.

**17-2**   The coach can expect a moderate to severe hamstring strain.

**17-3**   Because of the age of the athlete, the coach should consider the possibility of a growth problem. If a growth problem, it is most likely a slipped femoral epiphysis. The coach must refer this athlete immediately to a physician for x-ray examination.

**17-4**   This athlete has sustained a hip pointer or contusion to the skin and musculature in the region of the iliac crest. The athlete most likely will experience severe pain, muscle spasm, and an inability to rotate his trunk or flex his hip without pain.

## REVIEW QUESTIONS AND CLASS ACTIVITIES

1. What signs and symptoms are seen in each of the three degrees of quadriceps contusions? How are they managed?
2. What complications can occur if a thigh contusion is mishandled?
3. Why do hamstring strains often become recurrent?
4. Where do fractures occur most often in the femur? How are they recognized? What emergency care must be given?
5. What muscles are most often injured in a groin strain? How is this type of injury managed?
6. What type of hip problems occur in the young athlete?
7. Describe hip pointer prevention and care.

 **Dynamic Human CD**

For more information on skeletal anatomy of the pelvis, hip, and thigh click on:

- Skeletal
- Anatomy
- Gross anatomy
- Pelvic girdle
- Then, Lower limbs
- Femur

To take a closer look at the muscles that are involved in knee movement click on:

- Muscular
- Anatomy
- Body regions
- Thigh

To look at the muscular rehabilitation following healing of a fractured femur click on:

- Skeletal
- Clinical Concepts
- Fractured femur

### REFERENCES

1. Best TM, Garrett WE Jr: Hamstring strains: expediting return to play, *Physician Sportsmed* 24(8):52, 1996.
2. Boyd KT, Peirce NS, Batt ME: Common hip injuries in sport, *Sports Med* 24(4):273, 1997.
3. DePalma B: Rehabilitation of groin, hip, and thigh injuries. In Prentice WE, editor: *Rehabilitation techniques in sports medicine*, ed 3, Boston, MA, 1999, WCB/McGraw-Hill.
4. Hacutt JE: General types of injuries. In Birrer RB, editor: *Sports*

*medicine for the primary care physician,* ed 2, Boca Raton, Fla, 1994, CRC Press.

5. Hagerstown MT: Groin pain, *Sports Med* 18:133, 1996.

6. Hasselman CT et al: When groin pain signals an adductor strain, *Physician Sportsmed* 18(2):54, 1990.

7. Jackson DL: Stress fracture of the femur, *Physician Sportsmed* 19:39, 1991.

8. Johnson DL, Klabunde LA: The elusive slipped capital femoral epiphysis, *J Ath Train* 20(2):124, 1995.

9. Kaeding CC: Quadriceps strains and contusions, *Physician Sportsmed* 23 (1):59, 1995.

10. Levandowski R, Difliori JP: Thigh injuries. In Birrer RB, editor: *Sports medicine for the primary care physician,* ed 2, Boca Raton, Fla, 1994, CRC Press.

11. Paletta GA et al: Injuries about the hip and pelvis in the young athlete. In Michile LJ, editor: *The young athlete. Clinics in sports medicine,* vol 14, no 3, Philadelphia, 1995, WB Saunders.

12. Roos HP: Hip pain in sport, *Sports Med Arthroscop Rev* 5(4):292, 1997.

13. Weicker GG, Munnings F: How to manage hip and pelvis injuries in adolescents, *Physician Sportsmed* 21:72, 1993.

## ANNOTATED BIBLIOGRAPHY

Boyd KT, Peirce NS, Batt ME: *Common hip injuries in sports, Sports Med* 24(4):273, 1997.

    *Provides a detailed discussion of hip and pelvic anatomy and sports injuries.*

Torg JS, Shephard RJ, editors: *Current therapy in sports medicine,* ed 3, St Louis, 1995, Mosby.

    *A detailed sports medicine text with extensive coverage of thigh, hip, and pelvic injuries.*

## WEBSITES

Cramer First Aider: http://www.ccsd.k12.wy.us/CCHS_web/sptmed/fstaider.htm

World Ortho: http://www.worldortho.com

    *Use the search engine in this site to locate relevant information.*

Wheeless' Textbook of Orthopaedics: http://www.medmedia.com/med.htm

    *An excellent page for injuries, anatomy, and x rays.*

Karolinska Institute Library: Musculoskeletal Disease: http://www.mic.ki.se/Disease/c5.htm

American Orthopaedic Society for Sports Medicine: http://www.sportsmed.org

# The Shoulder Complex

*When you finish this chapter you will be able to:*

- Identify the bones, articulations, stabilizing ligaments, and musculature of the shoulder complex.
- Explain how shoulder injuries may be prevented.
- Describe the process for assessing injuries to the shoulder.
- Identify specific injuries that occur around the shoulder joint and describe plans for management.

The anatomy of the shoulder complex allows for a great degree of mobility. To achieve this mobility, stability of the complex is sometimes compromised and instability of the shoulder frequently leads to injury, particularly in those sports that involve overhead activity.[1] Sport activities such as throwing, swimming, or serving in tennis or volleyball place a great deal of stress on the supporting structures (Figure 18-1). Consequently, injuries related to overuse in the shoulder are commonplace in the athlete.[4]

Dynamic movement and stabilization of the shoulder complex require integrated function of the rotator cuff muscles, the joint capsule, and the muscles that stabilize and position the scapula.

## ANATOMY

### Bones

The bones that comprise the shoulder complex and shoulder joint are the clavicle, scapula, and humerus (Figure 18-2). These three bones form the four major articulations associated with the shoulder complex: the sternoclavicular joint, the acromioclavicular joint, the glenohumeral joint, and the scapulothoracic joint.

### Stabilizing Ligaments

A series of ligaments at each of the four articulations act collectively to provide stability to the shoulder complex (Figure 18-3).[18]

Shoulder complex articulations:
- Sternoclavicular
- Acromioclavicular
- Glenohumeral
- Scapulothoracic

The clavicle articulates with the sternum to form the sternoclavicular joint, the only direct connection between the upper extremity and the trunk. The sternoclavicular joint is extremely weak because of its bony arrangement, but it is held securely by the sternoclavicular ligament that pulls the clavicle downward and toward the sternum, in effect anchoring it. The clavicle is permitted to move up and down, forward and backward, in combination, and in rotation.

The acromioclavicular joint is a gliding articulation of the lateral end of the clavicle with the acromion process of the scapula. This junction is rather weak. The acromioclavicular ligament along with the coracoclavicular ligament helps to maintain the position of the clavicle relative to the acromion. The coracoacromial ligament connects the coracoid to the acromion. This ligament along with the acromion forms the coracoacromial arch.

At the glenohumeral joint (the true shoulder joint), the round head of the humerus articulates with the shallow glenoid cavity of the scapula. The position of the glenohumeral joint is maintained by the surrounding glenohumeral ligaments that form the joint capsule and by the rotator cuff muscles.

The scapulothoracic joint is not a true joint; however, the movement of the scapula on the wall of the thoracic cage is critical to shoulder joint motion. Contraction of the scapular muscles that attach the scapula to the axial skeleton is critical in stabilizing the scapula, thus providing a base on which a highly mobile joint can function.

## Muscles

The muscles that cross the glenohumeral joint produce dynamic motion and establish stability to compensate for a bony and ligamentous

**Figure 18-1**

Overhead throwing-type activities can produce a number of shoulder problems.

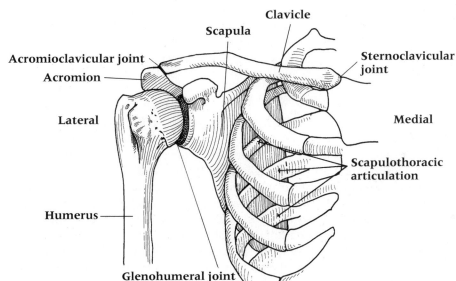

**Figure 18-2**

Skeletal anatomy of the shoulder complex

Clavicle

Scapula

Acromioclavicular joint

Acromion

Sternoclavicular joint

Lateral

Medial

Scapulothoracic articulation

Humerus

Glenohumeral joint

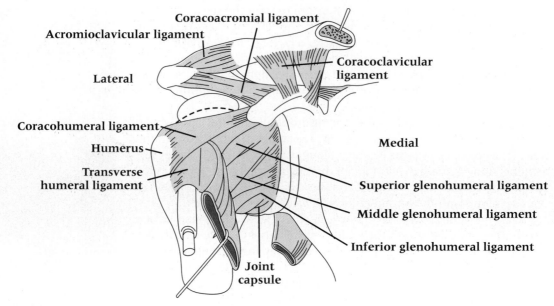

Coracoacromial ligament

Acromioclavicular ligament

Coracoclavicular ligament

Lateral

Coracohumeral ligament

Humerus

Medial

Transverse humeral ligament

Superior glenohumeral ligament

Middle glenohumeral ligament

Inferior glenohumeral ligament

Joint capsule

**Figure 18-3**

Shoulder complex articulations and ligaments

Glenohumeral joint movements:
- Flexion
- Extension
- Abduction
- Adduction
- External rotation
- Internal rotation

arrangement that allows for a great deal of mobility (Figure 18-4).[18] Movements at the glenohumeral joint include flexion, extension, abduction, adduction, and rotation. The muscles acting on the glenohumeral joint can be separated into three groups. The first group consists of muscles that originate on the axial skeleton and attach to the humerus, including the latissimus dorsi and the pectoralis major. The second group originates on the scapula and attaches to the humerus, including the deltoid, the teres major, the coracobrachialis, and the rotator cuff (subscapularis, supraspinatus, infraspinatus, teres minor). A third group of muscles attaches the axial skeleton to the scapula and includes the levator scapula, the trapezius, the rhomboids, and the serratus anterior and posterior. The scapular muscles are important in providing dynamic stability to the shoulder complex.[10]

## PREVENTION OF SHOULDER INJURIES

Proper physical conditioning is of major importance in preventing many shoulder injuries. As with all preventive conditioning, the program should be directed toward general body development and development of specific body areas for a given sport. If a sport places extreme, sustained demands on the arms and shoulders or if the shoulder is at risk for sudden traumatic injury, extensive conditioning must be used. All the muscles involved in movement of the shoulder complex should be strengthened through a full range of motion.

Proper warm-up must be performed gradually before dynamic arm movements are attempted. This warm-up causes a general increase in body temperature and is followed by sport-specific stretching of selected muscles.

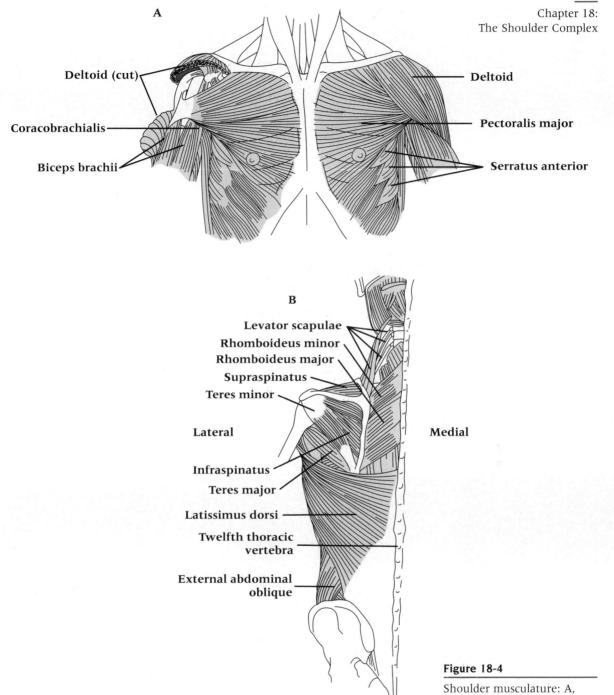

**A**

Deltoid (cut)

Coracobrachialis

Biceps brachii

Deltoid

Pectoralis major

Serratus anterior

**B**

Levator scapulae
Rhomboideus minor
Rhomboideus major
Supraspinatus
Teres minor

Lateral

Medial

Infraspinatus
Teres major

Latissimus dorsi

Twelfth thoracic
vertebra

External abdominal
oblique

**Figure 18-4**

Shoulder musculature: A,
Anterior; B, Posterior

**Figure 18-5**

Phases of throwing from left to right: wind-up, cocking, acceleration, deceleration, follow-through

All athletes in collision and contact sports should be instructed and drilled on how to fall properly. They must be taught not to try to catch themselves with an outstretched arm. Performing a shoulder roll is a safer way to absorb the shock of the fall. Specialized protective equipment such as shoulder pads must be properly fitted to avoid some shoulder injuries in tackle football.

### Using Correct Throwing Technique

To prevent overuse shoulder injuries, it is essential that athletes be correctly taught the appropriate techniques of throwing a baseball or football, throwing a javelin, serving or spiking a volleyball, and serving or hitting an overhead smash in tennis. If the thrower uses faulty technique, the joints are affected by atypical stresses that result in trauma to the joint and its surrounding tissues.[1]

Relative to the shoulder complex, throwing involves five distinct phases: wind-up, cocking, arm acceleration, arm deceleration, and follow-through (Figure 18-5).

Throwing phases:
- Wind-up
- Cocking
- Acceleration
- Deceleration
- Follow-through

#### Wind-up Phase

The wind-up or preparation phase lasts from the first movement until the ball leaves the gloved hand. During this phase the lead leg strides forward. Both shoulders abduct, externally rotate, and horizontally abduct.

#### Cocking Phase

The cocking phase begins when the hands separate and ends when maximum external rotation of the humerus has occurred. During this phase the foot comes in contact with the ground.

#### Acceleration Phase

The acceleration phase lasts from maximum external rotation until ball release. The humerus abducts, horizontally abducts, and internally rotates at velocities approaching 8000° per second. The scapula elevates, abducts, and upward rotates.

### Deceleration Phase

The deceleration phase lasts from ball release until maximum shoulder internal rotation. During this phase the external rotators of the rotator cuff contract eccentrically to decelerate the humerus. The rhomboids contract eccentrically to decelerate the scapula.

### Follow-through Phase

The follow-through phase lasts from maximum shoulder internal rotation until the end of the motion when there is a balanced position.

## ASSESSING THE SHOULDER COMPLEX

The shoulder complex is one of the most difficult regions of the body to evaluate.[13] One reason for this difficulty is that the biomechanical demands placed on these structures during overhand accelerations and decelerations are not yet clearly understood. It is essential that the coach understands the athlete's major complaints and the possible mechanisms of the injury.

### History

The following questions in regard to the athlete's complaints can help the coach determine the nature of the injury:

- What happened to cause this pain?
- Have you ever had this problem before?
- What is the duration and intensity of the pain?
- Where is the pain located?
- Is there crepitus during movement or numbness or distortion in temperature such as a cold or warm feeling?
- Is there a feeling of weakness or a sense of fatigue?
- What shoulder movements or positions seem to aggravate or relieve the pain?
- If therapy has been given before, what, if anything, offered pain relief (e.g., cold, heat, massage, or analgesic medication)?

### Observation

The athlete should be generally observed while walking and standing. Observation during walking can reveal asymmetry of arm swing or a lean toward the painful shoulder. The athlete is next observed from the front, side, and back while in a standing position. The coach looks for postural asymmetries, bony or joint deformities, or muscle spasm or guarding patterns.

### Anterior Observation

- Are both shoulder tips even with one another, or is one depressed?
- Is one shoulder held higher because of muscle spasm or guarding?
- Is the lateral end of the clavicle prominent (indicating acromioclavicular sprain or dislocation)?

- Is one lateral acromion process more prominent than the other (indicating a possible glenohumeral dislocation)?
- Does the clavicular shaft appear deformed (indicating possible fracture)?
- Is there loss of the normal lateral deltoid muscle contour (indicating glenohumeral dislocation)?
- Is there an indentation in the upper biceps region (indicating rupture of biceps tendon)?

### Lateral Observation

- Is there thoracic kyphosis or are the shoulders slumped forward (indicating weakness of the erector muscles of the spine and tightness in the pectoral region)?
- Is there forward or backward arm hang (indicating possible scoliosis)?

### Posterior Observation

- Is there asymmetry such as a low shoulder, uneven scapulae, or winging of one scapular wing and not the other (indicating postural scoliosis)?
- Is the scapula protracted because of constricted pectoral muscles?
- Is there a distracted or winged scapula on one or both sides? (A winged scapula on both sides could indicate a general weakness of the serratus anterior muscles; if only one side is winged, the long thoracic nerve may be injured.)

## Palpation

Palpation of the bony structures should be done with the coach standing in front of and then behind the athlete. Both shoulders are palpated at the same time for pain sites and deformities. Palpation of the muscles around the shoulder detects point tenderness, abnormal swelling or lumps, muscle spasm or guarding, and trigger points. The shoulder is then also palpated anteriorly and posteriorly.

## Special Tests

A number of special tests can help to determine the nature of an injury to the shoulder complex.[13] The shoulder's active and passive range of motion should be noted and compared to the opposite side. Strength of the shoulder musculature should be assessed by resisted manual muscle testing. Both the muscles that act on the glenohumeral joint and those that act on the scapula should be tested.

Following are descriptions of other tests used to assess shoulder instability, shoulder impingement, and muscle weakness.

### Apprehension Test (Crank Test)

With the arm abducted 90 degrees, the shoulder is slowly and gently externally rotated as far as the athlete will allow. The athlete with a history

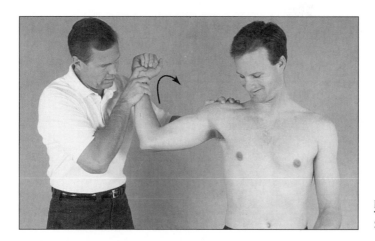

**Figure 18-6**

Shoulder apprehension test

of anterior glenohumeral instability shows great apprehension that is reflected by a facial grimace before an endpoint can be reached. At no time should the coach force this movement (Figure 18-6).

### Tests for Shoulder Impingement

Forced flexion of the humerus in the overhead position may cause impingement of soft tissue structures between the humeral head and the coracoacromial ligament. A second test involves horizontal adduction with forced internal rotation of the humerus that also produces impingement (Figure 18-7). A positive sign is indicated if the athlete feels pain and reacts with a grimace.[11]

### Test for Supraspinatus Muscle Weakness

The empty can test for supraspinatus muscle strength has the athlete bring both arms into 90 degrees of forward flexion and 30 degrees of horizontal abduction (Figure 18-8). In this position the arms are internally rotated as far as possible, thumbs pointing downward. A downward

One test for supraspinatus weakness is the empty can test.

**Figure 18-7**

Shoulder impingement tests

**Figure 18-8**

Empty can test

pressure is then applied by the coach. Weakness and pain can be detected as well as comparative strength between the two arms.

## RECOGNITION AND MANAGEMENT OF SHOULDER INJURIES

### Clavicle Fractures

**Cause of injury**   Clavicular fractures (Figure 18-9) are one of the most frequent fractures in sports. Fractures of the clavicle result from a fall on the outstretched arm, a fall on the tip of the shoulder, or a direct impact.

**Signs of injury**   The athlete with a fractured clavicle usually supports the arm on the injured side and tilts his or her head toward that side, with the chin turned to the opposite side. During inspection the injured clavicle appears a little lower than the unaffected side. Palpation may also reveal swelling, point tenderness, and mild deformity.

**Care**   The clavicular fracture is cared for immediately by applying a shoulder immobilizer and by treating the athlete for shock, if necessary (Figure 18-10). If x-ray examination reveals a fracture, a closed reduction should be attempted by the physician followed by immobilization with a clavicle strap (Figure 18-11). Immobilization should be maintained for 6 to 8 weeks. Following this period of immobilization, gentle isometric and mobilization exercises should begin with the athlete using a sling for an additional 3 to 4 weeks to provide protection. Occasionally, clavicle fractures may require operative management.[6]

**Figure 18-9**

Clavicular fracture

**Figure 18-10**

Shoulder immobilizer

**Figure 18-11**

Protective sling for clavicular fracture

## Fractures of the Humerus

**Cause of injury**   Fractures of the humerus (Figure 18-12) happen occasionally in sports, usually as the result of a direct blow, a dislocation, or the impact received by falling onto the outstretched arm.

**Signs of injury**   A fracture of the humerus is difficult to recognize by visual inspection alone; x-ray examination gives the only positive proof. Some of the more prevalent signs that may be present are pain, inability to move the arm, swelling, point tenderness, and discoloration of the superficial tissue.

**Care**   Recognition of humeral shaft fractures requires immediate application of a splint or immediate support with a sling, treatment for shock, and referral to a physician. The athlete with a fracture to the humerus will be out of competition for approximately 2 to 6 months depending on the location and severity of the fracture.[1]

**Figure 18-12**

Humeral fracture

**Figure 18-13**

Sternoclavicular sprain and
dislocation

**Figure 18-14**

Mechanism of
acromioclavicular joint sprain

## Sternoclavicular Joint Sprain

**Cause of injury**   A sternoclavicular sprain (Figure 18-13) is a relatively uncommon occurrence in sports. The mechanism of the injury is either an indirect force transmitted through the humerus, the shoulder joint, and the clavicle, or a direct impact to the clavicle. Usually the clavicle is displaced upward and forward.

**Signs of injury**   Sprain to the sternoclavicular joint can be described in three degrees. A grade 1 sprain is characterized by little pain and disability, with some point tenderness but no joint deformity. A grade 2 sprain displays subluxation of the sternoclavicular joint with visible deformity, pain, swelling, point tenderness, and an inability to abduct the shoulder in full range or to bring the arm across the chest, indicating disruption of stabilizing ligaments. The grade 3 sprain, which is the most severe, presents a picture of complete dislocation with gross displacement of the clavicle at its sternal junction, swelling, and disability, indicating complete rupture of the sternoclavicular ligament.

**Care**   RICE should be used immediately, followed by immobilization (refer to Figure 18-11). Immobilization is usually maintained for 3 to 5 weeks, followed by graded reconditioning exercises.[16] There is a high incidence of recurrence of sternoclavicular sprains.

## Acromioclavicular Joint Sprain

**Cause of injury**   The acromioclavicular joint is extremely vulnerable to sprains, especially in collision sports.[2] The primary mechanisms are a fall on an outstretched arm or a direct impact to the tip of the shoulder that forces the acromion process downward, backward, and inward while the clavicle is pushed down against the rib cage (Figure 18-14).

**Signs of injury**   In a grade 1 acromioclavicular sprain, there is point tenderness and discomfort during movement at the junction between the acromion process and the outer end of the clavicle. There is no deformity, indicating only mild stretching of the acromioclavicular ligaments.

A grade 2 sprain shows definite displacement and prominence of the lateral end of the clavicle when compared to the unaffected side. There is point tenderness during palpation of the injury site, and the athlete is unable to fully abduct through a full range of motion or to bring the arm completely across the chest.

A grade 3 sprain involves rupture of the acromioclavicular and coracoclavicular ligaments with dislocation of the clavicle. Such an injury has gross deformity and prominence of the distal clavicle, severe pain, loss of movement, and instability of the shoulder complex.

**Care**   Immediate care of the acromioclavicular sprain involves three basic procedures: (1) application of cold and pressure to control local hemorrhage, (2) stabilization of the joint by a shoulder immobilizer (refer to Figure 18-10), and (3) referral to a physician for definitive diagnosis and treatment.[2] Immobilization ranges from 3 to 4 days with a grade 1 to approximately 2 weeks with a grade 3. With all grades, an aggressive rehabilitation program involving joint mobilization, flexibility exercises, and strengthening exercises should begin immediately following the recommended period of protection.[2] Progression should be as rapid as the athlete can tolerate without increased pain or swelling.

## Glenohumeral Dislocations

**Cause of injury**   The most common glenohumeral dislocation is one in which the head of the humerus is forced out of its joint capsule in an anterior direction past the glenoid labrum and then downward to rest under the coracoid process. The mechanism for an anterior dislocation is abduction, external rotation, and extension that forces the humeral head out of the glenoid cavity (Figure 18-15).[15] An arm tackle in football or rugby or abnormal forces created in executing a throw can produce a sequence of events resulting in dislocation. On a rare occasion the humerus dislocates in an inferior direction.

Once an athlete has suffered a glenohumeral dislocation, he or she faces a high probability of recurrence because of chronic instability.[14]

**Signs of injury**   The athlete with an anterior dislocation displays a flattened deltoid contour. Palpation of the axilla reveals prominence of the humeral head. The athlete carries the affected arm in slight abduction and external rotation and is unable to touch the opposite shoulder with the hand of the affected arm. There is often moderate pain and disability.

**Care**   Initial management of the shoulder dislocation requires immediate immobilization in a position of comfort using a sling; immediate reduction by a physician; and control of the hemorrhage by cold packs. After the dislocation has been reduced and immobilized, muscle reconditioning should be initiated as soon as possible.[15] Protective sling immobilization should continue for approximately 1 week after reduction (refer to Figure 18-10). The athlete is instructed to begin a strengthening

18–1
_____

***Critical Thinking*** Exercise

A soccer player is tripped to the ground on a hard tackle and lands on the tip of her left shoulder. She complains of pain both in the tip of her shoulder and in her chest. She has difficulty lifting her arm above her shoulder because of the pain.

**?**  What injury diagnosis might result from this mechanism of injury?

18–2
_____

***Critical Thinking*** Exercise

A gymnast has a recurrent anterior dislocation of the glenohumeral joint. He is extremely worried that his shoulder will dislocate again.

**?**  What types of activities should the coach concentrate on during rehabilitation to help reduce the likelihood of a subsequent dislocation?

One test for glenohumeral instability is the apprehension test.

**Figure 18-15**

Anterior shoulder dislocation

program, progressing as quickly as pain allows. Protective shoulder braces may help limit shoulder motion (Figure 18-16).[7]

### Shoulder Impingement Syndrome

**Cause of injury**   Shoulder impingement involves a mechanical compression of the supraspinatus tendon, the subacromial bursa, and the long head of the biceps tendon, all of which are located under the coracoacromial arch (Figure 18-17).[12] Repetitive compression eventually leads to irritation and inflammation of these structures. Impingement most often occurs in repetitive overhead activities such as throwing, swimming, serving a tennis ball, or spiking a volleyball.[12]

**Figure 18-16**

Protective braces for the shoulder prevent overhead motion

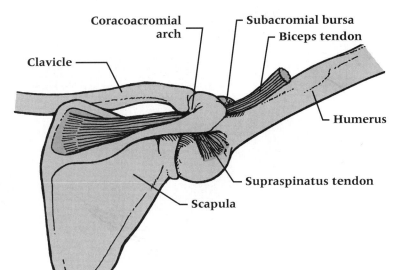

Coracoacromial arch

Subacromial bursa

Biceps tendon

Clavicle

Humerus

Supraspinatus tendon

Scapula

**Posterior view**

**Figure 18-17**

Shoulder impingement
compresses soft tissue
structures under the
coracoacromial arch.

**Signs of injury**  The athlete complains of diffuse pain around the acromion whenever the arm is in an overhead position. The external rotators are generally weaker than the internal rotators. There may be some tightness in the posterior and inferior joint capsule. There usually is a positive impingement test, and the empty can test may increase pain.[17]

**Care**  Management of impingement involves restoring normal biomechanics to the shoulder joint in an effort to maintain space under the coracoacromial arch during overhead activities. RICE can be used to modulate pain initially. Exercises should concentrate on strengthening the rotator cuff muscles, on strengthening those muscles that produce movement of the scapula, and on stretching posterior and inferior joint capsule. The activity that caused the problem in the first place should be modified so that the athlete has initial control over the frequency and the level of the activity with a gradual and progressive increase in intensity.[8]

## Rotator Cuff Strains

**Cause of injury**  The most common rotator cuff tendon strain involves the supraspinatus muscle, although any of the rotator cuff tendons are subject to injury (Figure 18-18). The mechanism of rotator cuff strains involves dynamic rotation of the arm at a high velocity as occurs during overhead throwing or any other activity in which there is rotation of the humerus.[19] Most rotator cuff tears occur in the supraspinatus in individuals with a long history of shoulder impingement or instability and are relatively uncommon in athletes under the age of 40.[5] Tears of the rotator cuff muscles are almost always near their insertion on the humerus.

18–3
*Critical Thinking* Exercise

A volleyball player consistently experiences pain when serving the ball overhead. She also indicates that most of the time when she spikes a ball at the net she experiences pain. During an evaluation the coach observes that when the humerus is flexed and internally rotated, the pain is worse.

**?**  What is most likely causing the pain when the athlete's shoulder is placed in this overhead position?

Shoulder impingement involves a mechanical compression of the supraspinatus tendon, the subacromial bursa, and the long head of the biceps tendon under the coracoacromial arch.

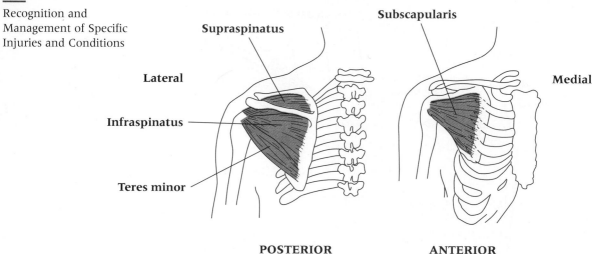

**Lateral**

**Supraspinatus**

**Subscapularis**

**Medial**

Infraspinatus —

Teres minor —

**POSTERIOR**   **ANTERIOR**

**Figure 18-18**

Rotator cuff muscles

Rotator cuff muscles:
- Subscapularis
- Supraspinatus
- Infraspinatus
- Teres minor

**Signs of injury**   Like other muscle strains, rotator cuff strains present pain with muscle contraction, some tenderness on palpation, and loss of strength because of pain. A tear or complete rupture of one of the rotator cuff tendons produces an extremely disabling condition in which pain, loss of function, swelling, and point tenderness are symptoms. In the case of a complete tear of the supraspinatus tendon, both the impingement test and the empty can test are positive.[19]

**Care**   RICE can be used to modulate pain initially. Exercises should concentrate on progressive strengthening of the rotator cuff muscles. The frequency and level of the activity should be reduced initially with a gradual and progressive increase in intensity.[9]

## Shoulder Bursitis

**Cause of injury**   The shoulder joint is subject to chronic inflammatory conditions resulting from trauma or from overuse.[3] Bursitis may develop from a direct impact, from a fall on the tip of the shoulder, or as a result of shoulder impingement. The bursa that is most often inflamed is the subacromial bursa (Figure 18-19).

**Signs of injury**   The athlete has pain when trying to move the shoulder, especially in abduction or with flexion, adduction, and internal rotation. There is also tenderness to palpation in the area just under the acromion. Impingement tests are positive.

**Care**   The use of cold packs and antiinflammatory medications to reduce inflammation is necessary. If impingement is the primary mechanism precipitating bursitis, then, as previously discussed, measures should be taken to correct this activity.[3] The athlete must maintain a consistent program of exercise, with emphasis placed on maintaining a full range of motion, so that muscle contractures and adhesions do not immobilize the joint.

Subcoracoid bursa

Subacromial bursa

Synovial capsule

Lateral          Medial

**Figure 18-19**

Synovial capsule and bursae of the shoulder

## Biceps Tenosynovitis

**Cause of injury**   Tenosynovitis of the biceps muscle is common among athletes engaged in overhead activities. Biceps tenosynovitis is prevalent among pitchers, tennis players, volleyball players, and javelin throwers. The repeated stretching of the biceps in these highly ballistic activities may eventually cause an inflammation of both the tendon and its synovial sheath.[1]

**Signs of injury**   There is tenderness in the anterior upper arm. There may also be some swelling, increased warmth, and crepitus caused by the inflammation. The athlete may complain of pain when performing dynamic overhead throwing activities.

**Care**   Biceps tenosynovitis is best cared for by complete rest for several days, combined with daily applications of cold to reduce inflammation. Antiinflammatory medications are also beneficial in reducing inflammation. After the inflammation is controlled, a gradual program of strengthening and stretching the biceps muscle should be initiated.[16]

## Contusions of the Upper Arm

**Cause of injury**   Contusions of the upper arm are frequent in contact sports. Although any muscle of the upper arm is subject to bruising, the area most often affected is the lateral aspect, primarily the brachialis muscle and portions of the triceps and biceps muscles. Repeated contusions to the lateral aspect of the upper arm can lead to myositis ossificans, more commonly known as linebacker's arm or blocker's exostosis. Myositis ossificans is calcifications or bone fragments that occur in a muscle or in soft tissues adjacent to bone.[14]

**Signs of injury**   Bruises to the upper arm area can be particularly handicapping, causing pain and tenderness, increased warmth, discoloration, and difficulty in achieving full extension and flexion of the elbow.

**Care**   RICE should be applied for a minimum of 24 hours after injury. In most cases this condition responds rapidly to treatment, usually within a few days. The key to treatment is to provide protection to the contused area to prevent repeated episodes that increase the likelihood of myositis ossificans.[16] It is also important for the athlete to maintain a full range of motion through stretching of the contused muscle.

18–4

***Critical Thinking*** Exercise

A football offensive lineman contuses his upper arm while blocking.

**?**  What should the coach be mainly concerned about and how can this be avoided?

## SUMMARY

- For the shoulder complex to have such a great degree of mobility, some compromise in stability had to be made; thus, the shoulder is highly susceptible to injury. Many sport activities that involve repetitive overhead movements place a great deal of stress on the shoulder joint.

- Four major articulations are associated with the shoulder complex: the sternoclavicular joint and ligament, the acromioclavicular joint and ligament, the glenohumeral joint and ligament, and the scapulothoracic joint.

- The muscles acting on the shoulder joint consist of those that originate on the axial skeleton and attach to the humerus, those that originate on the scapula and attach to the humerus, and a third group that attaches the axial skeleton to the scapula.

- When evaluating injuries to the shoulder complex, the coach must take into consideration all four joints. A number of special tests can provide insight relative to the nature of a particular injury.

- Fractures may occur to the clavicle or humerus, whereas sprains may occur at the sternoclavicular, acromioclavicular, or glenohumeral joints.

- Shoulder dislocations are relatively common, with an anterior dislocation the most likely to occur. After a dislocation has been reduced and immobilized, muscle reconditioning should be initiated as soon as possible.

- Shoulder impingement most often occurs in athletes involved with overhead activities. Shoulder impingement involves a mechanical compression of the supraspinatus tendon, the subacromial bursa, and the long head of the biceps tendon under the coracoacromial ligament.

- A number of injuries, including rotator cuff strain, bursitis, contusions, and biceps tenosynovitis, are all common injuries to the shoulder complex in athletes.

---

*Solutions to Critical Thinking* Exercises

**18-1** Falling on the tip of the shoulder is a typical mechanism of injury for a sprain of the acromioclavicular joint, the sternoclavicular joint, or both. It is also possible that a clavicular fracture has occurred.

**18-2** Exercises should be designed to strengthen the muscles of the rotator cuff in particular and the muscles that allow the scapula to provide a stable base of support. Exercises that

stress neuromuscular control should begin immediately in the rehabilitation program.

**18-3** This athlete's pain is likely caused by mechanical impingement or compression of the supraspinatus tendon, the subacromial bursa, or the long head of the biceps under the coracoacromial arch as the arm moves into a fully abducted or flexed position. The space under the arch becomes even more compressed as the humerus is internally rotated, which occurs during the follow-through.

**18-4** The biggest concern is that following repeated contusions myositis ossificans may develop in the biceps or brachialis. This can be prevented by having the athlete wear a protective pad to prevent subsequent contusion.

## REVIEW QUESTIONS AND CLASS ACTIVITIES

1. What are the bony and soft-tissue structures associated with the shoulder complex?
2. What four major joints make up the shoulder complex?
3. How can shoulder injuries be prevented?
4. Discuss the throwing motion and the injuries that can occur in each phase.
5. What causes clavicular fractures? How are they cared for?
6. Discuss the mechanism of injury of sternoclavicular and acromioclavicular ligament sprains.
7. What is the common mechanism of an anterior glenohumeral dislocation? How is it cared for?
8. What structural anatomic problems need to be addressed when treating shoulder impingement?
9. Briefly describe the history of a rotator cuff tear.
10. How does an athlete develop bursitis in the shoulder?
11. What is myositis ossificans and how can you prevent its development?
12. How may an athlete develop biceps tenosynovitis?

### Dynamic *Human* CD

For more information on skeletal anatomy of the shoulder click on:

- Skeletal
- Anatomy
- Gross anatomy
- Pectoral girdle
- Clavicle
- Then, Scapula
- Then, Upper limbs
- Humerus
- Then, Radius/ulna

To take a closer look at the muscles that are involved in shoulder movement click on:

- Muscular
- Anatomy
- Body regions
- Pectoral girdle
- Then, Upper arms

To look at the effect of a dislocated shoulder on the muscles and ligaments of the shoulder click on:

- Skeletal
- Clinical concepts
- Dislocated shoulder

## REFERENCES

1. Andrews J, Wilk K: *The athlete's shoulder,* New York, 1994, Churchill Livingstone.
2. Bach B, VanFleet T, Novak P: Acromioclavicular joint injuries: controversies in treatment, *Physician Sportsmed* 20(12):87, 1992.
3. Botte MJ, Abrams RA: Recognition and treatment of shoulder bursitis, *Sports Med Dig* 14:81, 1992.
4. Burkhart SS, Morgan CD, Kibler B: Shoulder injuries in overhead athletes: the "dead arm" revisited, *Clin Sports Med* 19(1):125, 2000.
5. Cavallo RJ, Speer KP: Shoulder instability and impingement in throwing athletes, *Med Sci Sports Exerc* 30(4 suppl):S18, 1998.
6. Craig E: Fractures of the clavicle. In Rockwood C, Masten F, Wirth M: *The shoulder,* Philadelphia, 1998, WB Saunders.
7. DeCarlo M et al: Evaluation of shoulder instability braces, *J Sport Rehab* 5(2):143, 1996.
8. Gross ML et al: Overworked shoulders, *Physician Sportsmed* 22:81, 1994.
9. Kibler WB: Shoulder rehabilitation: principles and practice, *Med Sci Sports Exerc* 30(4 suppl):S40, 1998.
10. Kibler WB: The role of the scapula in athletic shoulder function, *Am J Sports Med* 26(2):325, 1998.
11. Masten F, Arntz C: Subacromial impingement. In Rockwood C, Masten F, Wirth M: *The shoulder,* Philadelphia, 1998, WB Saunders.
12. Myers JB: Conservative management of shoulder impingement syndrome in the athletic population, *J Sport Rehab* 8(3):230, 1999.
13. Norris T: History and physical examination of the shoulder. In Nicholas JA, Hershman EB, editors: *The upper extremity in sports medicine,* St Louis, 1995, Mosby.
14. Pagnani M, Warren R: Instability of the shoulder. In Nicholas JA, Hershman EB, editors: *The upper extremity in sports medicine,* St Louis, 1995, Mosby.
15. Sawa T: An alternate conservative management of shoulder dislocations and subluxations, *J Ath Train* 27(4):366, 1992.
16. Schneider R, Prentice W: Rehabilitation of shoulder injuries. In Prentice W: *Rehabilitation techniques in sports medicine,* Boston, 1999, WCB/McGraw-Hill.
17. Watson K: Impingement and rotator cuff lesions. In Nicholas JA, Hershman EB, editors: *The upper extremity in sports medicine,* St Louis, 1995, Mosby.
18. Wilk KE, Arrigo CA, Andrews JR: Current concepts: the stabilizing structures of the glenohumeral joint, *J Orthop Sports Phys Ther* 25(6):364, 1997.
19. Wolin PM, Tarbet JA: Rotator cuff injury: addressing overhead overuse, *Physician Sportsmed* 25(6):54, 1997.

## ANNOTATED BIBLIOGRAPHY

Andrews J, Wilk K: *The athlete's shoulder,* New York, 1994, Churchill Livingstone.

*Concentrates on both conservative and surgical treatment of shoulder injuries occurring specifically in the athletic population.*

Nicholas JA, Hershman EB, editors: *The upper extremity in sports medicine,* St Louis, 1995, Mosby.

*The text has a great deal of information on the recognition, evaluation, and management of shoulder injuries, in addition to the elbow, wrist, and hand.*

Rockwood C, Masten F, Wirth M: *The shoulder,* Philadelphia, 1998, WB Saunders.

*A complete two-volume set that covers essentially every subject relative to the shoulder complex.*

**WEBSITES**

Cramer First Aider: http://www.ccsd.k12.wy.us/CCHS_web/sptmed/fstaider.htm

World Ortho: http://www.worldortho.com

*Use the search engine in this site to locate relevant information.*

Wheeless' Textbook of Orthopaedics: http://www.medmedia.com/med.htm

*An excellent page for injuries, anatomy, and x rays.*

Karolinska Institute Library: Musculoskeletal Disease: http://www.mic.ki.se/Disease/c5.htm

American Orthopaedic Society for Sports Medicine: http://www.sportsmed.org

MedFacts Sports Doc: http://www.medfacts.com

Anatomy of the Shoulder Tutorial http://www.ncl.ac.uk~nccc/tutorials/shoulder/

# The Elbow, Forearm, Wrist, and Hand

*When you finish this chapter you will be able to:*

- Describe the bony, ligamentous, and muscular anatomy of the elbow, forearm, wrist, and hand.
- List considerations for preventing injuries to the elbow, forearm, wrist, and hand.
- Discuss assessment of common elbow, forearm, wrist, and hand injuries.
- Discuss the possible causes and signs of various injuries that can occur in the elbow, forearm, wrist, and hand.
- Explain the procedures that can be used in caring for elbow, forearm, wrist, and hand injuries.

# ANATOMY OF THE ELBOW JOINT

## Bones

The elbow complex is composed of three bones: the humerus, the radius, and the ulna (Figure 19-1). The distal end of the humerus forms the medial and lateral epicondyles. The olecranon process of the ulna articulates with the trochlea and olecranon fossa on the posterior humerus. The radial head articulates with the capitellum of the ulna. Three separate joints collectively form the elbow complex, the humerosulnar joint, the humeroradial joint, and the radioulnar joint. Flexion and extension occur at the humeroulnar and humeroradial joints. Pronation and supination of the forearm occur at the radioulnar joint.

## Ligaments

The ulnar (medial) collateral ligament is most important for stability of the elbow and extends from the medial epicondyle to the proximal ulna. The annular ligament extends from the ulna, forming a sling around the radial head thus allowing free rotation of the radius. The radial (lateral) collateral ligament extends from the lateral epicondyle and attaches primarily to the annular ligament (refer to Figure 19-1).

## Muscles

The muscles of the elbow consist of the biceps barchii and the brachialis and brachioradialis muscles, all of which are flexors of the elbow. Exten-

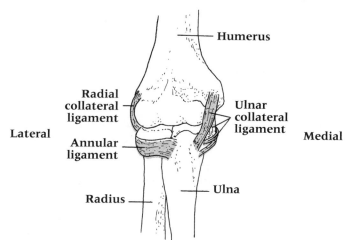

**Figure 19-1**

Bones and ligaments of the
elbow

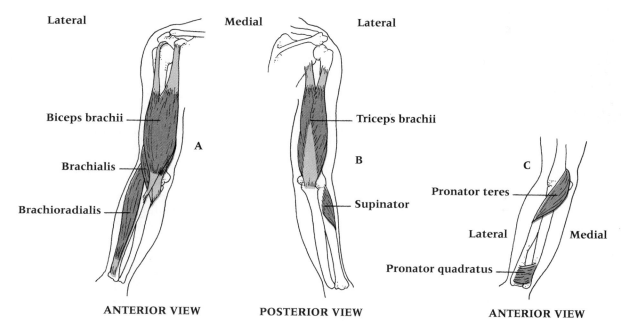

**Figure 19-2**

Muscles of the elbow joint:
A, Anterior view; B, Posterior
view; C, Forearm pronators

sion is controlled by the triceps brachii muscle. The biceps brachii and
supinator muscles allow supination of the forearm; the pronator teres
and pronator quadratus act as pronators (Figure 19-2).

## ASSESSING ELBOW INJURIES

### History

As with all sports injuries, the coach must first understand how the injury occurred. The following questions aid in evaluation of the elbow:

- Is the pain or discomfort caused by a direct trauma such as falling on an outstretched arm or landing on the tip of a bent elbow?
- Can the problem be attributed to sudden overextension of the elbow or to repeated overuse of a throwing-type motion?
- Are there movements or positions of the arm that increase or decrease the pain?
- Has a previous elbow injury been diagnosed or treated?
- Is there a feeling of locking or a grating during movement?

The location and duration should be ascertained. Like shoulder pain, elbow pain or discomfort may be from internal organ dysfunction or referred from a nerve root irritation or nerve impingement.

NOTE: Elbow pain may not be directly associated with an elbow injury but rather may be referred pain from the neck or shoulder.

### Observation

The athlete's elbow should be observed for obvious deformities and swelling. The following should be observed:

- The carrying angle, flexion, and extensibility of the elbow should be observed.
- If the carrying angle is abnormally increased or abnormally decreased, an injury may be present (Figure 19-3).
- A carrying angle that is too great or too little may indicate a bony or growth plate fracture.
- The athlete is next observed for the extent of elbow flexion and extension (Figure 19-4). The elbows are compared. A decrease in normal flexion, an inability to extend fully, or a beyond-normal extension may be a sign of joint problems (Figure 19-5).

### Palpation

Pain sites and deformities are determined through careful palpation of the epicondyles, olecranon process, distal aspect of the humerus, and proximal aspect of the ulna.

**Figure 19-3**

Testing for elbow carrying angle and the extent of cubitus valgus and cubitus varus

**Figure 19-4**

Testing for elbow flexion and
extension

**Figure 19-5**

Observing elbow
hyperextension

Soft tissue to be palpated includes the muscles and muscle tendons,
joint capsule, and ligaments surrounding the joint.

## PREVENTION OF ELBOW INJURIES

As with injury prevention in other areas of the body, elbow injury prevention requires year-round conditioning consisting of strength, endurance,
and flexibility activities. Because of the elbow's sensitivity to overuse problems, it is essential that sport-specific techniques be carefully carried out.[4]

## RECOGNITION AND MANAGEMENT OF INJURIES
## TO THE ELBOW

The elbow is subject to injury in sports because of its broad range of motion, weak lateral bone arrangement, and relative exposure to soft tissue
damage in the vicinity of the joint.[1] Many sports place excessive stress on
the elbow joint. Locking of the elbow in gymnastics or using implements
such as racquets, golf clubs, and javelins can cause injuries. The throwing
mechanism in baseball pitching can injure the elbow during both the acceleration and follow-through phases.[7]

The two most common
mechanisms of elbow injury:
• Throwing
• Falling on the outstretched
hand

### Olecranon Bursitis

**Cause of injury**   The olecranon bursa (Figure 19-6), lying between the
end of the olecranon process and the skin, is the most frequently injured

bursa in the elbow. The superficial location of the olecranon bursa makes it prone to acute or chronic injury, particularly as the result of direct blows.[10]

**Signs of injury**   The inflamed bursa produces pain, marked swelling, and point tenderness. Occasionally, swelling will appear almost spontaneously and without the usual pain and heat.

**Care**   If the condition is acute, a cold compress should be applied for at least 1 hour. Chronic olecranon bursitis requires a program of superficial therapy. In rare cases aspiration by a physician hastens healing. Although seldom serious, olecranon bursitis can be annoying and should be well protected by padding while the athlete is engaged in competition.

**Figure 19-6**

Olecranon bursitis

### Elbow Sprains

**Cause of injury**   Sprains to the elbow are usually caused by hyperextension or a force that bends or twists the lower arm outward, causing injury to the medial collateral ligament as occurs in throwing.[8]

**Signs of injury**   The athlete complains of pain and the inability to throw or grasp an object. There is a point tenderness over the medial collateral ligament.

**Care**   Immediate care for elbow sprain consists of cold and a pressure bandage for at least 24 hours with sling support fixed at 90 degrees of flexion. A coach's main concern should be to progressively aid the elbow in regaining a full range of motion, followed by active exercises until full mobility and strength have returned.

### Lateral Epicondylitis

**Cause of injury**   *Lateral epicondylitis* is one of the most common problems of the elbow occurring in sports. *Tennis elbow* is another name for lateral epicondylitis stemming from a backhand stroke involving overextending the wrist. The cause of lateral epicondylitis is repetitive extension of the wrist, which eventually causes irritation and inflammation to the insertion of the extensor muscle of the lateral epicondyle.[16]

**Signs of injury**   The athlete complains of an aching pain in the region of the lateral epicondyle during and after activity (Figure 19-7). The pain gradually becomes worse with weakness in the hand and wrist. Inspection reveals tenderness at the lateral epicondyle and pain on resisted dorsiflexion of the wrist and full extension of the elbow.

**Care**   Treatment includes immediate use of RICE, nonsteroidal antiinflammatory drugs (NSAIDs), and analgesics as needed. Rehabilitation includes range-of-motion exercises, progressive resistance exercises, deep friction massage, hand grasping while in supination, and avoiding pronation movements. Mobilization and stretching may be used within pain-free limits. The athlete may wear a counterforce or neoprene elbow sleeve for 1 to 3 months (Figure 19-8). The athlete must be taught proper skill techniques and the proper use of equipment to avoid recurrence of the injury.

### Medial Epicondylitis

**Cause of injury**   Irritation and inflammation of the medial epicondyle may result from a number of different sport activities that re-

**Figure 19-7**

Typical pain sites in the elbow region

quire repeated forceful flexions of the elbow. It has also been referred to as pitcher's elbow, racquetball elbow, golfer's elbow, and javelin-thrower's elbow.[12]

**Signs of injury**  Pain occurs around the medial epicondyle of the humerus during forceful wrist flexion and may radiate down the arm. There is usually point tenderness and in some cases mild swelling. Passive movement of the wrist seldom elicits pain, although active movement does.

**Care**  Conservative management of moderate to severe epicondylitis usually includes use of rest, cryotherapy, or heat through the application of ultrasound. Analgesics and antiinflammatory agents may be prescribed. A counterforce brace applied just below the bend of the elbow is highly beneficial in reducing elbow stress (refer to Figure 19-8). For more severe cases elbow splinting and complete rest for 7 to 10 days may be warranted.

## Elbow Osteochondritis Dissecans

Although osteochondritis dissecans is more common in knees it also can occur in elbows.

**Cause of injury**  The cause of osteochondritis dissecans is unknown; however, impairment of the blood supply can lead to fragmentation and separation of a portion of the articular cartilage and bone, creating loose bodies within the joint.[11]

**Signs of injury**  The adolescent athlete usually complains of sudden pain and locking of the elbow joint. Range of motion returns slowly over a few days. Swelling, pain, and crepitation also may occur.

**Care**  Repeated episodes of locking may warrant surgical removal of the loose bodies. If they are not removed, traumatic arthritis can eventually occur.

## Ulnar Nerve Injuries

**Cause of injury**  Because of the exposed position of the medial humeral condyle, the ulnar nerve is subject to a variety of problems. The

**Figure 19-8**

Counterforce brace for treatment of elbow and epicondylitis

Athletes with a pronounced cubitus valgus are prone to injuring the ulnar nerve.

Recognition and
Management of Specific
Injuries and Conditions

---

**paresthesia**
Lack of sensation.

---

19–1

*Critical Thinking* Exercise

A female javelin thrower complains of pain on the medial aspect of her elbow that is also referred distally to the forearm. The athlete senses an intermittent numbness, a burning sensation, and tingling in the fingers.

**?** What condition does this athlete have, and how could it have occurred?

Neurovascular problems are a possibility when an elbow is dislocated or fractured.

---

athlete with a pronounced outward angle of the elbow may develop a nerve friction problem. The ulnar nerve can also become recurrently dislocated because of a structural deformity or can become impinged by a ligament during flexion-type activities.

**Signs of injury**   Rather than being painful, ulnar nerve injuries usually respond with a **paresthesia** to the fourth and fifth fingers. The athlete complains of burning and tingling in the fourth and fifth fingers.

**Care**   The management of ulnar nerve injuries is conservative; aggravation of the nerve, such as placing direct pressure on it, is avoided. When stress on the nerve cannot be avoided, surgery may be performed to transpose it anteriorly to the elbow.[19]

## Dislocation of the Elbow

**Cause of injury**   Dislocation of the elbow has a high incidence in sports activity and most often is caused either by a fall on the outstretched hand with the elbow in a position of hyperextension or by a severe twist while the elbow is in a flexed position (Figure 19-9).[17]

**Signs of injury**   The bones of the forearm (ulna and radius) may be displaced backward, forward, or laterally. The appearance of the most common dislocation is a deformity of the olecranon process wherein it extends backward, well beyond its normal alignment with the upper arm.

Elbow dislocations involve rupturing and tearing of most of the stabilizing ligamentous tissue accompanied by profuse internal bleeding and subsequent swelling. There is severe pain and disability. The complications of such a trauma may include injury to the major nerves and blood vessels.[3]

**Care**   The primary responsibility is to provide the athlete with an immobilizing splint and to refer the athlete immediately to a physician for reduction as soon as possible. In most cases the physician administers an anesthetic before reduction to relax the muscles. After reduction, the physician often immobilizes the elbow in a position of flexion and applies a sling suspension, which should be used for approximately 3 weeks. A

---

**Figure 19-9**

A fall on the outstretched hand can produce an elbow dislocation and/or fracture.

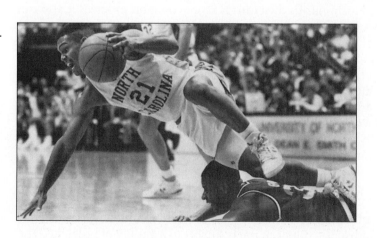

dislocated elbow, like a fracture, may also have possible neurovascular problems.[17]

### Fractures of the Elbow

**Cause of injury**   An elbow fracture can occur in almost any sports event and is usually caused by a fall on the outstretched hand or the flexed elbow or by a direct blow to the elbow. Children and young athletes have a much higher rate of this injury than do adults. A fracture can take place in any one or more of the bones that comprise the elbow. A fall on the outstretched hand quite often fractures the humerus above the condyles or the bones of the forearm or wrist.

**Signs of injury**   An elbow fracture may or may not result in visible deformity. There usually is hemorrhage, swelling, and muscle spasm in the injured area.

**Care**   Because of the seriousness of an elbow fracture, careful immediate care must be rendered. Following the application of cold and a sling support, the athlete must be referred immediately for medical attention. A fractured elbow is associated with rapid swelling that may cause a condition called Volkmann's contracture, an extremely serious and often irreversible condition.

### Volkmann's Contracture

**Cause of injury**   It is essential that athletes sustaining a serious elbow injury have the circulation monitored often throughout the day and night. Swelling, muscle spasm, or a bone displacement can put pressure on the brachial artery and inhibit blood circulation to the forearm, wrist, and hand. Such inhibition of circulation can lead to muscle contracture and permanent muscle paralysis.[1]

**Sign of injury**   The first indication of this problem is pain in the forearm that becomes progressively greater when the fingers of the affected arm are passively extended.

**Care**   Volkmann's contracture is a major problem requiring immediate referral for emergency treatment. The coach must remember that with this injury, time is of the essence.

*Volkmann's contracture is a major complication of a serious elbow injury.*

## ANATOMY OF THE FOREARM

### Bones

The bones of the forearm are the ulna and the radius (Figure 19-10). The ulna, which may be thought of as a direct extension of the humerus, is long, straight, and larger at its upper end than at its lower end. The radius, considered an extension of the hand, is thicker at its lower end than at its upper end.

### Joints

The forearm has three articulations: the superior, middle, and distal radioulnar joints.

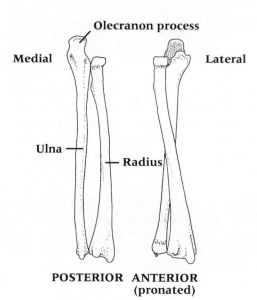

**Figure 19-10**

Bones of the elbow

## Muscles

The forearm muscles consist of flexors and pronators, positioned anteriorly and attached to the medial epicondyle, and of extensors and supinators, which lie posteriorly and are attached to the lateral epicondyle (Figure 19-11). The flexors of the wrist and fingers are separated into superficial muscles and deep muscles.

## ASSESSING FOREARM INJURIES

### History

The following questions are asked in the evaluation of forearm injuries:

- What caused the injury (e.g., blunt trauma, throwing, or chronic overuse)?
- What were the symptoms at the time of injury? Did symptoms occur later?
- Were symptoms localized or diffused?
- Was there swelling or discoloration?
- Was there immediate loss of function?
- What treatment was given?

### Observation

The entire forearm is first visually inspected, including the wrist and elbow, looking for obvious deformities, swelling, and skin defects. The athlete then is observed pronating and supinating the forearm when a deformity is not present.

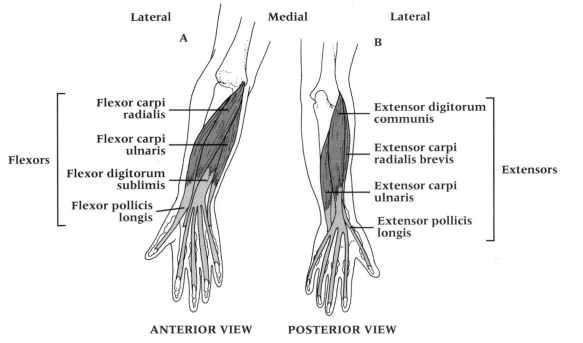

Flexor carpi radialis

Flexor carpi ulnaris

Flexors

Flexor digitorum sublimis

Flexor pollicis longis

Extensor digitorum communis

Extensor carpi radialis brevis

Extensors

Extensor carpi ulnaris

Extensor pollicis longis

**ANTERIOR VIEW**     **POSTERIOR VIEW**

**Figure 19-11**

Muscles of the forearm: A, Anterior view; B, Posterior view

## Palpation

The injured forearm is palpated at distant sites and the point of injury. Palpation can reveal tenderness, edema, fracture deformity, change in skin temperature, a false joint, bone fragments, or a lack of continuity between bones.

## RECOGNITION AND MANAGEMENT OF INJURIES TO THE FOREARM

Lying between the elbow joint and the wrist and hand, the forearm is indirectly influenced by injuries caused by overuse and by direct external injuries.

## Contusion

**Cause of injury**   The forearm is constantly exposed to bruising in contact sports such as football. The ulnar side receives the majority of blows in arm blocks and consequently the greater amount of bruising. Bruises to this area may be classified as acute or chronic. The acute contusion can, on rare occasions, result in a fracture. The chronic contusion develops from repeated blows to the forearm with attendant multiple irritations.[13]

**Signs of injury**   Most often muscles or bones develop varying degrees of pain, swelling, and accumulation of blood (hematoma). Extensive scar tissue may replace the hematoma, and in some cases, a bony callus replaces the scar tissue.

**Care**    Care of the contused forearm requires proper attention in the acute stages by application of RICE for 20 minutes every 1½ waking hours, followed the next day by cold and exercise. Protection of the forearm is important for athletes who are prone to this condition. The best protection consists of a full-length sponge rubber pad for the forearm early in the season.

## Forearm Splints and Other Strains

Forearm strain occurs in a variety of sports; most such injuries come from repeated static contractions.

Forearm splints, like shin splints, commonly occur early and late in the sports season.

**Cause of injury**    Forearm splints occur most often in gymnastics. The reason for this problem is probably static muscle contractions of the forearm, such as those that occur when an athlete performs on the side horse. Constant static muscle contraction causes minute tears in the deep connective tissues of the forearm.

**Signs of injury**    The main symptom of forearm splints is a dull ache of the extensor muscles crossing the back of the forearm. Muscle weakness may accompany the dull ache. Palpation reveals an irritation of the deep tissue between the muscles. The cause of this condition is uncertain; like shin splints, forearm splints usually appear either early or late in the season, indicating poor conditioning or chronic fatigue.

**Care**    Care of forearm splints is symptomatic. If the problem occurs early in the season, the athlete should concentrate on increasing the strength of the forearm through resistance exercises; if it arises late in the season, emphasis should be placed on rest, cold, or heat and on use of a supportive wrap during activity.

## Fractures

**Cause of injury**    Fractures of the forearm (Figure 19-12) are particularly common among active children and youths. Forearm fractures occur as the result of a blow or a fall on the outstretched hand. Fractures to the ulna or the radius singly are much rarer than simultaneous fractures to both.

**Signs of injury**    The break usually presents all the features of a long-bone fracture: pain, swelling, deformity, and a false joint. The older the athlete, the greater the danger of extensive damage to soft tissue and the greater the possibility of paralysis from Volkmann's contractures.[13]

**Care**    To prevent complications, a cold pack must be applied immediately to the fracture site, the arm splinted and put in a sling, and the athlete referred to a physician. The athlete usually is incapacitated for about 8 weeks.

## Colles' Fracture

Colles' fracture (Figure 19-13), among the most common forearm fractures, involves the lower (distal) end of the radius.[13]

A

B

**Figure 19-12**

A, Fracture of the radius and ulna; B, Compound fracture of the ulna

**Cause of injury**   The cause of a Colles' fracture is usually a fall on the outstretched hand, forcing the forearm backward and upward into hyperextension.

**Signs of injury**   In most cases there is a visible deformity to the wrist. Sometimes no deformity is present, and the injury may be passed off as a bad sprain. Bleeding is profuse in this area, with the accumulated fluids causing extensive swelling in the wrist and, if unchecked, in the fingers and forearm. Ligamentous tissue is usually unharmed, but tendons may be torn away from their attachment, and there may possibly be median nerve damage.

**Care**   The main responsibility is to apply a cold compress, splint the wrist, put the limb in a sling, and then refer the athlete to a physician for x-ray examination and immobilization. Lacking complications, Colles' fracture will keep an athlete out of sports for 1 to 2 months.

**Figure 19-13**

Common appearance of the forearm in Colles' fracture

## ANATOMY OF THE WRIST, HAND, AND FINGERS

### Bones

The wrist is formed by the distal aspect of the radius and the ulna with a proximal row of four and a distal row of four carpal bones that articulate with five metacarpals. The metacarpal bones join the carpal bones above and the phalanges below, forming metacarpophalangeal (MCP) articulations. The four fingers each have a proximal, middle, and distal phalanx, whereas the thumb has only two phalanges (Figure 19-14A).

### Ligaments

The wrist is composed of many ligaments that bind the carpal bones to one another, to the ulna and radius, and to the proximal metacarpal bones. Of major interest in wrist injuries are the collateral ulnar ligament and collateral radial ligament. Crossing the volar aspect of the carpal

19–2

**_Critical Thinking_** Exercise

A young athlete falls off the parallel bars onto his outstretched left hand, forcing the wrist into hyperextension. There is a visible deformity to the wrist.

**?**  Describe the deformity presented and the actions that should be taken by the coach.

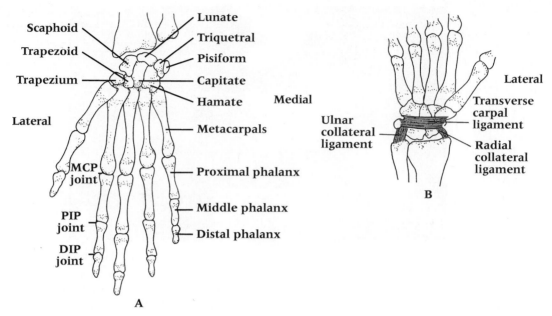

**Figure 19-14**

A, Bones of the wrist and hand; B, Ligaments of the wrist

bones is the transverse carpal ligament. This ligament serves as the roof of the carpal tunnel, in which the median nerve is often compressed (Figure 19-14B). The interphalangeal (PIP) joints have medial and lateral collateral ligaments and a thickened joint capsule on the palmer surface that is referred to as the *volar plate*.

## Muscles

The wrist and hand are a complex of extrinsic (originate outside of the hand) and intrinsic (originate in the hand) muscles. In general both the extrinsic and intrinsic muscles located on the medial aspect and front of the wrist and hand flex the wrist and fingers and the muscles on the posterior and lateral aspect of the wrist and hand extend the wrist and fingers (refer to Figure 19-11). Intrinsic muscles of the hand also abduct, adduct, and in the thumb create opposition, of the metacarpals.

## ASSESSMENT OF THE WRIST, HAND, AND FINGERS

### History

As with other conditions, the evaluator asks about the location and type of pain:

- What increases or decreases the pain?
- Has there been a history of trauma or overuse?
- What therapy or medications, if any, have been given?

**At rest**

**Normal fist**    **Clenched fist**

**Figure 19-15**

General normal attitudes of
the hand

## Observation

As the athlete is observed, arm and hand asymmetries are noted:

- Are there any postural deviations?
- Does the athlete hold the part in a stiff or protected manner?
- Is the wrist or hand swollen?

Hand usage such as writing or unbuttoning a shirt is noted. The general
attitude of the hand is observed (Figure 19-15). When the athlete is asked
to open and close the hand, the evaluator notes whether this movement
can be performed fully and rhythmically. Another general functional activity is to have the athlete touch the tip of the thumb to each fingertip
several times. The last factor to be observed is the color of the fingernails.
Nails that are very pale instead of pink may indicate a problem with blood
circulation.

## Palpation

The bones of the wrist region are palpated for pain and deformity. The examiner palpates each metacarpal bone, MCP joint, and each phalanx,
starting with the PIP joint and progressing to the distal interphalangeal
(DIP) joint. Each tendon is palpated as it crosses the wrist region. The examiner palpates the flexor muscles of the fingers and thumb. On the dorsal aspect, the examiner palpates the extension tendons and phalanges.

## RECOGNITION AND MANAGEMENT OF WRIST, HAND, AND FINGER INJURIES

### Wrist Sprain

**Cause of injury**    It is often very difficult to distinguish between a
wrist sprain and a tendon sprain in the carpal region. A sprain is by far
the most common wrist injury. It can occur from any abnormal, forced

Sprains are the most
common wrist injury in
sports and often the worst
managed.

**Figure 19-16**

Wrist injuries commonly
occur from falls on the
outstreched hand or from
repeated flexion, extension,
lateral, or rotary movement.

movement of the wrist. Falling on the hyperextended wrist is the most
common cause of wrist sprain, but violent flexion or torsion can also
cause injury (Figure 19-16).[14]

**Signs of injury** The athlete complains of pain, swelling, and difficulty moving the wrist. On examination there is tenderness, swelling,
and limited range of motion. All athletes having severe sprains should
be referred to a physician for x-ray examination to determine possible
fractures.

**Care**   Mild and moderate sprains should initially be given RICE, splinting, and analgesics. It is desirable to have the athlete start wrist-strengthening exercises almost immediately after the injury has occurred. Taping for support can benefit healing and help prevent further injury.

## Wrist Tendonitis

**Cause of injury**   Wrist tendonitis occurs in weight lifters, rowers, and participants in other sports that require the athlete to perform repetitive wrist accelerations and decelerations.[15]

**Signs of injury**   The athlete complains of pain with use or pain in passive stretching. There is tenderness and swelling over the tendon.

**Care**   Acute pain and inflammation are managed by ice massage for 10 minutes four times a day for the first 48 to 72 hours, antiinflammatory medication, and rest. A wrist splint may protect the injured tendon. When swelling has subsided range of motion is stressed. When pain and swelling have subsided, progressive resistance exercise can be instituted.

## Carpal Tunnel Syndrome

**Cause of injury**   The carpal tunnel is located on the anterior aspect of the wrist. The floor of the carpal tunnel is formed by the carpal bones and the roof by the transverse carpal ligament. A number of anatomical structures course through this limited space, including eight long finger flexor tendons, their synovial sheaths, and the median nerve. Carpal tunnel syndrome results from an inflammation of the tendons and synovial sheaths within this space, which ultimately leads to compression of the median nerve. Carpal tunnel syndrome most often occurs in athletes who engage in activities that require repeated wrist flexion, although it can also result from direct trauma to the anterior aspect of the wrist.[18]

**Signs of injury**   Compression of the median nerve usually results in both sensory and motor deficits. Sensory changes can result in tingling, numbness, and paresthesia in the arc of median nerve innervation over the thumb, index and middle fingers, and palm of the hand. The median nerve innervates the lumbrical muscles of the index and middle fingers and three of the thenar muscles. Thus weakness in thumb movement is associated with this condition.

**Care**   Initially, conservative treatment involving rest, immobilization, and nonsteroidal antiinflammatory medication is recommended. If the syndrome persists, injection with a corticosteroid and possible surgical decompression of the transverse carpal ligament may be necessary.[5]

**Figure 19-17**

Dislocation of the wrist

## Dislocation of the Lunate Bone

**Cause of injury**   Dislocation of the lunate is considered the most common dislocation of a carpal bone but is relatively infrequent in sports. Most occur from a forceful hyperextension of the wrist (Figure 19-17).[14]

**Signs of injury**   The primary signs of this condition are pain, swelling, and difficulty in executing wrist and finger flexion. There also

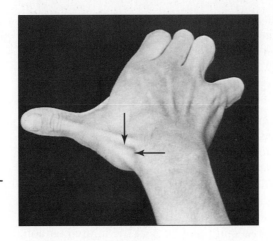

**Figure 19-18**

Anatomical snuffbox formed
by extensor tendons of the
thumb

may be numbness or even paralysis of the flexor muscles because of lunate pressure on the median nerve.

**Care**  This condition should be treated as acute, and the athlete should be sent to a physician for reduction of the dislocation. If it is not recognized early enough, bone deterioration may occur, requiring surgical removal. The usual time of disability and subsequent recovery is 1 to 2 months.

### Scaphoid Fracture

**Cause of injury**  The scaphoid bone is the most frequently fractured of the carpal bones. The injury is usually caused by a force on the outstretched hand, which compresses the scaphoid bone between the radius and the second row of carpal bones.[14]

**Signs of injury**  The signs of a recent scaphoid fracture include swelling in the area of the carpal bones and severe point tenderness over the scaphoid bone in the anatomical snuffbox (Figure 19-18).

**Care**  In an athlete with these signs, cold should be applied, the area splinted, and the athlete referred to a physician for x-ray study and casting. In most cases, cast immobilization lasts for approximately 6 weeks and is followed by strengthening exercises coupled with protective taping. Immobilization is discontinued for rehabilitation. The wrist needs protection against impact loading for an additional 3 months.

### Hamate Fracture

**Cause of injury**  A fracture of the carpal hamate bone, and in particular the hook of the hamate, can occur from a fall but more commonly occurs from contact when holding a sports implement such as the handle of a tennis racket, a baseball bat, a lacrosse stick, a hockey stick, or a golf club.

**Signs of injury**  Wrist pain and weakness and point tenderness are experienced. There is possibly tingling, numbness, and weakness in the

*Critical Thinking* Exercise

A basketball player stumbles and falls on an outstretched hand. She comes to the coach complaining of pain at the base of the thumb at the wrist. She is very point tender.

**?**  What specific injury might be causing her pain and what should the coach do?

little and ring fingers because the ulnar nerve may be compromised because of its close proximity to the hamate.

**Care** Casting of the wrist is usually the treatment of choice. The
hook of the hamate can be protected by wearing a doughnut pad to take
pressure off the area.

## Wrist Ganglion

**Cause of injury** A wrist ganglion (Figure 19-19) is considered by
many to be either a herniation of the joint capsule, of the synovial sheath
of a tendon, or a cystic structure. It usually appears slowly, after repeated
forced hyperextension of the wrist, and contains a clear, mucinous fluid.
The ganglion most often appears on the back of the wrist.[15]

**Signs of injury** The athlete complains of occasional pain with a
lump at the site. Pain increases with wrist extension. There is a cystic
structure that may feel soft, rubbery, or very hard.

**Care** An old method of treatment was first to break down the
swelling through digital pressure and then apply a felt pressure pad for a
time to encourage healing. A newer approach is the use of a combination
of aspiration and chemical cauterization, with subsequent application of
a pressure pad. Neither of these methods prevents the ganglion from recurring. Surgical removal is the best of the various methods of treatment.

**Figure 19-19**

Wrist ganglion

## Metacarpal Fracture

**Cause of injury** Fractures of the fifth metacarpal are associated with
boxing and the martial arts and are usually called a *boxer's fracture* (Figure 19-20). The cause of metacarpal fractures is commonly a direct axial
force caused by punching the wall or another person.[6]

**Signs of injury** There is point tenderness and likely a palpable defect in the shaft of the fifth metacarpal. Swelling is rapid.

**Care** An athlete with a suspected boxer's fracture should be referred to a physician for reduction and immobilization for a period lasting 3 to 4 weeks.

**Figure 19-20**

Fractures of the metacarpals

## Mallet Finger

**Cause of injury** The mallet finger is sometimes called *baseball finger*
or *basketball finger*. It is caused by a blow from a thrown ball that strikes
the tip of the finger, jamming and avulsing the extensor tendon from its
insertion along with a piece of bone.[2]

**Signs of injury** The athlete complains of pain at the distal interphalangeal joint. X-ray examination may show a bony avulsion from the dorsal
proximal distal phalanx. The athlete is unable to extend the finger, carrying
it at approximately a 30-degree angle. There is also point tenderness at the
site of the injury, and the avulsed bone often can be palpated (Figure 19-21).

**Care** RICE is given for the pain and swelling. If there is no fracture
the distal phalanx should immediately be splinted in a position of extension for a period of 6 to 8 weeks (Figure 19-22).

**19-4**

***Critical Thinking*** Exercise

A football player gets into a
fistfight on the field and injures
his right hand.

**?** What type of injury should
be suspected by the coach?

**Figure 19-21**

Mallet finger

## Boutonnière Deformity

**Cause of injury** The boutonnière, or buttonhole, deformity is caused by a rupture of the extensor tendon over the middle phalanx. Trauma occurs to the tip of the finger, which forces the DIP joint into extension and the PIP joint into flexion.[2]

**Signs of injury** The athlete complains of severe pain and inability to extend the DIP joint. There is swelling, point tenderness, and an obvious deformity.

**Care** Care of the boutonnière deformity includes cold application followed by splinting of the PIP joint in extension. NOTE: If this condition is inadequately splinted, the classic boutonnière deformity will develop (Figure 19-23). Splinting is continued for 5 to 8 weeks. While splinted, the athlete is encouraged to flex the distal phalanx.

## Jersey Finger

**Cause of injury** Jersey finger is a rupture of the flexor digitorum profundus tendon from its insertion on the distal phalanx. It most often occurs in the ring finger when the athlete tries to grab a jersy of an opponent, either rupturing the tendon or avulsing a small piece of bone.[9]

**Figure 19-22**

Splinting of a mallet finger

**Figure 19-23**

Boutonnière deformity

**Signs of injury**   Because the tendon is no longer attached to the distal phalanx the DIP joint cannot be flexed and the finger is in an extended position. There is pain and point tenderness over the distal phalanx.

**Care**   If the tendon is not surgically repaired the athlete will never be able to flex the DIP joint, causing weakness in grip strength; otherwise function is relatively normal. If surgery is done the course of rehabilitation requires about 12 weeks and there is often poor gliding of the tendon with the possibility of rerupture.

## Gamekeeper's Thumb

**Cause of injury**   A sprain of the ulnar collateral ligament of the MCP joint of the thumb is common among athletes, especially skiers and tackle football players. The mechanism of injury is usually a forceful abduction of the proximal phalanx, which is occasionally combined with hyperextension.[14]

**Signs of injury**   The athlete complains of pain over the ulnar collateral ligament with a weak and painful pinch. Inspection demonstrates tenderness and swelling over the medial aspect of the thumb.

**Care**   Because the stability of pinching can be severely reduced, proper immediate and follow-up care must be performed. If there is instability in the joints, the athlete should be immediately referred to an orthopedist. If the joint is stable, x-ray examination should be performed to rule out fracture. Splinting of the thumb should be applied for protection over a 3-week period or until it is pain free.

## Collateral Ligament Sprain

**Cause of injury**   A collateral ligament sprain of a finger is very common in sports such as basketball, volleyball, and football. A common cause of collateral sprains is an axial force to the tip of the finger, producing the "jammed" effect.

**Signs of injury**   Severe point tenderness exists at the joint site, especially in the region of the collateral ligaments. There may be a lateral or medial joint instability when the joint is in 150 degrees of flexion.

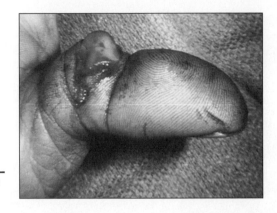

**Figure 19-24**

Compound dislocation of the thumb

**Care**    Care of a collateral sprain includes ice packs for the acute stage, x-ray examination, and splinting.

### Dislocations of the Phalanges

**Cause of injury**    Dislocations of the phalanges (Figure 19-24) occur frequently in sports and are caused mainly by a blow to the tip of the finger by a ball. The force of injury is usually directed upward from the palmar side, displacing either the first or second joint dorsally. The resultant problem is primarily a tearing of the supporting capsular tissue, accompanied by hemorrhaging. However, there may be a rupture of the flexor or extensor tendon and chip fractures in and around the dislocated joint.[9]

**Care**    Reduction of the dislocated thumb should be performed by a physician. To ensure the most complete healing of dislocated finger joints, splinting should be maintained for about 3 weeks in 30 degrees of flexion. Inadequate immobilization can cause an unstable joint and/or excessive scar tissue and possibly a permanent deformity.

Special consideration must be given to dislocations of the thumb and second or third joints of the fingers.[9] A properly functioning thumb is necessary for hand dexterity; consequently, *any injury to the thumb should be considered serious.* Thumb dislocations occur frequently at the second joint, resulting from a sharp blow to its tip with the trauma forcing the thumb into hyperextension and dislocating the second joint downward. Any dislocation of the third joint of the finger can lead to complications and requires the immediate care of an orthopedist. *All hand dislocations must be x-rayed to rule out fracture.*

### Subungual Hematoma

**Cause of injury**    A particularly common contusion of the finger is bruising of the distal phalanx, which results in a subungual hematoma (contusion of the fingernail).

**Signs of injury**    This is an extremely painful condition because of the accumulation of blood underneath the fingernail.

**Care**   The athlete should place the finger in ice water until the hemorrhage ceases, and the pressure of blood should then be released (Figure 19-25). There are two common methods for releasing the pressure of the subungual hematoma.

1. The injured finger should first be coated with an antiseptic solution. A sharp scalpel point or small-gauge drill is used to penetrate the injured nail through a rotary action. If the hematoma extends as far as the end of the nail, it may be best to release the blood by slipping the scalpel tip under the end of the nail.

2. A paper clip is heated to red-hot temperature and then laid on the surface of the nail with moderate pressure, melting a hole through the nail to the accumulation of blood in the nail bed.

### Phalanx Fractures

**Cause of injury**   Phalanx fractures can occur from a variety of actions: The fingers are stepped on, hit by a ball, or twisted.[6]

**Signs of injury**   The athlete complains of pain and swelling in a finger. Tenderness is felt at the point of fracture.

**Care**   The finger suspected of fracture should be splinted in flexion around a gauze roll or a curved splint to avoid full extension. Flexion splinting reduces the deformity by relaxing the flexor tendons. Fracture of the distal phalanx is less complicated than fracture of the middle or proximal phalanx.

### SUMMARY

**Figure 19-25**

Releasing blood from beneath the nail in a subungual hematoma

- The humeroradial and humeroulnar joints of the elbow allow the movements of flexion and extension, and the radioulnar joint allows forearm pronation and supination.

- Olecranon bursitis occurs from falling on the tip of the elbow.

- The ulnar collateral ligament is injured as a result of a valgus force from the repetitive trauma of overhead throwing.

- Medial epicondylitis is also called golfer's elbow, raquetball elbow, or pitcher's elbow and occurs because of repetitive forced flexion of the wrist.

- Lateral epicondylitis or tennis elbow occurs with repetitive wrist extension.

- Elbow dislocations result from elbow hyperextension from a fall on an extended arm, with the radius and ulna dislocating posteriorly. The degree of stability present determines the course of rehabilitation. If the elbow is stable, a brief period of immobilization is followed by rehabilitation.

- Fractures in the elbow may occur from a direct blow or from falling on an outstretched hand. They may be treated by casting or in some cases by surgical reduction and fixation.

- The forearm is composed of two bones, the ulna and the radius, and the flexors and extensors of the wrist. Sports injuries to the region commonly consist of contusions, chronic forearm splints, acute strains, and fractures.

- Injuries to the wrist usually occur as the result of a fall on an outstretched hand or repeated movements of flexion, extension, and/or rotation. Common injuries are sprains, tendonitis, carpal tunnel syndrome, lunate dislocation, scaphoid fracture, hamate fracture, and wrist ganglion.

- Injuries to the hand and fingers occur frequently in sports activities. Common injuries include boxer's fracture, mallet finger, boutonnière deformity, jersey finger, gamekeeper's thumb, sprains, dislocations and fractures of the phalanges, and subungual hematoma.

*Solutions to Critical Thinking* Exercises

**19-1** This javelin thrower has sustained an ulnar nerve injury. Because of a pronounced elbow cubitus valgus, the ulnar nerve recurrently subluxates. Because of ligamentous laxity, there is nerve impingement and compression.

**19-2** This injury is a Colles' fracture, which is caused by the fracture displacement of the distal radius. The coach applies an ice compress, a splint, and a sling. The athlete is then referred to a physician for an x ray and definitive treatment.

**19-3** This is likely a scaphoid fracture. The wrist and thumb should be immobilized in a splint and she should be sent to a physician for an x ray.

**19-4** The coach should suspect a fracture of a metacarpal bone. The injury may appear as an angular or rotational deformity. RICE and analgesics are given along with an x-ray examination. The injury is splinted for about 4 weeks, and early range-of-motion exercises are prescribed.

## REVIEW QUESTIONS AND CLASS ACTIVITIES

1. Describe the procedures for assessing an elbow injury.
2. Describe the mechanism and management of elbow sprains.
3. How does the elbow develop medial and lateral epicondylitis?
4. What are the symptoms and signs of elbow osteochondritis dissecans?
5. Describe a dislocated elbow—its cause, appearance, and care.
6. Compare forearm splints and shin splints. How does each occur?
7. What is the difference between a wrist strain and a wrist sprain?
8. Describe the Colles' fracture of the forearm—its cause, appearance, and care.
9. How does carpal tunnel syndrome develop and how would you care for it?
10. Discuss injuries that can occur to the lunate, scaphoid, and hamate bones in the wrist.
11. What is the difference between a mallet finger, a boutonnière deformity, and jersey finger?
12. What is the gamekeeper's thumb and how should it be treated?
13. Should a dislocated finger be reduced by an athletic trainer?
14. How should a subungual hematoma be managed?

## Dynamic Human CD

For more information on skeletal anatomy of the elbow, wrist, hand, and fingers click on:

- Skeletal
- Anatomy
- Gross anatomy
- Upper limbs
- Humerus
- Then, Radius/ulna
- Then, Hand

To take a closer look at the muscles that are involved in elbow, wrist, hand, and finger movement click on:

- Muscular
- Anatomy
- Body regions
- Pentoral girdle
- Then, Upper arms
- Then, Body regions
- Forearm

To look at the effect of carpal tunnel syndrome on various msucles click on:

- Nervous
- Clinical Concepts
- Carpal Tunnel Syndrome

### REFERENCES

1. Andrews JR, Whiteside JA: Common elbow problems in the athlete, *J Orthop Sports Phys Ther* 17(6):289, 1993.

2. Bach AW: Finger joint injuries in active patients: pointers for acute and late-phase management, *Physician Sportsmed* 27(3):89, 1999.

3. Blackard D, Sampson J: Management of an uncomplicated posterior elbow dislocation, *J Ath Train* 32(1):63, 1997.

4. Buettner CM, Leaver-Dunn D: Prevention and treatment of elbow injuries in adolescent pitchers, *Ath Ther Today* 5(3):19, 2000.

5. Case WS: Carpal tunnel syndrome, *Physician Sportsmed* 33(1): 27, 1995.

6. Caso JT, Hastings H: Metacarpal and phalangeal fractures in athletics. In Rettig AC, editor: *Hand and wrist. Clinics in sports medicine,* vol 17, no 3, Philadelphia, 1998, WB Saunders.

7. Ellenbecker TS et al: Medial elbow joint laxity in professional baseball pitchers, *Am J Sports Med* 26(3): 420, 1998.

8. Field LD, Savoie FH: Surgical treatment of ulnar collateral ligament injuries, *Ath Ther Today* 5(3):25, 2000.

9. Fincher AL: Taking finger injuries seriously, *Ath Ther Today* 4(3):45, 1999.

10. Frostick SP, Mohammad M, Ritchie DA: Sport injuries of the elbow, *Br J Sports Med* 33(5):301, 1999.

11. Hall TL, Galea AM: Osteochondritis dissecans of the elbow: diagnosis, treatment, and prevention, *Physician Sportsmed* 27(2):75, 1999.

12. Hannafin JA: How I manage tennis and golfer's elbow, *Physician Sportsmed* 24(2):63, 1996.

13. Lord JL: Forearm injuries. In Birrer RB, editor: *Sports medicine for the primary care physician*, ed 2, Boca Raton, Fla, 1994, CRC Press.

14. Schneider AM: *Rehabilitation of wrist, hand, and finger injuries.* In Prentice WE, editor: Rehabilitation techniques in sports medicine, ed 3, Boston, 1999, WCB/McGraw-Hill.

15. Servi JT: Wrist pain from overuse, *Physician Sportsmed* 25(12):41, 1997.

16. Sevier TL, Wilson JK: Treating lateral epicondylitis, *Sports Med* 28(5):375, 1999.

17. Uhl TL: Uncomplicated elbow dislocation rehabilitation, *Ath Ther Today* 5(3):31, 2000.

18. Zimmerman G: Carpal tunnel syndrome, *J Ath Train* 29(1):22, 1994.

19. Zulia P, Prentice W: Rehabilitation of elbow injuries. In Prentice W, editor: *Rehabilitation techniques in sports medicine*, ed 3, Boston, 1999, WCB/McGraw-Hill.

## ANNOTATED BIBLIOGRAPHY

Clark GL et al, (editors): *Hand rehabilitation: a practical guide*, ed 2, New York, 1997, Churchill Livingstone.

*A major reference devoted to treatment goals and purposes, indications, precautions for therapy, nonoperative therapy, postoperative therapy, postoperative complications, and evaluation.*

McCabe S, Goldman S: *The hand wrist and arm source book*, New York, 1999, Lowell House.

*A very well written and presented health reference for the nonspecialist general reader, which provides all the details necessary to understand both injuries and common problems of hand injuries.*

Rettig AC, editor: *Hand and wrist injuries. Clinics in sports medicine*, vol 17, no 3, Philadelphia, 1998, WB Saunders.

*A monograph covering all aspects of sports injuries to the hands and wrists.*

**WEBSITES**

World Ortho: http://www.worldortho.com

*Use the search engine in this site to locate relevant information.*

Wheeless' Textbook of Orthopaedics: http://www.medmedia.com/med/htm

*An excellent page for injuries, anatomy, and x rays.*

Karolinska Institute Library: Musculoskeletal Disease: http://www.mic.ki.se/Disease/c5.htm

American Orthopaedic Society for Sports Medicine: http://www.sportsmed.org

MedFacts Sports Doc: http://www.medfacts.com

Electronic Textbook of Hand Surgery: http://www.e-hand.com/default.htm

Tennis Elbow Central: http://www.tennis-elbow.net/

The Physician and Sportsmedicine: Elbow Injuries: http://www.physsportsmed.com/issues/may_96/ nirschl.htm

Elbow Injuries: http://www.swmed.edu/home_pages/library/consumer/elbow.htm

Braces and Supports for tennis elbow and elbow pain: http://orthobionics.com/elbow/index.htm

MEDLINEplus: Elbow Injuries and Disorders: http://medlineplus.nlm.nih.gov/medlineplus/elbowinjuries

# The Spine

*When you finish this chapter you will be able to:*

■ Describe the anatomy of the cervical, thoracic, and lumbar spine.

■ Explain how the nerve roots from the spinal cord combine to form specific peripheral nerves.

■ Describe measures to prevent injury to the spine.

■ Describe a process to assess injuries of the cervical and lumbar spine.

■ Identify specific injuries that can occur to the various regions of the spine.

Regions of the spinal column:
• Cervical
• Thoracic
• Lumbar
• Sacrum
• Coccyx

Movements of the vertebral column:
• Flexion
• Extension
• Lateral flexion
• Rotation

T he spine is one of the most complex regions of the body. It contains a multitude of bones, joints, ligaments, and muscles, all of which are collectively involved in spinal movement. The relationship of the spinal cord and the peripheral nerves and their proximity to the vertebral column add to the complexity of this region. Injury to the cervical spine has potentially life-threatening implications. Low back pain is one of the most common ailments known to humans. Thus some understanding of the anatomy, assessment techniques, and specific injuries of the spine is essential for the coach.

## ANATOMY OF THE SPINE

### Bones

The spine, or vertebral column, is composed of thirty-three individual bones called *vertebrae*. Twenty-four are classified as movable, or true, and nine are classified as immovable, or false. The movable vertebrae are the cervical vertebrae, thoracic vertebrae, and lumbar vertebrae. The false vertebrae, which are fixed by fusion, form the sacrum and the coccyx. The design of the spine allows a high degree of flexibility forward and laterally and limited mobility backward. Rotation around a central axis in the areas of the neck and the lower back is also permitted.

#### The Cervical Spine

Because of the vulnerability of the cervical spine to sports injuries, coaches should have a general knowledge of the cervical spine anatomy

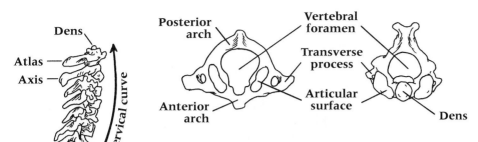

**ATLAS**
**First cervical vertebra**

**AXIS**
**Second cervical vertebra**

**Figure 20-1**

Anatomy of the cervical spine, atlas, and axis

and its susceptibility to sports injuries.[1,5] The cervical spine consists of seven vertebrae, with the first two differing from the other true vertebrae (Figure 20-1). These first two are called the *atlas* and the *axis,* respectively, and they function together to support the head on the spinal column and to permit cervical rotation.

### The Thoracic Spine

The thoracic spine consists of twelve vertebrae (Figure 20-2). Thoracic vertebrae have long transverse processes and prominent but thin spinous processes. Thoracic vertebrae 1 through 10 articulate with the ribs. There is very little movement in the thoracic vertebrae.

### The Lumbar Spine

The lumbar spine is composed of five vertebrae (Figure 20-3). They are the major support of the low back and are the largest and thickest of the vertebrae, with large spinous and transverse processes. Movement occurs in all the lumbar vertebrae; however, there is much less flexion than extension. Rotation is important in the lumbar region.

### The Sacrum

The sacrum is formed by the fusion of five vertebrae and, with the two hip bones, constitutes the pelvis (Figure 20-4). The sacrum articulates with the ilium to form the sacroiliac joints. During both sitting and standing the body's weight is transmitted through these joints. A complex of ligaments serves to make these joints very stable.

### The Coccyx

The coccyx, or tailbone, is the most inferior part of the vertebral column and consists of four or more fused vertebrae (refer to Figure 20-4). The gluteus maximus muscle attaches to the coccyx posteriorly.

## Intervertebral Articulations and Disks

Intervertebral articulations are between vertebral bodies. Between each of the cervical, thoracic, and lumbar vertebrae lie fibrocartilaginous

20-1

*Critical Thinking* Exercise

While doing a back evaluation on a soccer player, the coach finds that backward bending is limited, yet the movement diminishes pain; straight leg raising is limited and painful; forward bending is extremely limited and increases pain; and back pain is diminished when lying down, but increased in sitting.

? What types of exercises should the coach recommend to the athlete that should routinely be done during a rehabilitation program?

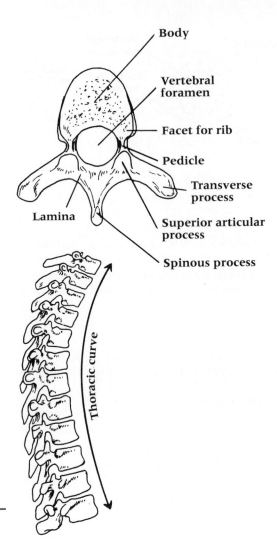

**Figure 20-2**

Anatomy of the thoracic
spine and vertebrae

**Figure 20-3**

Anatomy of the lumbar spine

intervertebral disks (Figure 20-5). Each disk is composed of the annulus fibrosus and the nucleus pulposus. The annulus fibrosus forms the periphery of the intervertebral disk and is composed of strong, fibrous tissue. In the center is the semifluid nucleus pulposus, compressed under pressure. The disks act as important shock absorbers for the spine.

### Ligaments

The major ligaments that join the various vertebral parts are the anterior longitudinal, the posterior longitudinal, and the supraspinous (Figure 20-6). The interspinous, supraspinous, and intertransverse ligaments stabilize the transverse and spinous processes, extending between adjacent vertebrae. The sacroiliac joint is maintained by the extremely strong dorsal sacral ligaments. The sacrotuberous and the sacrospinous ligaments maintain the position of the sacrum relative to the ischium.

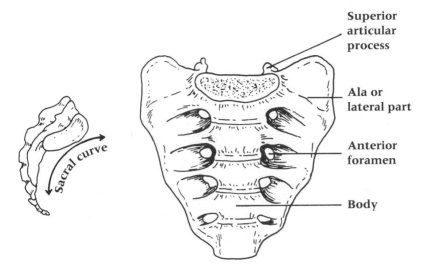

**Superior articular process**

**Ala or lateral part**

**Anterior foramen**

**Body**

Sacral curve

**Figure 20-4**

Anatomy of the sacrum and coccyx

## Muscles

The muscles that extend the spine and rotate the vertebral column can be classified as either superficial or deep (Figure 20-7). The superficial muscles, or erector spinae, extend from the vertebrae to ribs. The erector spinae are a group of paired muscles made up of three columns, or bands: the longissimus group, the iliocostalis group, and the spinalis group. Each of these groups is further divided into regions: the cervicis region in the neck, the thoracis region in the middle back, and the lumborum region in the low back. Generally the erector spinae muscles extend the spine.

**Figure 20-5**

Intervertebral disk

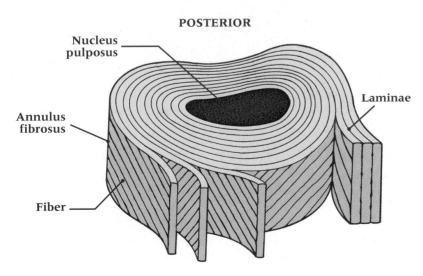

**POSTERIOR**

**Nucleus pulposus**

**Annulus fibrosus**

**Fiber**

**Laminae**

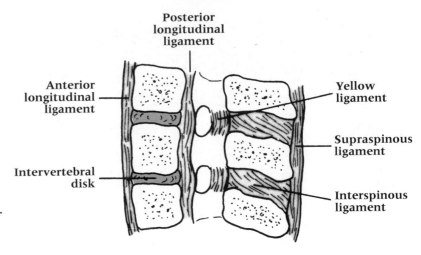

**ANTERIOR**

Posterior
longitudinal
ligament

Anterior
longitudinal
ligament

Intervertebral
disk

Yellow
ligament

Supraspinous
ligament

Interspinous
ligament

**Figure 20-6**

Major ligaments of the
lumbar spine

**Figure 20-7**

Deep and superficial muscles
of the spine

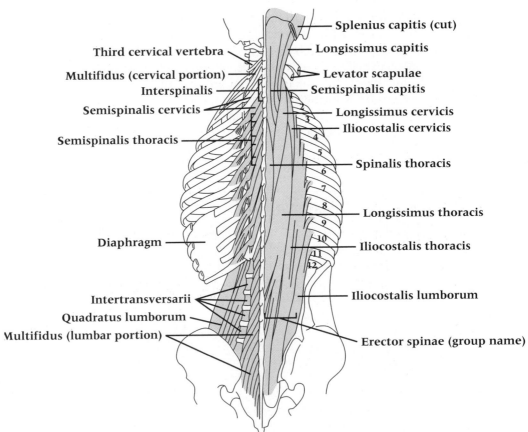

Third cervical vertebra

Multifidus (cervical portion)

Interspinalis

Semispinalis cervicis

Semispinalis thoracis

Diaphragm

Intertransversarii

Quadratus lumborum

Multifidus (lumbar portion)

Splenius capitis (cut)

Longissimus capitis

Levator scapulae

Semispinalis capitis

Longissimus cervicis

Iliocostalis cervicis

Spinalis thoracis

Longissimus thoracis

Iliocostalis thoracis

Iliocostalis lumborum

Erector spinae (group name)

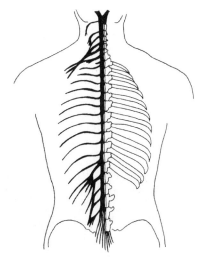

**Figure 20-8**

Relationship of cord and spinal nerves to the vertebral column

The deep muscles extend from one vertebra to another. The deep muscles include the interspinals, multifidus, rotatores, thoracis, and the semispinalis cervicis. These muscles extend and rotate the spine.

### Spinal Cord and Spinal Nerves

The spinal cord is that portion of the central nervous system that is contained within the vertebral canal of the spinal column. It extends from the cranium to the first or second lumbar vertebra. The lumbar roots and the sacral nerves form a horselike tail called the cauda equina.

Thirty-one pairs of spinal nerves extend from the sides of the spinal cord: eight cervical, twelve thoracic, five lumbar, five sacral, and one coccygeal (Figure 20-8).

## PREVENTING INJURIES TO THE SPINE

### Cervical Spine

#### Strength

Acute traumatic injuries to the spine can be potentially life threatening, particularly if the cervical region of the spinal cord is involved. Thus the athlete must do everything possible to minimize the chance of injury. Strengthening the musculature of the neck is critical. The neck muscles can function to protect the cervical spine by resisting excessive hyperflexion, hyperextension, or rotational forces. During participation the athlete should be in a constant state of readiness to "bull" the neck when making contact with an opponent. This protection is accomplished by elevating both shoulders and isometrically contracting the muscles surrounding the neck. Protective cervical collars can also help limit movement of the cervical spine. Athletes with long, weak necks are especially at risk. Tackle football players and wrestlers must have highly stable necks. Specific strengthening exercises are essential for the development

Long-necked football players and wrestlers are at risk and need to establish neck stability through strengthening exercises.

of stability. A variety of different exercises that incorporate isotonic, isometric, or isokinetic contractions can be used.

### Flexibility

In addition to strong muscles, the athlete's neck should have a full range of motion. Ideally the athlete should be able to place the chin on the chest and to extend the head back until the face is parallel with the ceiling. There should be at least 40 to 45 degrees of lateral flexion and enough rotation to allow the chin to reach a level even with the tip of the shoulder. Flexibility is increased through stretching exercises and strength exercises that are in full range of motion. When flexibility is restricted, manual static stretching can be beneficial.

### Using Proper Technique

Athletes involved in collision sports—in particular football and rugby, which involve tackling an opponent—must be taught and required to use techniques that reduce the likelihood of cervical injury. The head, especially one in a helmet, should not be used as a weapon. Football helmets do not protect players against neck injury. In the illegal spearing situation, the athlete uses the helmet as a weapon by striking the opponent with its top. Most serious cervical injuries in football result from deliberate axial loading while spearing.[16] Coaches cannot stress enough to the athlete the importance of using appropriate tackling techniques. In other sports, such as diving, wrestling, and bouncing on a trampoline, the athlete's neck can be flexed at the time of contact. Energy of the forward-moving body mass cannot be fully absorbed, and fracture or dislocation or both can occur. Diving into shallow water causes many catastrophic neck injuries. Many of the same forces are applied in wrestling. In such trauma, paraplegia, quadriplegia, or death can result.

## Lumbar Spine

Low back pain is caused by many factors, many of which can be prevented by using proper body mechanics when sitting, lying, standing, or bending (Focus Box 20-1).

### Strength and Flexibility

Coaches need to be aware of any postural anomalies that the athletes possess. With this knowledge, a coach can establish individual corrective programs. Basic conditioning should include an emphasis on trunk flexibility. Every effort should be made to produce maximum range of motion in rotation and in both lateral and forward flexion. Both strength and flexibility should be developed in the spinal extensors (erector spinae). Abdominal strength is essential to ensure proper postural alignment.[2]

### Using Proper Technique

In weightlifters, the chance of injury to the lumbar spine can be minimized by using proper lifting techniques. Incorporating appropriate

**20-1** *Focus Box*

**Recommended Postures and Practices for Preventing Low Back Pain**

**Sitting**

1. Do not sit for long periods.
2. Avoid sitting forward on a chair with back arched.
3. Sit on a firm, straight-backed chair.
4. The low back should be slightly rounded or positioned firmly against the back of the chair.
5. The feet should be flat on the floor with knees above the level of the hips (if unable to adequately raise the knees, the feet should be placed on a stool).
6. Avoid sitting with legs straight and raised on a stool.

**Standing**

1. If standing for long periods:
   a. Shift position from one foot to the other.
   b. Place one foot on a stool.
2. Stand tall, flatten low back, and relax knees.
3. Avoid arching back.

**Lifting and carrying**

1. To pick up an object:
   a. Bend at knees and not the waist.
   b. Do not twist to pick up an object—face it squarely.
   c. Tuck in buttocks and tighten abdomen.
2. To carry an object:
   a. Hold object close to body.
   b. Hold object at waist level.
   c. Do not carry object on one side of the body—if it must be carried unbalanced, change from one side to the other.

**Sleeping**

1. Do not stay in one position too long.
2. The bed should be flat and firm yet comfortable.
3. Do not sleep on the abdomen.
4. Do not sleep on the back with legs fully extended.
5. If sleeping on the back, a pillow should be placed under the knees.
6. Ideally, sleep on the side with the knees drawn up.
7. Arms should never be extended overhead.
8. The least strain on the back is in the fully recumbent position with the hips and knees at angles of 90 degrees. In the case of a chronic or a subacute low back condition, a firm mattress affords better rest and relaxation of the lower back. Placing a ¾-inch plywood board underneath the mattress gives a firm, stable surface for the injured back. Sleeping on a water bed often relieves low back pain. The value of a water bed is that it supports the body curves equally, decreasing abnormal pressures to any one body area.

breathing techniques that involve inhaling and exhaling deeply during lifting can help stabilize the spine. Weight belts can also help stabilize the lumbar spine. Spotters can greatly enhance safety by helping lift and lower the weight.

## ASSESSMENT OF THE SPINE

Assessment of injuries to the spine is somewhat more complex than assessment of the joints of the extremities because of the number of articulations involved in spinal movement.[13,14] It is also true that injury to the spine, or in particular the spinal cord, may have life-threatening or life-altering implications. Thus the coach must be able to rule out spinal injury by asking the appropriate questions.[1]

### History

The most critical part of the evaluation is to rule out the possibility of spinal cord injury.[5] Questions that address this possibility should first establish the mechanism of injury.

- What do you think happened?
- Did you hit someone with or land directly on the top of your head?
- Were you knocked out or unconscious? Any time an impact is sufficient to cause unconsciousness, the potential for injury to the spine exists.
- Do you have any pain in your neck?
- Do you have tingling, numbness, or burning in your shoulders, arms, or hands?
- Do you have equal muscle strength in both hands?
- Are you able to move your ankles and toes? Any sensory or motor changes bilaterally may indicate some spinal cord injury.

*A yes response to any of these questions necessitates extreme caution when moving the athlete.* **In cases of suspected cervical spine injury, if the coach is going to make a mistake, the error should be made in being overly cautious.** Emergency care of the athlete with suspected cervical spine injury was discussed in detail in Chapter 7.

Once cervical spine injury has been ruled out, other general questions may provide some indication as to the nature of the problem.

- Where is the pain located?
- What kind of pain do you have?
- What were you doing when the pain began?
- Were you standing, sitting, bending, or twisting?
- Did the pain begin immediately?
- How long have you had this pain?
- Do certain movements or positions cause more pain?
- Can you assume a position that gets rid of the pain?

- Is there any tingling or numbness in the arms or legs?
- Is there any pain in the buttocks or the back of the legs?
- Have you ever had any back pain before?
- What position do you usually sleep in? How do you prefer to sit?

It is important to remember that pain in the back may be caused by many different conditions. The source may be musculoskeletal or visceral, or it may be referred.

## Observation

Observing the posture and movement capabilities of the athlete during the evaluation can help clarify the nature and extent of the injury. General observations relative to posture include the following:

- Is the athlete willing to move the head and neck freely?
- Are the shoulders level and symmetrical?
- Is the head tilted to one side?
- Is one scapula lower or more prominent than the other?
- Is the trunk bent or curved to one side?
- Is the space between the body and arm greater on one side?
- Is one hip more prominent than the other?
- Are the hips tilted to one side?
- Are the ribs more pronounced on one side?
- Does one arm hang longer than the other?
- Does one arm hang farther forward than the other?
- Is one patella lower than the other?

## Palpation

Palpation should be performed with the athlete lying prone and the spine as straight as possible. The head and neck should be slightly flexed. In cases of low back pain, a pillow placed under the hips might make the athlete more comfortable. The spinous processes and transverse process of each vertebra along with the sacrum and coccyx should be palpated for spots of tenderness or increases in pain. The musculature on each side of the spine should also be palpated for tenderness or guarding. Palpation should progress from proximal to distal. It should be remembered that referred pain can produce tender areas away from the site of injury.

## Special Tests

Special tests for the lumbar spine should be performed in standing, sitting, supine, side-lying, and prone positions.[8] Special tests include testing both the cervical and lumbar spines in forward bending, backward bending, side bending, and rotation. Any increase in pain or restriction in movement indicates the existence of some condition or injury that should be referred for further evaluation.[8]

**Figure 20-9**

Straight leg raising test: pain
in SLR test may indicate a
problem in the sciatic nerve,
sacroiliac joint, or lumbar
spine.

A

B

**Figure 20-10**

A, Sacral compression; B,
Sacral distraction; both tests
can help determine if there is
a problem in the sacroiliac
joint.

### Straight Leg Raises

Straight leg raising applies pressure to the sacroiliac joint and may indicate a problem either in the sciatic nerve, the sacroiliac joint, or the lumbar spine (Figure 20-9).

### Compression and Distraction Tests

Sacroiliac compression and distraction tests are useful in determining if there is a problem in the sacroiliac joint (Figure 20-10).

## RECOGNITION AND MANAGEMENT OF CERVICAL SPINE INJURIES AND CONDITIONS

Because the neck is so mobile, it is extremely vulnerable to a wide range of sports injuries.[21] Although relatively uncommon, severe sports injury to the neck can produce catastrophic impairment of the spinal cord (Figure 20-11). The neck is also prone to subtle injuries stemming from stress, tension, and postural malalignments.

### Cervical Fractures

**Cause of injury** Fortunately, neck fractures are relatively uncommon in athletics. Nevertheless, the coach must constantly be prepared to handle such a situation should it arise. **Axial loading** of the cervical vertebrae from a force to the top of the head combined with flexion of the

**axial loading**

A blow to the top of the
athlete's head while in
flexion.

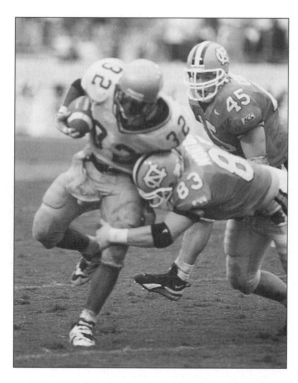

**Figure 20-11**

The possibility of cervical neck injury is always present in sport.

neck can result in an anterior compression.[17] If the head is also rotated when making contact, a dislocation may occur along with the fracture. Those sports having the highest incidence of neck fractures are gymnastics, ice hockey, diving, football, and rugby.[18]

**Signs of injury**   The athlete may have one or more of the following signs of cervical fracture: neck point tenderness and restricted movement, cervical muscle spasm, cervical pain and pain in the chest and extremities, numbness in trunk and/or limbs, weakness or paralysis in limbs and/or trunk, a loss of bladder and/or bowel control.

**Care**   An unconscious athlete should be treated as if a serious neck injury is present until this possibility is ruled out by the physician. Extreme caution must be used in moving the athlete.[1] The coach must always be aware that an athlete can sustain a catastrophic spinal injury from improper handling and transportation (see Chapter 7 for a detailed description of the emergency care of spinal injuries).

## Cervical Dislocations

**Cause of injury**   Cervical dislocations are not common, but they do occur much more frequently in sports than do fractures. Dislocations usually result from violent flexion and rotation of the head, as occurs in pool diving accidents.

**Signs of injury**   For the most part, a cervical dislocation produces many of the same signs as a fracture. Both can result in considerable pain, numbness, and muscle weakness or paralysis. The most easily discernible

A unilateral cervical dislocation can cause the neck to tilt toward the dislocated side, with tight muscles on the elongated side and relaxed muscles on the tilted side.

difference is the position of the neck in a dislocation: a unilateral dislocation causes the neck to be tilted toward the dislocated side with extreme
muscle tightness on the elongated side and a relaxed muscle state on the
tilted side.

**Care**  Because a dislocation of a cervical vertebrae has a greater likelihood of causing injury to the spinal cord, even greater care must be exercised when moving the patient. The procedures described in Chapter 7
should be applied to cervical dislocations.

### Acute Muscle Strains of the Neck and Upper Back

**Cause of injury**  In a strain of the neck or upper back, the athlete has
usually turned the head suddenly or has forced flexion, extension, or rotation. Muscles involved are typically the upper trapezius, sternocleidomastoid,
the scalenes on the front of the neck, and the splenius capitis and cervicis.

**Signs of injury**  Localized pain, point tenderness, and restricted motion are present. Muscle guarding resulting from pain is common, and
there is a reluctance to move the neck in any direction.

**Care**  Care usually includes use of RICE immediately after the strain
occurs and use of a cervical collar (Figure 20-12). Follow-up management may include range-of-motion exercises followed by isometric exercises progressing to full-range isotonic strengthening exercises. In addition, cold or superficial heat and analgesic medications are used as
prescribed by the physician.

### Cervical Sprain (Whiplash)

**Cause of injury**  A cervical sprain can occur from the same mechanism as the strain but usually results from a more violent motion. More
commonly, a cervical sprain occurs when the head snaps suddenly, such

**Figure 20-12**

Wearing a soft cervical collar
helps reduce pain and spasm
in an athlete with an injured
neck.

as when the athlete is tackled or blocked while unprepared (Figure 20-13). Frequently muscle strains occur with ligament sprains. A sprain of the neck produces tears in the supporting tissue of the anterior or posterior longitudinal ligaments, the interspinous ligament, or the supraspinous ligament.

**Signs of injury**   The sprain displays all the signs of the strained neck but the symptoms persist longer. There may also be tenderness over the transverse and spinous processes that serve as sites of attachment for the ligaments. Pain may not be experienced initially but always appears the day after the trauma.

**Care**   As soon as possible, the athlete should have a physician evaluation to rule out the possibility of fracture, dislocation, or disk injury. A soft cervical collar may be applied to reduce muscle spasm. RICE is used for 48 to 72 hours while the injury is in the acute stage of healing. In an athlete with a severe injury, the physician may prescribe 2 to 3 days of bed rest along with analgesics and antiinflammation agents. Therapy might include cold or heat and massage. Mechanical traction may also be prescribed to relieve pain and muscle spasm.

**Figure 20-13**

Whiplash injury

### Acute Torticollis (Wryneck)

**Cause of injury**   Acute torticollis is a very common condition, more frequently called wryneck or stiffneck. The athlete usually complains of pain on one side of the neck when awakening. Wryneck happens when a small piece of synovial membrane lining the joint capsule is impinged or trapped between the cervical vertebrae. This problem can also occasionally follow exposure to a cold draft of air or holding the head in an unusual position over time.

**Signs of injury**   During inspection, there is palpable point tenderness and muscle spasm. Head movement is restricted to the side opposite the irritation with marked muscle guarding. X-ray examination rules out a more serious injury.

**Care**   Cold or heat and massage may be used to modulate pain in an attempt to break a pain-spasm-pain cycle. Gentle traction, rotation, and lateral bending, first in the pain-free direction then in the direction of pain, can help reduce the guarding. The athlete may find it helpful to wear a soft cervical collar for comfort (refer to Figure 20-12). This muscle guarding generally lasts for 2 to 3 days, during which the athlete progressively regains motion.

### Pinched Nerve (Brachial Plexus Injury)

**Cause of injury**   A pinched nerve resulting from stretching or compression of the brachial plexus is the most common of all cervical neurological injuries in the athlete.[12] Other terms commonly used to indicate this condition are *stinger* or *burner*.[19] The primary mechanism of injury is the stretching of the brachial plexus of nerves when the neck is forced laterally to the opposite side while the shoulder is depressed, as occurs with a shoulder block in football.

20–2

*Critical Thinking* Exercise

When making a tackle a football player experiences burning and tingling with a loss of strength in his left arm.

?   What condition has most likely occurred and how should the coach manage this problem?

**Signs of injury** The athlete complains of a burning sensation, numbness and tingling, and pain extending from the shoulder down to the hand, with some loss of function of the arm and hand that lasts for several minutes. Rarely, symptoms may persist for several days. Neck range of motion is usually normal. Repeated brachial plexus nerve stretch injuries may result in permanent damage.[11]

**Care** Once the symptoms have completely resolved and there are no associated neurological symptoms, the athlete may return to full activity. Thereafter the athlete should begin strengthening and stretching exercises for the neck musculature. A football player should be fitted with shoulder pads and a cervical neck roll to limit neck range of motion during impact.

## RECOGNITION AND MANAGEMENT OF LUMBAR SPINE INJURIES AND CONDITIONS

### Low Back Pain

**Cause of injury** Low back pain is one of the most common and disabling ailments known to humans. In sports, back problems are common and are most often the result of either congenital anomalies, mechanical back defects caused mainly by faulty posture, or trauma to the back including sprains, strains, or contusions.

**Signs of injury** With repeated episodes of injury, the athlete may develop recurrent or chronic low back pain. Gradually this problem can lead to muscular weakness and impairment of sensation and reflex responses. The older the athlete, the more prone he or she is to developing chronic low back pain. The incidence of this condition at the high school level is low, but it becomes progressively greater with increasing age.

**Care** The athlete, like everyone else in the population, can prevent low back pain by avoiding unnecessary stresses and strains associated with standing, sitting, lying, working, or exercising.[2] Care should be taken to avoid postures and positions that can cause injuries (refer to Focus Box 20-1).

### Lumbar Vertebrae Fracture and Dislocation

**Cause of injury** Fractures in the lumbar region of the vertebral column are not serious in terms of bone injury, but they pose dangers when related to spinal cord damage. Lumbar vertebrae fractures of the greatest concern in sports are compression fractures and fractures of the transverse and spinous processes.

The compression fracture may occur as a result of hyperflexion of the trunk. Falling from a height and landing on the feet or buttocks may also produce a compression fracture. Fractures of the transverse and spinous processes result most often from a kick or other direct impact to the back. Dislocations of the lumbar vertebrae in sports are rare, occurring only when there is an associated fracture.

**Signs of injury** Recognition of the compression fracture is difficult without an x-ray examination. A basic evaluation may be made with a knowledge of the history and point tenderness over the affected vertebrae. Fractures of the transverse and spinous processes may be directly palpable. There will be point tenderness and some localized swelling along with muscle guarding to protect the area.

**Care**   If the symptoms and signs associated with a fracture are present, the injured athlete should be x-rayed. Transporting and moving the athlete should be done on a spine board as described in Chapter 7 to minimize movement of the fractured segment.

### Low Back Muscle Strains

**Cause of injury**   There are two mechanisms of the typical low back strain in sports activities.[4] The first happens from a sudden extension, usually in combination with trunk rotation. The second is the chronic strain commonly associated with faulty posture.

**Signs of injury**   Evaluation should be performed immediately after injury to rule out the possibility of fracture. Discomfort in the low back may be diffused or localized in one area. Pain is present on active extension and with passive flexion.

**Care**   Initially, cold packs and/or ice massage should be used to decrease muscle guarding. An elastic wrap or an abdominal support corset-type brace helps compress the area (Figure 20-14). A graduated program of stretching and strengthening begins slowly during the acute stage. Injuries of moderate-to-severe intensity may require complete bed rest to help break the pain–muscle spasm cycle.

### Lumbar Sprains

**Cause of injury**   Sprains may occur in any of the ligaments in the lumbar spine. The most common sprain occurs when the athlete is

**Figure 20-14**

An abdominal brace helps support the lumbar area.

bending forward and twisting while lifting or moving some object. Lumbar sprain can occur with a single episode or with chronic repetitive stress that becomes progressively worse with activity.

**Signs of injury**  The pain is localized and is located just lateral to the spinous process. Pain becomes sharper with certain movements or postures, and the athlete limits movement in painful ranges. Flexion, extension, and rotational movements of the vertebrae can increase pain.

**Care**  Initial treatment should include RICE to reduce pain. Strengthening exercises for abdominals and back extensors and stretching in all directions should be limited to a pain-free range. An abdominal brace or support should be worn to limit movement during early return to activity. As with sprains to other joints in the body, some time is required for healing.

### Back Contusions

**Cause of injury**  Back contusions rank third to strains and sprains in incidence. Because of its surface area, the back is quite vulnerable to bruises in sports. Football produces the greatest number of these injuries. A significant impact to the back can cause serious injury to the kidneys. Contusion of the back must be distinguished from a vertebral fracture. In some instances this distinction is possible only through an x-ray examination.

**Signs of injury**  The bruise causes local pain, muscle spasm, and point tenderness. A swollen, discolored area may be visible also.

**Care**  Cold and pressure should be applied immediately for approximately 72 hours or longer along with rest. Ice massage combined with gradual stretching benefits soft-tissue contusion in the region of the low back. Recovery usually ranges from 2 days to 2 weeks.

### Sciatica

**Cause of injury**  The term *sciatica* has been incorrectly used as a general term to describe all low back pain without reference to exact causes. **Sciatica** is an inflammatory condition of the sciatic nerve that can accompany recurrent or chronic low back pain. This nerve is particularly vulnerable to torsion or direct blows that tend to impose abnormal stretching and pressure on it as it emerges from the spine.[7]

**sciatica** (sigh **at** tika)
Inflammatory condition of the sciatic nerve; commonly associated with peripheral nerve root compression.

**Signs of injury**  Sciatica may begin either abruptly or gradually. It produces a sharp shooting pain that follows the nerve pathway along the posterior and medial thigh. There may also be some tingling and numbness along its path. The nerve may be extremely sensitive to palpation. Straight leg raising usually intensifies the pain.

**Care**  In the acute stage, rest is essential. The cause of the inflammation must be identified and treated. If there is a disk protrusion, lumbar traction may be appropriate. Because recovery from sciatia usually occurs within 2 to 3 weeks, surgery should be delayed to see if symptoms resolve. Oral antiinflammatory medication may help reduce inflammation.

## Herniated Lumbar Disk

**Cause of injury**   The mechanism of a disk injury is the same as that of the lumbar sprain—forward bending and twisting that places abnormal strain on the lumbar region. This movement produces herniation or bulging of the nucleus pulposus of a disk on a nerve root (Figure 20-15).[10] The pain associated with disk herniation is substantial. The disk most often injured lies between the L4 and the L5 vertebrae.

**Signs of injury**   A herniated lumbar disk usually creates centrally located pain that radiates on one side to the buttocks and down the back of the leg or pain that spreads across the back. Symptoms are worse on rising in the morning. Onset may be sudden or gradual, with pain increasing after the athlete sits and then tries to resume activity. Posture exhibits a slight forward bend with side bending away from the side of pain. Straight leg raising increases pain.

**Care**   Initially, rest and ice should be used to help modulate pain. Backward bending or extension makes the athlete more comfortable. As pain and posture return to normal, back extensor and abdominal strengthening should be used.[6] Sometimes the symptoms resolve with time. But signs of nerve damage may necessitate surgery.

## Spondylolysis and Spondylolisthesis

**Cause of condition**   Spondylolysis refers to a degeneration of the vertebrae and, more commonly, a defect in the articular processes of the vertebrae (Figure 20-16A).[20] It is often attributed to a congenital

**Figure 20-15**

Intervertebral disk syndrome

Spondylolisthesis is considered to be a complication of a spondylolysis.

**Figure 20-16**

A, Spondylolysis; B, Spondylolisthesis

weakness with the defect occurring as a stress fracture. It is more common among boys.[9] Sports movements that characteristically hyperextend the spine, such as arching the back in gymnastics, lifting weights, blocking in football, serving in tennis, spiking in volleyball, and using the butterfly stroke in swimming, are most likely to cause this condition.[20]

Spondylolisthesis is a complication of spondylolysis often resulting in hypermobility of a vertebral segment.[7] Spondylolisthesis has the highest incidence with L5 slipping on S1 (Figure 20-16B). A direct blow or sudden twist or chronic low back strain may cause the defective vertebra to displace itself forward on the sacrum.

**Signs of condition**   The athlete complains of persistent aching pain or stiffness across the low back, with increased pain after, not usually during, physical activity. The athlete feels the need to change positions frequently or "pop" the low back to reduce the pain. There may be tenderness localized to one segment.

**Care**   Initially, bracing and occasionally bed rest for 1 to 3 days helps to reduce pain. The major focus in rehabilitation should be directed toward exercises that control or stabilize the hypermobile segment.[15] Progressive trunk-strengthening exercises, especially through the midrange, should be incorporated. Braces are most helpful during high-level activities. It may be necessary for the athlete to avoid vigorous activity.

## RECOGNITION AND MANAGEMENT OF SACROILIAC JOINT DYSFUNCTION

The sacroiliac is the junction formed by the ilium and the sacrum, and it is fortified by strong ligaments that allow little motion to take place. Because the sacroiliac joint is a synovial joint, disorders can include sprain, inflammation, hypermobility, and hypomobility.[3]

### Sacroiliac Sprain

**Cause of injury**   A sprain of the sacroiliac joint may result from twisting with both feet on the ground, stumbling forward, falling backward, stepping too far down and landing heavily on one leg, or forward bending with the knees locked during lifting.[14]

**Signs of injury**   A sprain of the sacroiliac joint may have palpable pain and tenderness directly over the joint with some associated muscle guarding. Hip levels may appear to be asymmetrical.

**Care**   Ice can be used to reduce pain. A supportive brace is also helpful in an acute sprain. Strengthening exercises should be incorporated to improve stability to a hypermobile joint.

### Coccyx Injuries

**Cause of injury**   Coccygeal injuries in sports are prevalent and occur primarily from direct impact, which may result from forcibly sitting down, falling, or being kicked by an opponent. Injuries to the coccyx may include sprains, contusions, or fractures.

**20-3**

*Critical Thinking* Exercise

A gymnast constantly hyperextends her low back. She complains of stiffness and persistent aching pain across the low back with increased pain after but not during practice. The athlete feels that she needs to change positions frequently or self-manipulate her low back to reduce the pain. She is beginning to develop pain in her buttock and some muscle weakness in her leg.

**?**   What type of injury should the coach suspect? Can anything be done about it?

**20-4**

*Critical Thinking* Exercise

During a takedown move a wrestler falls down hard on his buttocks in a sitting position. He complains of intense localized pain at the tip of his spine.

**?**   What has most likely been injured?

**Signs of injury**   Pain in the coccygeal region is often prolonged and at times chronic. There is tenderness over the bone, and the athlete has difficulty sitting.

**Care**   Treatment consists of analgesics and a ring seat to relieve the pressure on the coccyx while sitting. It should be noted that pain from a fractured coccyx may last for many months. Once a coccygeal injury has healed, the athlete should be protected against reinjury by appropriately applied padding.

## SUMMARY

- The spine, or vertebral column, is composed of thirty-three individual vertebrae. The design of the spine allows for flexion, extension, lateral flexion, and rotation. The movable vertebrae are separated by intervertebral disks, and position is maintained by a series of muscular and ligamentous supports. The spine can be divided into three different regions: the cervical, thoracic, and lumbar regions. The sacrum and coccyx are fused vertebrae within the vertebral column.

- The spinal cord is that portion of the central nervous system that is contained within the vertebral canal of the spinal column. Thirty-one pairs of spinal nerves extend from the sides of the spinal cord.

- Acute traumatic injuries to the spine can be potentially life threatening, particularly if the cervical region of the spinal cord is involved. Thus the athlete must do everything possible to minimize injury. Strengthening of the musculature of the neck is critical. In addition to strong muscles, the athlete's neck should have a full range of motion. Athletes involved in collision sports must be taught and required to use techniques that reduce the likelihood of cervical injury.

- Low back pain is one of the most common and disabling ailments known to humans. The athlete, like everyone else in the population, can prevent low back pain by avoiding unnecessary stresses and strains associated with standing, sitting, lying, working, or exercising. Care should be taken to avoid postures and positions that can cause injuries.

- The most critical part of assessment of the spine is to rule out the possibility of spinal cord injury. Observing the posture and movement capabilities of the athlete during the evaluation can help clarify the nature and extent of the injury.

- Because the cervical and lumbar regions of the spine are so mobile, they are extremely vulnerable to a wide range of sports injuries, including fractures, dislocations, strains, sprains, contusions, lesions of the intervertebral disks, herniations, injuries to spinal nerves, and degenerative conditions.

## *Solutions to Critical Thinking* Exercises

**20-1** Given this set of existing conditions, the coach should have the athlete engage in extension exercises to strengthen the back extensors, stretch the abdominals, and reduce the pressure on the intervertebral disks.

**20-2** It is most likely that the athlete has a brachial plexus injury that is sometimes called a stinger or burner. Normally the symptoms resolve on their own over several minutes. The coach might consider having the athlete wear a cervical collar.

**20-3** The gymnast likely has a spondylolisthesis that has resulted in hypermobility of a vertebral segment. Initially, rest will help to reduce pain. The major focus in rehabilitation should be directed toward exercises that control or stabilize the hypermobile segment. Progressive trunk-strengthening exercises, especially to the abdominal muscles through the midrange, should be incorporated. A brace can be helpful during practice.

**20-4** The wrestler has most likely contused his coccyx. Fractures of this bone are relatively uncommon. It may be necessary to apply a protective pad over the injured area.

## REVIEW QUESTIONS

1. Identify the various regions of the spine.
2. What is the relationship between the spinal cord and the nerve roots?
3. Discuss the various considerations in prevention of cervical injuries.
4. Describe the special tests used in evaluating the lumbar and sacroiliac portions of the spine.
5. What can be done to minimize the incidence of low back pain?
6. Describe the mechanism of injury for a herniated disk.
7. How does a spondylolysis become a spondylolisthesis?
8. What is the usual mechanism for injury to the sacroiliac joint?

 **Dynamic Human CD**

For more information on skeletal anatomy of the spine click on:

- Skeletal
- Anatomy
- Gross anatomy
- Vertebral column
- Thoracic cage
- Then, Pelvic girdle

To take a closer look at the muscles that are involved in spine movement click on:

- Muscular
- Anatomy
- Body regions
- Head and neck
- Then, Abdomen and back

To look at the effect of flexion and extension movements on a herniated disk click on:

- Skeletal
- Clinical concepts
- Herniated disk

## REFERENCES

1. Anderson C: Neck injuries, backboard, bench, or return to play, *Physician Sportsmed* 21(8):23, 1993.
2. Carpenter DM, Nelson BW: Low back strengthening for the prevention and treatment of low back pain, *Med Sci Sports Exerc* 31(1):18, 1999.
3. Cibulka M: The treatment of the sacroiliac joint component to low back pain, *Phys Ther* 72(12):917, 1992.
4. DeRosa C, Poterfield J: A physical therapy model for the treatment of low back pain, *Phys Ther* 72(4):261, 1992.
5. Fourre M: On-site management of cervical spine injuries, *Physician Sportsmed* 19:4, 1991.
6. Hammann L: Functional back rehabilitation, *Ath Ther Today* 5(2):22, 2000.
7. Herring S, Weinstein S: Assessment and neurological management of athletic low back injury. In Nicholas J, Herschman E: *The lower extremity and spine in sports medicine*, St Louis, 1995, Mosby.
8. Hooker D: Back rehabilitation. In Prentice W: *Rehabilitation techniques in sports medicine*, Boston, 1999, WCB/McGraw-Hill.
9. Johnson R: Low back pain in sports: managing spondylolysis in young athletes, *Physician Sportsmed* 21(4):53, 1993.
10. Lord M, Carson W: Management of herniated lumbar disks in the athlete, *Sports Med Digest* 16:1, 1994.
11. Markey K, Benedetto M, Curl W: Upper trunk and brachial plexopathy, *Am J Sports Med* 21(5):650, 1993.
12. Rapport L, O'Leary P, Cammisa F: Diagnosis and treatment of cervical spine injuries. In Nicholas J, Herschman E: *The lower extremity and spine in sports medicine*, St Louis, 1995, Mosby.
13. Rodriquez J: Clinical examination and documentation. In Hochschuler S, Cotler H, Guyer R: *Rehabilitation of the spine: science and practice*, St Louis, 1993, Mosby.
14. Saunders D: *Evaluation, treatment, and prevention of musculoskeletal disorders*, Bloomington, Minn, 1985, Educational Opportunities.
15. Stone JA: Back stabilization exercises, *Ath Ther Today* 4(3):23, 1999.
16. Storey MD: Anterior neck trauma, *Physician Sportsmed* 17(9):85, 1993.
17. Torg JS et al: The axial load teardrop fracture, *Am J Sports Med* 19(4):355, 1991.
18. Torg J, Fay C: Cervical spinal stenosis with cord neurapraxia and transient quadriplegia. In Torg J: *Athletic injuries to the head, neck, and face*, St Louis, 1991, Mosby.
19. Vereschagin KS et al: Burners, *Physician Sportsmed* 1(9):96, 1991.
20. Weber MD, Woodall WR: Spondylogenic disorders in gymnasts, *JOSPT* 14(1)s:6, 1991.
21. Wilkerson JE, Maroon JC: Cervical spine injuries in athletes, *Physician Sportsmed* 18(3):57, 1990.

## ANNOTATED BIBLIOGRAPHY

Braggins S: *Back care: a clinical approach,* Philadelphia, 2000, Churchill Livingstone.

> *A comprehensive text that focuses on all aspects of treatment and rehabilitation of the spine.*

Nicholas J, Herschman E: *The lower extremity and spine in sports medicine,* St Louis, 1995, Mosby.

> *This two-volume text discusses all aspects of injury to the extremities and the spine. The section on evaluation and treatment of spinal conditions is concise but thorough.*

Torg JS, editor: *Head and neck injuries. Clinics in sports medicine,* vol 6, no 1, Philadelphia, 1991, WB Saunders.

> *In-depth coverage of head and neck injuries stemming from sports activities.*

White A, Schofferman J: *Spine care: diagnosis and conservative treatment,* vol. 1, St Louis, 1995, Mosby.

> *A two-volume set that looks at both conservative and surgical management of back injuries.*

## WEBSITES

World Ortho: http://www.worldortho.com

> *Use the search engine in this site to locate relevant information.*

Wheeless' Textbook of Orthopaedics: http://www.medmedia.com/med/htm

> *An excellent page for injuries, anatomy, and x rays.*

Karolinska Institute Library: Musculoskeletal Disease: http://www.micki.se/Disease/c5.htm

American Orthopaedic Society for Sports Medicine: http://www.sportsmed.org

Spinal Cord 101: http://www.goes.com/billr/html/_spinal_cord_101.html

The Cleveland Clinic Foundation: Spinal Cord Trauma: http://www.anes.ccf.org:8080/PILOT/NEURO/sci.htm

Spine-Health: http://www.spine-health.com

> *Written and updated by a multispecialty team of medical professionals. It provides a comprehensive overview of causes and treatments for low back pain, and a variety of services and in-depth features.*

The Back Page: http://www.thebackpage.net

> *Comprehensive information on low back and neck pain.*

# The Thorax and Abdomen

*When you finish this chapter you will be able to:*
- Describe the anatomy of the thorax and abdomen.
- Identify the location and function of the heart and lungs.
- Identify the location and function of the abdominal viscera.
- Describe the techniques for assessing thoracic and abdominal injuries.
- Identify various injuries to the structures of the thorax.
- Describe various injuries and conditions in structures of the abdomen.

T his chapter covers major sports injuries to the thorax and abdomen. In an athletic environment, injuries to the thorax and abdomen have a lower incidence than injuries to the extremities and the spine. However, unlike the musculoskeletal injuries to the extremities discussed to this point, injuries to the heart, lungs, and abdominal viscera can be potentially serious and even life threatening if not recognized and managed appropriately. It is imperative for the coach to be familiar with anatomy and the more common injuries seen in the abdomen and thorax (Figure 21-1).

## ANATOMY OF THE THORAX

The thoracic cage protects the heart and lungs.

The thorax is that portion of the body commonly known as the chest, which lies between the base of the neck and the diaphragm. It is contained within the thoracic vertebrae and the twelve pairs of ribs that give it its shape (Figure 21-2). Its main function is to protect the vital respiratory and circulatory organs and to assist the lungs in inspiration and expiration during the breathing process.[13]

The ribs are flat bones that are attached to the thoracic vertebrae in the back and to the sternum in the front. The upper seven ribs are called sternal or true ribs, and each rib is joined to the sternum by a separate costal cartilage. The eighth, ninth, and tenth ribs (false ribs) have cartilages that join each other and the seventh rib before uniting with the sternum. The eleventh and twelfth ribs (floating ribs) remain unattached to the sternum but do have muscle attachments. The intercostal muscles,

**Figure 21-1**

Collision sports can
produce serious trunk
injuries.

which lie between the ribs, and the diaphragm muscle, which separates
the thoracic cavity from the abdominal cavity, function in inspiration and
expiration (Figure 21-3).

## ANATOMY OF THE ABDOMEN

The abdominal cavity lies between the diaphragm and the pelvis and is
bounded by the margin of the lower ribs, the abdominal muscles, and the
vertebral column. The abdominal muscles—the rectus abdominis, the external and internal obliques, and the transverse abdominis—collectively
produce trunk flexion and rotation, but more important, they function to
protect the underlying abdominal viscera (Figure 21-4).[13]

**Figure 21-2**

The thoracic cage

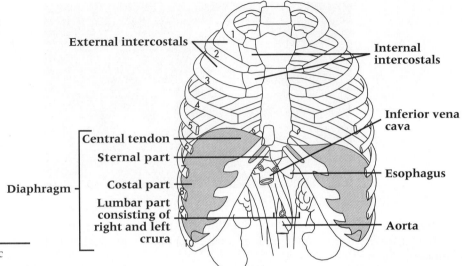

**Figure 21-3**

Anatomy of the thoracic
muscles

**Figure 21-4**

The abdominal musculature

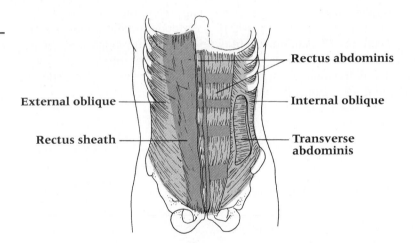

Solid internal organs are
more at jeopardy from an
injury than are hollow
organs.

Abdominal viscera are part of
the urinary, digestive,
reproductive, and lymphatic
systems.

The abdominal viscera are composed of both hollow and solid organs. The solid organs are the kidneys, spleen, liver, pancreas, and adrenal glands. The hollow organs include the stomach, intestines, gallbladder, and urinary bladder (Figure 21-5). Organs in the abdominal cavity may be classified as part of the urinary system, the digestive system, the reproductive system, or the lymphatic system.[13]

## PREVENTING INJURIES TO THE THORAX AND ABDOMEN

Injuries to the thorax may be prevented by wearing appropriate protective equipment, particularly in collision sport activities. In football, for example, shoulder pads are usually designed to extend to at least below the level of the sternum. Rib protectors may be worn to cover the entire thoracic cage if necessary (Figure 21-6).

**Figure 21-5**

Abdominal viscera

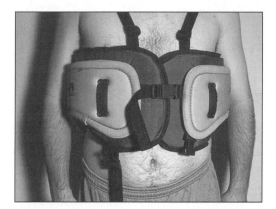

**Figure 21-6**

Protective rib belt

The muscles of the abdomen should be strengthened to provide protection to the underlying viscera. A consistent regimen of sit-up exercises done in various positions can markedly increase the strength and size of the abdominal musculature.

Making sure that the hollow organs, in particular the stomach and bladder, are emptied before competition can reduce the chance of injury to those structures. Meals should be eaten at least 3 to 4 hours before competition to allow foods to clear the stomach. Urinating immediately before stepping onto the field or court protects the bladder from injury.

## ASSESSMENT OF THE THORAX AND ABDOMEN

Injuries to the thorax and abdomen can produce potentially life-threatening situations. An injury that may seem relatively insignificant at first may rapidly develop into one that requires immediate and appropriate medical attention. Thus, for the coach evaluating an injury, the initial primary survey should focus on those signs and symptoms that indicate some life-threatening condition. The injured athlete should be continually monitored by the coach to identify any disruption of normal breathing or circulation or any indication of internal hemorrhage that could precipitate shock.

## History

The questions asked to determine a history in the case of thoracic and abdominal injuries are somewhat different than those questions pertinent to musculoskeletal injuries of the extremities.[12] The primary mechanism of injury should be determined first.

- What happened to cause this injury?
- Was there direct contact or a direct blow?
- What position were you in?
- What type of pain is there (sharp, dull, localized, etc.)?
- Was there immediate or gradual pain?
- Do you feel any pain other than in the area where the injury occurred?
- Have you had any difficulty breathing?
- Are certain positions more comfortable than others?
- Do you feel faint, lightheaded, or nauseous?
- Do you feel any pain in your chest?
- Did you hear or feel a pop or crack in your chest?
- Have you had any muscle spasms?
- Have you noticed any blood in your urine?
- Is there any difficulty or pain in urinating?
- Was the bladder full or empty?
- How long has it been since you have eaten?

## Observation

If the athlete is observed immediately following injury, check for normal breathing and respiratory patterns.

- Most important, is the athlete breathing at all?
- Is the athlete having difficulty breathing deeply, or is the athlete struggling to catch the breath?
- Does breathing cause pain?
- Is the athlete holding the chest wall?
- Is there symmetry in movement of the chest during breathing?
- If the wind was knocked out, did normal breathing return rapidly or was there prolonged difficulty? This difficulty may indicate a more severe injury.
- What is the body position of the athlete?
- Is there protrusion or swelling of any portion of the abdomen? This may indicate internal bleeding.
- Does the thorax appear to be symmetrical? Rib fractures can cause one side to appear different.

**Figure 21-7**

Checking asymmetry of chest
wall during breathing

- Are the abdominal muscles tight and guarding?
- Is the athlete holding or splinting a specific part of the abdomen?

It is important to monitor vital signs, including pulse, respiration, and blood pressure. A rapid, weak pulse and/or a significant drop in blood pressure is an indication of some potentially serious internal injury often involving loss of blood.

### Palpation

#### Thorax

The hands should first be placed on either side of the chest wall to check for symmetry in chest wall movement during deep inspiration and expiration and to begin to isolate areas of tenderness (Figure 21-7). Once a tender area is identified, the coach should palpate along the rib and in the space between the ribs to locate a specific point of tenderness.

#### Abdomen

To palpate the abdominal structures, the athlete should be supine with the arms at the sides and the abdominal muscles relaxed (Figure 21-8). Uninjured areas should be palpated first with the tips of the fingers to feel for any tightness or rigidity. An athlete with an abdominal injury voluntarily contracts the abdominal muscles to guard or protect the tender area. If there is bleeding or irritation inside the abdominal cavity, the abdomen will exhibit what is referred to as "boardlike rigidity" and cannot be voluntarily relaxed.[12] Pressure on the abdominal organs may elicit referred pain in predictable patterns away from the source.[14]

## RECOGNITION AND MANAGEMENT OF THORACIC INJURIES

### Rib Contusions

**Cause of injury**   A blow to the rib cage can contuse intercostal muscles between the ribs or, if severe enough, produce a fracture. Because the intercostal muscles are essential for breathing, when they are bruised, both expiration and inspiration become very painful.

**Figure 21-8**

Palpating the abdomen for
guarding or rigidity

**Signs of injury**  Characteristically the pain is sharp during breathing, there is point tenderness, and pain is elicited when the rib cage is compressed. X-ray examination should be routine in such an injury.

**Care**  RICE and antiinflammatory agents are commonly used. As with most rib injuries, contusions to the thorax are self-limiting, responding best to rest and cessation of sports activities.

### Rib Fractures

**Cause of injury**  Rib fractures are not uncommon in sports and have their highest incidence in collision sports.[10] Fractures can be caused either by direct impact, as by a kick, or by compression of the rib cage, as may occur in football or wrestling. Ribs five through nine are the most commonly fractured. There is always the possibility that a rib fracture can cause damage to or puncture the underlying lung.

A rib fracture may be indicated by a severe, sharp pain during breathing.

**Signs of injury**  The rib fracture is usually quite easily detected. The athlete complains of severe pain during inspiration and point tenderness with sharp pain during palpation.

**Care**  The athlete should be referred to the team physician for x-ray examination if there is any indication of fracture. The rib fracture is usually managed with support and rest. Simple fractures heal within 3 to 4 weeks. A rib brace can offer the athlete some rib cage stabilization and comfort (Figure 21-9).

### Costal Cartilage Injury

**Cause of injury**  Costal cartilage injuries have a higher incidence than do fractures. This injury can occur from a direct blow to the thorax or indirectly from a sudden twist or a fall on a ball, compressing the rib cage. A costal cartilage injury displays signs similar to the rib fracture, with the exception that pain is localized in the junction of the rib cartilage and rib (Figure 21-10).

**Signs of injury**  The athlete complains of sharp pain during sudden movement of the trunk and of difficulty in breathing deeply. Palpation

**Figure 21-9**

A commercial rib brace can
provide moderate support to
the thorax.

reveals point tenderness with swelling. In some cases there is a rib deformity and a complaint that the rib makes a crackling noise (crepitus) as it
moves in and out of place.

**Care**   As with a rib fracture, the costal cartilage injury is managed
by rest and immobilization by rib brace. Healing takes anywhere from 1
to 2 months, precluding any sports activities until the athlete is symptom
free.

### Intercostal Muscle Injuries

**Cause of injury**   The muscles of the thorax are all subject to contusions and strains in sports. The intercostals are especially vulnerable.
Traumatic injuries occur most often from direct blows or sudden torsion
of the athlete's trunk.

**Signs of injury**   Like other muscle strains, pain occurs on active motion. However, injuries to muscles in this region are particularly painful
during inspiration and expiration, laughing, coughing, or sneezing.

**Care**   Care requires immediate application of cold and compression
for approximately 1 hour. After hemorrhaging has been controlled, immobilization should be used to make the athlete more comfortable (refer
to Figure 21-9).

### Injuries to the Lungs

**Cause of injury**   Fortunately, injuries to the lungs resulting from
sports trauma are rare.[16] However, because of the seriousness of this type
of injury, the coach must be able to recognize the basic signs. The most

**Figure 21-10**

Costal cartilage injury

Lung injuries can result in:
• Pneumothorax
• Tension pneumothorax
• Hemothorax
• Traumatic asphyxia

**A. Pneumothorax**  **B. Tension pneumothorax**  **C. Hemothorax**

**Figure 21-11**

A, Pneumothorax; B, Tension pneumothorax; C, Hemothorax

serious of the conditions are pneumothorax, tension pneumothorax, hemothorax, and traumatic asphyxia.

*Pneumothorax* is a condition in which the pleural cavity surrounding the lung becomes filled with air that has entered through an opening in the chest (Figure 21-11A).[1] As the pleural cavity fills with air, the lung on that side collapses.

A *tension pneumothorax* occurs when the pleural cavity on one side fills with air and displaces the lung and the heart toward the opposite side, thus compressing the opposite lung (Figure 21-11B).

*Hemothorax* is the presence of blood within the pleural cavity (Figure 21-11C). It results from the tearing or puncturing of the lung or pleural tissue, involving the blood vessels in the area.

*Traumatic asphyxia* occurs as the result of a violent blow to or a compression of the rib cage, causing a cessation of breathing.[6] A condition of this type demands immediate mouth-to-mouth resuscitation and medical attention.

**Signs of injury**   Signs may include breathing difficulty or shortness of breath; chest pain on the side of the injury; coughed up blood; cyanosis (bluish skin); and, potentially, shock. With a total collapse of the lung, medical attention is required immediately.

**Care**   Each of these conditions is a medical emergency requiring immediate physician attention. Thus the athlete must be transported to the emergency room as quickly as possible.

## Sudden Death Syndrome in Athletes

Common causes of sudden death syndrome:
- Hypertrophic cardiomyopathy
- Anomalous origin of the coronary artery
- Marfan's syndrome

**Cause of condition**   The most common cause of exercise-induced sudden death in an athlete is some congenital cardiovascular abnormality. The three most prevalent conditions are hypertrophic cardiomyopathy, anomalous origin of the coronary artery, and Marfan's syndrome.[7]

**Signs of condition**   Common symptoms and signs associated with cardiac causes of sudden death may include chest pain or discomfort during exertion, heart palpitations or flutters, syncope, nausea, profuse sweating, heart murmurs, shortness of breath, general malaise, and fever.[3]

**Care**   This condition is a life-threatening emergency situation that requires immediate access of the rescue squad.[3] The coach should be prepared to perform CPR until the rescue squad arrives (see Chapter 7).

### Breast Problems

**Cause of injury**   Violent up-and-down and lateral movements of the breasts, such as are encountered in running and jumping, can bruise and strain the breast, especially in large-breasted women. Constant uncontrolled movements of the breast over time can stretch the Cooper's ligament, which supports the breast at the chest wall, leading to premature sagging of the breasts. "Runner's nipples," in which the shirt rubs the nipples and causes an abrasion, can be prevented by placing an adhesive bandage over each nipple before participation. "Bicyclist's nipples" can also occur as the result of a combination of cold and evaporation of sweat, causing the nipples to become painful. Wearing a windbreaker can prevent this problem.

**Care**   Wearing a well-designed bra that has minimum elasticity and allows little vertical or horizontal breast movement is most desirable (refer to Figure 6-14).[11] Breast injuries usually occur during physical contact with either an opponent or equipment. In sports such as fencing or field hockey, female athletes should protect themselves by wearing plastic cup protectors.

## RECOGNITION AND MANAGEMENT
## OF ABDOMINAL INJURIES

Although abdominal injuries comprise only about 10 percent of sports injuries, they can require long recovery periods and can be life threatening.[12] The abdominal area is particularly vulnerable to injury in all contact sports. A blow can produce superficial or even deep internal injuries, depending on its location and intensity.[2] In internal injuries of the abdomen that occur in sports, the solid organs are most often affected. Strong abdominal muscles give good protection when they are tensed, but when relaxed, the underlying organs may be easily injured. It is very important to protect the trunk region properly against the traumatic forces of collision sports. Good conditioning is essential, as is the use of proper protective equipment and the application of safety rules.

### Injuries to the Abdominal Wall

**Cause of injury**   Abdominal muscle strains occur with sudden twisting of the trunk or reaching overhead. The rectus abdominus is the most commonly strained abdominal muscle. Potentially these types of injuries can be incapacitating.

Contusions to the abdominal wall occur because of compressive forces. Although not very common, when they do happen, they are more likely to occur in collision sports such as football or ice hockey; however, any sports implement or high-velocity projectile can cause injury. Hockey goalies and baseball catchers are vulnerable to injury without their protective torso pads. The extent and type of injury varies depending on whether the force is blunt or penetrating.

**Signs of injury**   An abdominal muscle strain or contusion of the rectus abdominis muscle can be disabling. A severe blow may cause a hematoma that develops under the fascial tissue surrounding this muscle. The pressure that results from hemorrhage causes pain and tightness in the region of the injury.

**Care**   Initially, ice and an elastic compression wrap should be used. The coach should also look for signs of possible internal injury. Treatment should be conservative, and exercise should be kept within pain-free limits.

### Hernia

Inguinal hernias occur in males; femoral hernias occur in females.

**Cause of injury**   The term *hernia* refers to the protrusion of abdominal viscera through a portion of the abdominal wall. Hernias resulting from sports most often occur in the groin area.[8] Inguinal hernias (Figure 21-12A), which occur in men (more than 75%), and femoral hernias (Figure 21-12B), most often occurring in women, are the most prevalent types. The inguinal hernia results from an abnormal enlargement of the opening of the inguinal canal through which the vessels and nerves of the male reproductive system pass. In contrast, the femoral hernia arises in the canal that transports the vessels and nerves that go to the thigh and lower limb.[4]

When intraabdominal tension is produced in these areas, muscles produce contraction around these canal openings. If the muscles fail to react, abdominal contents may be pushed through the opening.

**Signs of injury**   A hernia may be recognized by the following: previous history of a blow or strain to the groin area that produced pain and prolonged discomfort; superficial protrusion in the groin area that is increased by coughing; or, reported feeling of weakness and pulling sensation in the groin area.[5]

**Care**   Most physicians think that any athlete who has a hernia should be prohibited from engaging in hard physical activity until surgical repair has been made. Mechanical devices, designed to prevent hernial protrusion, are for the most part unsuitable in sports because of the friction and irritation they produce. Exercise has been thought by many to be beneficial to a mild hernia, but such is not the case. Exercise will not affect the stretched inguinal or femoral canals positively.

**Figure 21-12**

A, Inguinal hernia. B, Femoral hernia.

### Blow to the Solar Plexus

**Cause of injury**   A blow to the middle portion of the abdomen, or solar plexus, produces a transitory paralysis of the diaphragm (wind knocked out). There should always be some concern that a blow hard enough to knock out the wind could also cause internal organ injury.

**Signs of injury**   Paralysis of the diaphragm stops respiration and leads to anoxia. When the athlete is unable to inhale, short-term panic may result. These symptoms are usually transitory. It is necessary to allay such fears and instill confidence in the athlete.

**Care**   In dealing with an athlete who has had the wind knocked out of him or her, the coach should adhere to the following procedures: help the athlete overcome apprehension by talking in a confident manner; loosen the athlete's belt and the clothing around the abdomen; have the athlete bend the knees; and encourage the athlete to relax by initiating short inspirations and long expirations.

Because of the fear of not being able to breathe, the athlete may hyperventilate. Hyperventilation is an increased rate of ventilation that results in increased levels of oxygen. It causes a variety of physical reactions such as dizziness, a lump in the throat, pounding heart, or fainting. The coach should have the athlete breath slowly into a paper bag to increase levels of carbon dioxide.

## Stitch in the Side

**Cause of injury**   A stitch in the side is the name given an idiopathic condition that occurs in some athletes. The cause is obscure, although several hypotheses have been advanced. Among these causes are the following: constipation, intestinal gas, overeating, diaphragmatic spasm as a result of poor conditioning, lack of visceral support because of weak abdominal muscles, distended spleen, breathing techniques that lead to a lack of oxygen in the diaphragm, and ischemia of either the diaphragm or the intercostal muscles.

**Signs of injury**   A stitch in the side is a cramplike pain that develops on either the left or right costal border during hard physical activity. Sports that involve running apparently produce this condition.

**Care**   Immediate care of a stitch in the side demands relaxation of the spasm, for which two methods have proved beneficial. First, the athlete is instructed to stretch the arm on the affected side as high as possible. If this is inadequate, flexing the trunk forward on the thighs may prove of some benefit.

Athletes with recurrent abdominal spasms may need special study. Identification of poor eating habits, poor elimination habits, or an inadequate athletic training program may explain the athlete's particular problem. A stitch in the side, although not considered serious, may require further evaluation by a physician if abdominal pains persist.

## Injury of the Spleen

**Cause of injury**   Injuries to the spleen are uncommon but occur most often because of a fall or a direct blow to the left upper quadrant of the abdomen when some existing medical condition has caused enlargement of the spleen. Infectious mononucleosis is the most likely cause of spleen enlargement.

**Signs of injury**   The gross indications of a ruptured spleen must be recognized so that an immediate medical referral can be made. Indications include a history of a severe blow to the abdomen and possibly signs of shock, abdominal rigidity, nausea, and vomiting. There may be a reflex pain occurring approximately 30 minutes after injury, called Kehr's sign, which radiates to the left shoulder and one-third of the way down the left

***Critical Thinking*** Exercise

A wrestler is engaged in a strenuous off-season weight-lifting program. Recently he has begun to experience pain in his groin. Whenever he strains hard to lift a weight, and especially if he holds his breath, the pain appears. He is concerned that he has developed a hernia.

**?** What symptoms and signs should the coach look for to indicate that the athlete does have a hernia?

A blow to the solar plexus can lead to transitory paralysis of the diaphragm and to unconsciousness.

***Critical Thinking*** Exercise

A cross country runner complains of a recurring stitch in the side. She has a cramplike pain that develops on the left costal angle during a hard run. She indicates that when she stops running the cramp disappears but seems to come back if she starts to run again.

**?** What can the coach recommend to help this runner alleviate this problem?

Infectious mononucleosis can cause spleen enlargement.

Athletes who complain of
external pain in the
shoulders, trunk, or pelvis
after a severe blow to the
abdomen or back may be
describing referred pain from
an injury to an internal
organ.

21–3

*Critical Thinking* Exercise

A football receiver jumps to
catch a high pass thrown over
the middle. A defensive back
hits the receiver in the low
back. The athlete does not
seem to have a specific injury.
After the game he notices
blood in his urine and becomes
worried.

? Is blood in the urine a cause
for concern, and what should
the coach do to manage it?

Kidney and bladder
contusions can cause
hematuria.

Hepatitis can cause
enlargement of the liver.

21–4

*Critical Thinking* Exercise

A soccer player is kicked in the
abdomen above the umbilicus.
Initially she had the wind
knocked out of her. Now, she is
complaining of pain and her
abdomen is tight on palpation.

? What should the coach be
most concerned about, and
what organs may potentially be
involved?

arm.[9] A ruptured spleen can hemorrhage profusely into the abdominal cavity, causing the athlete to die of internal bleeding days or weeks after the injury.

**Care**    Conservative nonoperative treatment is recommended initially along with a week of hospitalization.[9] At 3 weeks, the athlete can engage in light conditioning activities and at 4 weeks can fully return to activity as long as no symptoms appear. If surgical repair is necessary, the athlete will require 3 months to recover, whereas removal of the spleen will require 6 months before the athlete can return to activity.

### Kidney Contusion

**Cause of injury**    The kidneys are seemingly well protected within the abdominal cavity. However, on occasion, contusions and even ruptures of these organs occur. The kidney may be susceptible to injury because of its normal distention by blood. An external force applied to the back of the athlete causes abnormal extension of an engorged kidney, resulting in injury.[2]

**Signs of injury**    An athlete who has received a contusion of the kidney may display signs of shock, nausea, vomiting, rigidity of the back muscles, and hematuria (blood in the urine). As with injuries to other internal organs, kidney injury may cause referred pain. Pain may radiate forward around the trunk into the lower abdominal region.

**Care**    Any athlete who reports having received a severe blow to the abdomen or back region should be instructed to urinate two or three times and to look for the appearance of blood in the urine. If there is any sign of hematuria, immediate referral to a physician must be made.[2] Medical care of the contused kidney usually consists of a 24-hour hospital observation, with a gradual increase of fluid intake. If the hemorrhage fails to stop, surgery may be indicated. Controllable contusions usually require 2 weeks of bed rest and close surveillance after activity is resumed. In questionable cases, complete withdrawal from one active playing season may be required.

### Liver Contusion

**Cause of injury**    In sports activities, liver injury is very rare. A hard blow to the right side of the rib cage can tear or seriously contuse the liver, especially if it is enlarged as a result of some disease such as hepatitis.

**Signs of injury**    Liver injury can cause hemorrhage and shock, requiring immediate surgical intervention. Liver injury commonly produces a referred pain that is just below the right scapula, right shoulder, substernal area, and on occasion, the anterior left side of the chest.

**Care**    A liver contusion requires immediate referral to a physician for diagnosis and treatment.

### Appendicitis

**Cause of injury**    Inflammation of the appendix can be chronic or acute. It is caused by a variety of factors, for example, a fecal obstruction. Its highest incidence is in males between the ages of fifteen and twenty-five. Appendicitis can be mistaken for a common gastric complaint. In its early stages, the appendix becomes red and swollen; in later stages it may become gangrenous, rupturing into the bowels and causing peritonitis. Bacterial infection is a complication of rupture of the inflamed appendix.

**Signs of injury** The athlete may complain of a mild-to-severe pain in the lower abdomen, associated with nausea, vomiting, and a low-grade fever ranging from 99° to 100° F (37° to 38° C). Later, the cramps may localize into a pain in the lower right side, and palpation may reveal abdominal rigidity and tenderness at a point between the anterior superior spine of the ilium and the umbilicus (McBurney's point).[15]

**Care** Surgical removal of the inflamed appendix is often necessary. If the bowel is not obstructed, there is no need to rush surgery. However, an obstructed bowel with an acute rupture is a life-threatening condition.

> Appendicitis is often mistaken for a common gastric problem.

### Injuries to the Bladder

**Cause of injury** On rare occasions a blunt force to the lower abdominal region may injure a urinary bladder that is distended by urine. The appearance of red blood cells within the urine (hematuria) is often associated with contusion of the bladder during running and has been referred to as a "runner's bladder."[17]

**Signs of injury** With any impact to the abdominal region, the possibility of internal damage must be considered, and after such trauma the athlete should be instructed to check periodically for blood in the urine. Bladder injury commonly causes referred pain to the lower trunk, including the upper thigh anteriorly. With a bladder rupture, the athlete will be unable to urinate.

### Scrotal/Testicular Contusion

**Cause of injury** As the result of their considerable sensitivity and particular vulnerability, the scrotum and the testicles may sustain a contusion that causes a very painful, nauseating, and disabling condition.

**Signs of injury** As is characteristic of any contusion or bruise, there is hemorrhage, fluid effusion, and muscle spasm, the degree of which depends on the intensity of the impact to the tissue.[5]

**Care** Immediately following a testicular contusion, the athlete is placed on his side and instructed to flex his thighs to his chest (Figure 21-13). As the pain diminishes, a cold pack is applied to the scrotum. Increasing or unresolved pain after 15 to 20 minutes requires prompt referral to a physician for evaluation.

> Injuries to the reproductive organs in sports are much more likely to occur in the male because the male genitalia are more exposed.

### Gynecological Injuries

In general the female reproductive organs have a low incidence of injury in sports. By far the most common gynecological injury in the female athlete involves a contusion to the external genitalia, or vulva, which includes the labia, clitoris, and the vestibule of the vagina. A hematoma

**Figure 21-13**

Body position following
scrotum contusion

results from the contusion, which most often occurs with a direct impact
to this area. A contusion of this area may also injure the pubis symphasis, producing ostitis pubis.

## SUMMARY

- The thorax is that portion of the body commonly known as the chest,
  which lies between the base of the neck and the diaphragm. Its main
  functions are to protect the vital respiratory and circulatory organs and
  to assist the lungs in inspiration and expiration during the breathing
  process. Within the thoracic cage lie the lungs and the heart.

- The abdominal cavity lies between the diaphragm and the bones of the
  pelvis and is bounded by the margin of the lower ribs, the abdominal
  muscles, and the vertebral column. The abdominal viscera are composed of both hollow and solid organs. Organs in the abdominal cavity may be classified as part of the urinary system, the digestive system,
  the reproductive system, or the lymphatic system.

- Injuries to the heart, lungs, and abdominal viscera can be potentially
  serious and even life threatening if not recognized and managed
  appropriately.

- For the coach evaluating an injury to the abdomen or thorax, the initial primary survey should focus on those signs and symptoms that indicate some life-threatening condition. Asking pertinent questions, observing body positioning, and palpation of the injured structures are
  critical in assessing the nature of the injury.

- Rib fractures and contusions, costal border injuries, muscle strains, and breast injuries are all common injuries to the chest wall.

- Injuries involving the lungs include pneumothorax, tension pneumothorax, hemothorax, and traumatic asphyxia.

- The most common cause of exercise-induced sudden death is some congenital cardiovascular abnormality. The three most prevalent conditions are hypertrophic cardiomyopathy, anomalous origin of the coronary artery, and Marfan's syndrome.

- Injuries to the abdominal wall include muscle strains, getting the wind knocked out, and the development of an inguinal or femoral hernia.

- With any injury to the abdominal region, internal injury to the abdominal viscera must be considered. Injuries to the liver, spleen, and kidneys are among the more common athletic injuries associated with the abdominal viscera.

- Injuries to the reproductive organs in sports are much more likely to occur in the male because the male genitalia are more exposed.

---

### *Solutions to Critical Thinking* Exercises

**21-1** Most often an athlete with a hernia has some previous history of a blow or strain to the groin area that produced pain and prolonged discomfort. There may be a superficial protrusion in the groin area that is increased by coughing, or the athlete may have a feeling of weakness and a pulling sensation in the groin area. An inguinal hernia results from an abnormal enlargement of the opening of the inguinal canal through which the abdominal contents may be pushed.

**21-2** The coach should try to modify this athlete's eating habits, which might be producing constipation or gas. Cramps can be caused by improper breathing techniques that may cause a lack of oxygen in the diaphragm and ischemia of either the diaphragm or the intercostal muscles. Cramps may also be caused by a diaphragmatic spasm that results from poor conditioning or a lack of visceral support because of weak abdominal muscles.

Athletes with recurrent abdominal spasms should have further evaluation by a physician if the abdominal pains persist.

**21-3** Any time blood appears in the urine there is cause for concern. In this case it is likely that the kidneys have been contused and the blood that appears in the urine will disappear over the next couple of days. Nevertheless, the athlete should be referred to the team physician for diagnosis.

**21-4** The coach should be concerned about the possibility of injury to an organ that can potentially lead to internal blood loss and eventually result in shock. It is possible that the spleen, liver, stomach, small intestine, pancreas, or gallbladder may be injured. It is also possible that there may be a contusion to the muscles of the abdominal wall that is causing muscle guarding.

## REVIEW QUESTIONS AND CLASS ACTIVITIES

1. Describe the anatomy of the thorax.
2. Differentiate among rib contusions, rib fractures, and costal border injuries.
3. Compare the signs of pneumothorax, tension pneumothorax, hemothorax, and traumatic asphyxia.
4. Identify the possible causes of sudden death syndrome among athletes.
5. List the abdominal viscera and other structures associated with the urinary system, the digestive system, the lymphatic system, and the reproductive system.
6. What muscles protect the abdominal viscera?
7. What conditions of the abdominal viscera produce pain in the abdominal region?
8. Contrast the signs of a ruptured spleen with signs of a severely contused kidney.
9. How do you manage an athlete who has had his or her wind knocked out?
10. Distinguish an inguinal hernia or a femoral hernia from a groin strain.
11. Describe the signs of a stitch in the side.

 **Dynamic Human CD**

For more information on skeletal anatomy of the thorax and abdomen click on:

- Skeletal
- Anatomy
- Gross anatomy
- Thoracic cage
- Then, 3D Viewer: Thoracic

To take a closer look at the muscles that are involved in thorax and abdomen movement click on:

- Muscular
- Anatomy
- Body regions
- Abdomen and back

To look at a transverse or cross-sectional view of the thorax and abdomen click on:

- Human body
- Explorations
- Visible human
- Thorax
- Then, Abdomen

To look at the anatomy of the various organs in the thorax and abdomen click on:

- Cardiovascular (Disk 1)
- Lymphatic (Disk 2)
- Digestive (Disk 2)
- Respiratory (Disk 2)
- Urinary (Disk 2)
- Reproductive (Disk 2)

## REFERENCES

1. Ciocca M: Pneumothorax in a weight lifter: the importance of vigilance, *Physician Sportsmed* 28(4):97, 2000.
2. Freitas JE: Renal imaging following blunt trauma, *Physician Sportsmed* 17(12):59, 1989.
3. Futterman LG, Myerburg R: Sudden death in athletes: an update, *Sports Med* 26(5):335, 1998.
4. Kemp S, Batt ME: The "sports hernia": a common cause of groin pain, *Physician Sportsmed* 26(1):36, 1998.
5. Lacroix VJ: A complete approach to groin pain, *Physician Sportsmed* 28(1):66, 2000.
6. Lee M, Wong S, Chu J: Traumatic asphyxia, *Ann Thoracic Surg* 51(1): 86, 1991.
7. Maron B et al: Blunt trauma to the chest leading to sudden death from cardiac arrest during sports activities, *N Engl J Med* 333(6):337, 1995.
8. Meyers WC et al: Management of severe lower abdominal or inguinal pain in high-performance athletes, *Am J Sports Med* 28(1):2, 2000.
9. Morden R, Berman B, Nagle C: Spleen injury in sports: avoiding splenectomy, *Physician Sportsmed* 20(4):126, 1992.
10. O'Kane J, O'Kane E, Marquet J: Delayed complication of a rib fracture, *Physician Sportsmed* 26(4):69, 1998.
11. Page KA, Steele JR: Breast motion and sports brassiere design: implications for future research, *Sports Med* 27(4):205, 1999.
12. Ryan JM: Abdominal injuries and sport, *Br J Sports Med* 33(3):155, 1999.
13. Saladin K: *Anatomy and Physiology*, Boston, 1998, McGraw-Hill.
14. Stopka CB, Zambito KL: Referred visceral pain: what every sports medicine professional needs to know, *Ath Ther Today* 4(1):29, 1999.
15. Tabor's cyclopedic medical dictionary, Philadelphia, 1997, FA Davis.
16. Wagner R, Sidhu G, Radcliffe W: Pulmonary contusion in contact sports, *Physician Sportsmed* 20(2): 126, 1992.
17. York J: Bladder trauma from jogging, *Physician Sportsmed,* 18(9): 116, 1990.

## ANNOTATED BIBLIOGRAPHY

Tabor's cyclopedic medical dictionary, Philadelphia, 2000, FA Davis.

*Despite the dictionary format, this is an excellent guide for the athletic trainer searching for clear, concise descriptions of various injuries and illnesses accompanied by brief recommendations for management and treatment.*

Saladin K: *Anatomy and physiology*, Boston, 1998, McGraw-Hill.

*This anatomy text helps to clarify anatomy of the various systems of the abdomen and thorax.*

## WEBSITES

Acute Appendicits: http://www.
healthanswers.com/database/
ami/converted/000256.html

Anatomy of the Human Body: http://
rpiwww.nidacc.tmc.edu/mmlearn/
anatomy.html

Chest Trauma: http://www.madsci.
com/manu/trau_che.htm#30

National Heart, Lung, and Blood Institute: http://www.nhlbi.nib.gov/
nhlbi/nhlbi.htm

Abdominal Injuries: http://www.hhp.
ufl.edu/ess/at/Abdomen Web/
Frontpage.htm

TRAUMA.ORG: http://www.trauma.
org/abdo/renal/management.html
*Abdominal trauma and goals of man-
agement*

American Thoracic Society-About ATS:
http://www.thoracic.org/

# The Head, Face, Eyes, Ears, Nose, and Throat

*When you finish this chapter you will be able to:*

- Describe the anatomy of the head, face, eyes, ears, nose, and throat.
- Explain how injuries to the head, face, eyes, ears, nose, and throat can be prevented.
- Discuss the assessment process in dealing with injuries to the head and face.
- Discuss recognition and management of concussions and mild head injuries.
- Recognize common injuries to the face, eyes, ears, nose, and throat.

Sports injuries to the head can be life threatening.

I njuries to the region of the head, face, eyes, ears, nose, and throat are common in sports. The severity of injuries to this region can vary from something as benign as a nosebleed to a severe concussion.

## PREVENTING INJURIES TO THE HEAD, FACE, EYES, EARS, NOSE, AND THROAT

Although injuries to the head and face are more prevalent in collision and contact sports, the potential for head injuries exists in all sports.[18] Wearing a helmet or protective headgear and in some instances a face mask in sports like football, ice hockey, lacrosse, wrestling, and baseball has dramatically reduced the incidence of injuries to the head, face, eyes, ears, and nose. Some have argued that if the face mask was eliminated in a sport like football, the number of cervical spine and head injuries would likely be reduced because the athlete would be less likely to use the head when making contact. However, it is certain that the incidence of injuries to the face, eyes, ears, and nose would significantly increase. A helmet can only do so much in preventing injury to the brain.

Unquestionably, the single most important consideration in reducing injuries to this region is teaching athletes to use correct techniques when initiating contact. All football helmets have written warnings that discourage the use of the head as a weapon. Coaches have a responsibility to make certain that athletes are taught and are using correct and safe techniques.

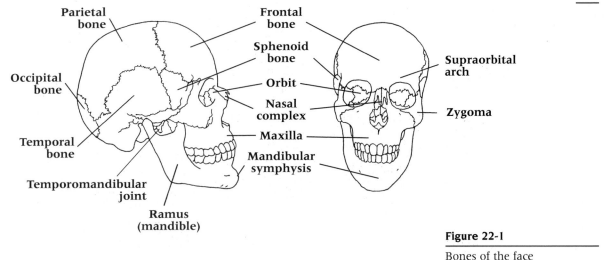

**Figure 22-1**

Bones of the face

## ANATOMY OF THE HEAD

### Bones

The skull is composed of twenty-two bones. With the single exception of the mandible, all of the bones are joined together in immovable joints called *sutures*. The cranial vault, which houses the brain, is enclosed by the cranium or skull and is made up of the frontal, ethmoid, sphenoid, two parietal, two temporal, and the occipital bones (Figure 22-1).

### The Brain

The brain is the part of the central nervous system that is contained within the bony cavity of the cranium and is divided into four sections. The *cerebrum* or *cortex* coordinates all voluntary muscle activities and interprets sensory impulses in addition to controlling higher mental functions including memory, reasoning, intelligence, learning, judgment, and emotions. The *cerebellum* controls movements of skeletal muscle and plays a critical role in the coordination of voluntary muscular movements. The *pons* controls sleep, posture, respiration, swallowing, and the bladder. The *medulla oblongata* is the lowest part of the brainstem and regulates heart rate, breathing, blood pressure, and coughing, sneezing, and vomiting.[15]

#### Meninges

The *meninges* are three membranes that protect the brain and the spinal cord. Outermost is the *dura mater*. A layer of fat that contains vital arteries and veins separates this membrane from the bony wall and forms the epidural space. The *arachnoid* lines the dura mater. The space between the arachnoid and the *pia mater*, the membrane that helps contain the spinal fluid, is called the subarachnoid space (Figure 22-2).[15]

*Cerebrospinal fluid* is contained between the arachnoid and the pia mater membrane and completely surrounds and suspends the brain. Its

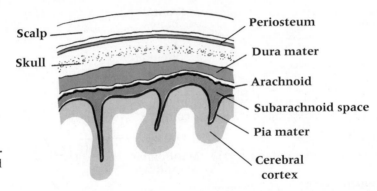

**Figure 22-2**

Cross-section of the head and
brain

main function is to act as a cushion, helping to diminish the transmission
of shocking forces.

## ASSESSING HEAD INJURIES

An athlete who receives either a direct blow to the head or body contact
that causes the head to snap forward, backward, or rotate to the side
must be carefully evaluated for injury to the brain. Injuries to the brain
may or may not result in unconsciousness; disorientation or amnesia;
motor, coordination, or balance deficits; and cognitive deficits.

### Dealing With An Unconscious Athlete

*All unconscious athletes
should be handled as if they
have a serious neck injury.*

On-the-field management of the unconscious athlete was discussed in detail in Chapter 7. The coach must be adept at recognizing and interpreting
the signs that an unconscious athlete presents. Priority first aid for any head
injury must always deal with any life-threatening condition, but in particular loss of breathing. When dealing with an unconscious athlete, the
coach must always suspect a cervical neck injury and manage the situation
accordingly as described in Chapter 7.[2] It is recommended that an athlete
who has been unconscious be removed from the field on a spine board.

   If no life-threatening conditions exist, the coach should note the
length of time that the athlete is unconscious, and not move the athlete
until consciousness is regained. Once the athlete regains consciousness,
or in cases in which the athlete may never have lost consciousness, the
coach should try to obtain a history from the athlete.

### History

An athlete who has sustained a head injury may or may not be able to
respond to questions about exactly what happened to cause the loss of
consciousness. Nevertheless the following questions should be asked:

- Do you know where you are?
- Can you tell me what happened to you?
- Can you remember if you have ever been knocked out before?
- Does your head hurt?

- Do you have any pain in your neck?
- Can you move your hands and feet?

## Observation

Because the coach is usually around the athlete both on and off the field, the coach has the advantage of knowing what the athlete's affect is normally like and how he or she normally acts. The following observations should be made:

- Is the athlete disoriented and unable to tell where he or she is, what time it is, what date it is, who the opponent is?
- Is there a blank or vacant stare? Does the athlete have difficulty keeping the eyes open?
- Is there slurred or incoherent speech?
- Are there delayed verbal and motor responses (slow to answer questions or follow instructions)?
- Is there gross disturbance to coordination (i.e., stumbling, inability to walk a straight line, can't touch finger to nose)?
- Is there an inability to focus attention and is the athlete easily distracted?
- Does there appear to be a memory deficit exhibited by repeated asking of the same questions or not knowing what happened?
- Does the athlete have normal cognitive function (serial 7s, assignment on a particular play)?
- Is there a normal emotional response from the athlete?
- How long was the athlete's affect abnormal?
- Is there a clear, straw-colored fluid in the ear canal? (cerebrospinal fluid leakage that occurs with skull fracture)

## Palpation

Palpation of the skull should be performed in a systematic manner to identify areas of point tenderness or deformity of the skull that may indicate the presence of a skull fracture.

## Special Tests

### Neurological Exam

A neurological exam consists of testing five major areas: cerebral testing to assess cognitive function, cranial nerve testing, cerebellar testing to assess coordination and motor function, sensory testing, and reflex testing. The neurological exam should be done by a trained health care professional.

### Eye Function

Abnormal function of the eyes is often related to head injury and the following observations should be made:

Checking for eye signs can yield important information about possible brain injury.

**Figure 22-3**

A Rhomberg test using a
tandem stance on a foam
surface

1. Pupils should be equal and reactive to light (PEARL).
   a. Dilated or irregular pupils. Checking pupil sizes may be
   particularly difficult at night and under artificial lights. To
   ensure accuracy, the athlete's pupil size should be compared
   with that of an official or another player present. It should be
   remembered, however, that some individuals normally have
   pupils that differ in size.[8]
   b. Inability of the pupils to accommodate rapidly to light
   variance. Eye accommodation should be tested by covering
   one eye with a hand. The covered eye normally dilates,
   whereas the uncovered pupil remains the same. When the
   hand is removed, the previously covered pupil normally
   accommodates readily to the light. A slow-accommodating
   pupil may be an indicator of cerebral injury.[8]
2. Check for ability of eyes to track smoothly. The athlete is asked
   to hold the head in a neutral position, eyes looking straight
   ahead. The athlete is then asked to follow the top of a pen or
   pencil, first up as far as possible, then down as far as possible.
   The eyes are observed for smooth movement and any signs of
   pain. Next, the tip of the pen or pencil is slowly moved from left
   to right to determine whether the eyes follow the tip smoothly
   across the midline of the face or whether they make involuntary
   movements. A constant involuntary back and forth, up and
   down, or rotary movement of the eyeball is called *nystagmus*.[8]
3. Blurred vision is determined by difficulty or inability to read a
   game program or the scoreboard.

### Balance Tests

If the athlete is capable of standing, a Rhomberg test can be used to assess static balance. The best on-the-field balance test uses a tandem
stance performed on a foam surface (Figure 22-3).[4] A positive sign is seen
when the athlete begins to sway, cannot keep the eyes closed, or obviously loses balance.

### Coordination Tests

A number of tests have been used to determine whether the head injury
has affected coordination. These tests include the finger-to-nose test,
heel-to-toe walking, and the standing heel-to-knee test. Inability to perform any of these tests may be indicative of injury to the cerebellum.

### Cognitive Tests

The purpose of cognitive testing is to establish the effects of head trauma
on various cognitive functions and obtain an objective measure to assess
the athlete's status and improvement.[5] Two commonly used on-the-field
cognitive tests are serial 7s, in which the athlete counts backward from
100 by 7, and naming the months in reverse order. Recently other cognitive tests also referred to as *neuropsychological assessments* have been developed for use in an off-the-field evaluation.

# RECOGNITION AND MANAGEMENT OF SPECIFIC HEAD INJURIES

Head injuries occur from direct and blunt forces to the skull. It is estimated that at least thirty to forty major head injuries and occasionally a death occur during sport-related activities each year.[6]

## Skull Fracture

**Cause of injury** Skull fractures occur most often from a blunt trauma, such as a baseball to the head, a shot to the head, or a fall from a height.

**Signs of injury** The athlete complains of severe headache and nausea. Palpation may infrequently reveal a defect such as a skull indention. There may be blood in the middle ear, blood in the ear canal, bleeding through the nose, discoloration around the eyes called "raccoon eyes," or behind the ear called a "Battle's sign." Cerebrospinal fluid (straw colored) may appear in the ear canal and nose.[16]

**Care** It must be noted that it is not the skull fracture itself that causes the most serious problem but complications that stem from intracranial bleeding, bone fragments embedded in the brain, and infection.[16] Such an injury requires immediate hospitalization and referral to a neurosurgeon.

## Concussion (Mild Head Injury)

**Cause of injury** Concussion has been traditionally defined as a clinical syndrome characterized by immediate and transient posttraumatic impairment of neural functions, such as alterations of consciousness, disturbance of vision, equilibrium, etc.[6] It is important to realize that in the athletic population, the majority of concussions do not involve loss of consciousness.[6]

Direct blows occur when the athlete is struck in the head by some object (i.e., a ball, a baseball bat, a lacrosse stick, or contact with another player). A direct blow may also occur when the athlete's moving head strikes some fixed object (i.e., the floor, a goal post), resulting in impact deceleration of the brain. A blow to the head can produce an injury to the brain either at the point of contact or on the opposite side, which is referred to as a *contrecoup* injury. Acceleration, deceleration, and particularly rotational forces produce shaking of the brain within the skull.[2]

Recently the term *mild head injury* (MHI) has gained popularity in the sports medicine community and is broadly defined as immediate, transient impairment of cerebral function.[10]

**Signs of injury** Signs of concussion or mild head injury are highly variable but generally may include headache, tinnitus (ringing in ears), nausea, irritability, confusion, disorientation, dizziness, loss of consciousness, **posttraumatic amnesia** (can't remember anything that occurred after the injury), retrograde amnesia (can't remember things that occurred before injury), concentration difficulty, blurred vision, photophobia (sensitivity to light), and sleep disturbance.[13]

> **posttraumatic amnesia**
> Inability of athlete to recall events since injury.

**TABLE 22-1** Guide to Classifying Four Levels of Cerebral Concussion

| Level | Consciousness | 3 C's: Cranial Nerves II, III, IV, VII, VIII<br>Cognition (Memory & Concentration)<br>Coordination (Balance & Finger/Feet Tasks) | Headache |
|---|---|---|---|
| Mild (Grade 0) | No loss | Mild confusion, but is asymptomatic within 10 min<br>Passes functional tests without recurrence of signs and symptoms | Possibly develops later |
| Mild (Grade 1) | No loss | *At least one of the following:*<br>Abnormal cranial nerve assessment <1 hour<br>Abnormal cognition <1 hour<br>Abnormal coordination <3 days | Probable; 10 min–2 days |
| Moderate (Grade 2) | Brief loss 10 sec–1 min or Altered <2 min | *At least one of the following:*<br>Abnormal cranial nerve assessment >1 hour<br>Abnormal cognition >1 hour<br>Abnormal coordination >3 days | Probable; 24 hrs–4 days |
| Severe (Grade 3) | Prolonged loss >1 min or altered >2 min | 2 of 3 C's abnormal for >24 hours | Most likely; >4 days |

In recent years, considerable debate has raged over a variety of classification systems that have been proposed for determining severity of concussion. To date no single system of classification has been universally endorsed. Table 22-1 provides a recommended guide for classifying four levels of cerebral concussion.

**Care**   Returning an athlete to competition following concussion often creates a difficult dilemma for the sports medicine team.[1] Certainly there is a difference between athletes who have a mild head injury—who have simply "had their bell rung," and those who have experienced a loss of consciousness. Nevertheless, returning an athlete who has experienced any type of injury to the brain to competition too early has the potential to become a very costly decision, one that could lead to death.[1]

**Any time an athlete loses consciousness for any reason, the athlete must be removed from further activity immediately.** If the athlete has sustained a head injury that causes unconsciousness, the coach must always suspect that the athlete may also have a cervical neck injury and must remove the athlete from the field using a spine board.[10]

The decision to allow an athlete with a mild head injury to return to play is more difficult and to date has been based primarily on the subjective judgment of the team physician. Recent studies have indicated that the recovery period following even a mild head injury may be longer than has been thought.[4] Athletes who have sustained a mild head injury should not be permitted to return to activity until all postconcussive symptoms including visual, motor, or sensory changes and difficulty with thought or memory have resolved. Permitting an athlete, particularly one in a contact sport, to return before symptoms resolve may place the athlete at risk.[1] **A coach should never allow an athlete who has sustained any type of head injury to return to activity until that athlete has been cleared by the team physician.** Table 22-2 provides guidelines that can help in decision-making for return to play following head injury.

Even after postconcussive symptoms have disappeared and the athlete has returned to play, there is still a danger in recurrent concussions, which can produce cumulative traumatic injury to the brain. If more than one concussion occurs during a season, decisions must be made as to whether to allow the athlete to continue to compete. Table 22-3 provides some recommendations for return to play after recurrent concussion.

## Second Impact Syndrome

**Cause of injury**    Second impact syndrome occurs as a result of rapid swelling of the brain following a second head injury that occurs before the symptoms of a previous head injury have resolved.[1] This second impact may be relatively minor and in some cases may not even involve a blow to the head. A blow to the chest or back may create enough force to snap the athlete's head and create acceleration and deceleration forces upon an already compromised brain. Second impact syndrome is most likely to occur in athletes less than 20 years of age.

**Signs of injury**    Often athletes do not even lose consciousness and may look "stunned." They may remain on their feet and be able to leave the playing field under their own power. However, within 15 seconds to several minutes, their condition worsens rapidly with loss of consciousness leading to coma, dilated pupils, loss of eye movement, and respiratory failure.[1] This is a life-threatening situation that has a mortality rate of approximately 50 percent.

**Care**    Second impact syndrome is a life-threatening emergency that must be dealt with within a matter of approximately 5 minutes by dramatic life-saving measures performed in an emergency care facility.[1] The best way to manage second impact syndrome is to prevent it from occurring. Thus decisions to allow an athlete to return to play following an initial head injury must be carefully made based on the absence of postconcussive symptoms.

## Cerebral Contusion

**Cause of injury**    A contusion of the cerebrum is a focal injury to the brain that involves small hemorrhages or *intracerebral bleeding* within either the cortex, the brainstem, or the cerebellum (Figure 22-4).[2] Brain contusions usually result from an impact injury in which the head strikes a stationary immovable object such as the floor.

**Critical Thinking** Exercise

A football player receives a grade 2 concussion. It is his second concussion this season.

**?**  What guidelines should be followed regarding his return to play?

**Critical Thinking** Exercise

A volleyball player is knocked to the ground and hits the back of her head on the court, briefly losing consciousness. A few minutes after regaining consciousness she appears to be absolutely normal with no residual signs of concussion.

**?**  Should the coach allow her to return to the game?

Second impact syndrome is a life-threatening emergency that must be dealt with immediately.

**Figure 22-4**

Intracranial hemorrhage

**TABLE 22-2** Guidelines for Immediate Management of Concussion (Refer to Table 22-1 for grade/level)

| | |
|---|---|
| Mild (Grade 0) | Remove from contest. Examine immediately and at 5-minute intervals for development of abnormal C's (cranial nerves, cognition, coordination) or other postconcussive symptoms at rest and with exertion. May return to contest if examination is normal and no symptoms develop for at least 20 minutes. |
| | If any symptoms develop within the initial 20 minutes, return on that day should not be permitted. |
| (Grade 1) | If the athlete is removed from participation as a result of developing symptoms, follow-up evaluations should be conducted daily. May return to *restricted* participation when the athletic trainer and team physician are assured the athlete has been asymptomatic at rest and with exertion for at least 2 days, followed by return to *unrestricted* participation if asymptomatic for 1 additional day. Neuropsychological assessment and balance/coordination testing are valuable criteria, especially if preseason baseline measures are available. |
| Moderate (Grade 2) | Remove from contest and prohibit return on that day. Examine immediately and at 5-minute intervals for signs of evolving intracranial pathology. Re-examine daily. May return to *restricted* participation when the athletic trainer and team physician are assured the athlete has been asymptomatic at rest and with exertion for at least 4 days, followed by return to *unrestricted* participation if asymptomatic for an additional 2 days. The performance during restricted participation should be used as a guide for making the decision for unrestricted participation. Neuropsychological assessment and balance/coordination testing are valuable criteria, especially if preseason baseline measures are available. |
| Severe (Grade 3) | Treat on field/court as if there has been a cervical spine injury. Examine immediately and at 5-minute intervals for signs of evolving intracranial pathology. Re-examine daily. Return to play is based on how quickly the athlete's initial symptoms resolve: |
| | 1) If symptoms totally resolve within the first week, athlete may return to *restricted* participation when the athletic trainer and team physician are assured the athlete has been asymptomatic at rest and with exertion for at least 10 days, followed by return to *unrestricted* participation if asymptomatic for an additional 3 days. |
| | 2) If symptoms fail to totally resolve within the first week, athlete may return to *restricted* participation when the athletic trainer and team physician are assured the athlete has been asymptomatic at rest and with exertion for at least 17 days, followed by return to *unrestricted* participation if asymptomatic for an additional 3 days. |
| | The performance during restricted participation should be used as a guide for making the decision for unrestricted participation. Neuropsychological assessment and balance/coordination testing are valuable criteria, especially if preseason baseline measures are available. |

*NOTE: "Asymptomatic" involves no abnormal C's and no headache.
Any second concussion sustained within a 3-month period of the first concussion requires that the athlete rest for twice the maximum number of days recommended for the respective severity level.

**Signs of injury**    Depending on the extent of trauma and the injury site, signs of injury may vary significantly. In most instances there is a loss of consciousness in an athlete who subsequently become very alert and talkative. A neurological exam is normal, however, symptoms such as headaches, dizziness, and nausea persist.

**TABLE 22-3** Guidelines for Return to Activity Following Initial and Subsequent Concussion

| Grade | First Concussion | Second Concussion | Third Concussion |
|---|---|---|---|
| 1 (mild) | Return to play if asymptomatic* | Return to play in 2 weeks if asymptomatic for 1 week | Terminate season; may return to play next season if asymptomatic |
| 2 (moderate) | Return to play if asymptomatic for 1 week | 1 month minimum restriction; may then return to play if asymptomatic for 1 week; consider terminating season | Terminate season; may return to play next year if asymptomatic |
| 3 (severe) | 1 month minimum restriction; may then return to play if asymptomatic for 1 week | Terminate season; may return to play next year if asymptomatic | |

*No headache or dizziness; no impaired orientation, concentration, or memory during rest or exertion.

**Care** Hospitalization with a variety of imaging tests is standard for a cerebral contusion. Treatment varies according to the clinical status of the athlete.[2] A decision to return to play can only be made by the physician when the athlete is asymptomatic and a computed tomography (CT) scan is normal.

## Epidural Hematoma

**Cause of injury** A blow to the head, often resulting from a skull fracture, can cause a tear of the meningeal arteries that are embedded in bony grooves in the skull (Figure 22-5). Because of arterial blood pressure, blood accumulation and the creation of an *epidural hematoma* are extremely fast.[5]

**Signs of injury** In most cases initially there is a loss of consciousness. In some cases, once consciousness is regained, the athlete may be lucid, with few or none of the symptoms of serious head injury. Gradually symptoms begin to worsen with severe head pains, dizziness, nausea, dilation of one pupil usually on the same side as the injury, or sleepiness. Later stages of cerebral hemorrhage are characterized by deteriorating consciousness, neck rigidity, depression of pulse and respiration, and convulsions. This is a life-threatening situation, necessitating urgent neurosurgical care.

**Care** A CT scan is necessary to diagnose an epidural hematoma. The pressure of an epidural hematoma must be surgically relieved as soon as possible to avoid the possibility of death or permanent disability.

## Subdural Hematoma

**Cause of injury** Acute *subdural hematomas* occur much more frequently than epidural hematomas. Subdural hematomas result from acceleration and deceleration forces that tear vessels that bridge the dura mater and the brain.[5] Subdural hematomas usually involve venous

**Figure 22-5**

Epidural hematoma

Signs of subdural hematoma may appear several hours after injury.

bleeding and thus signs of injury tend to appear more slowly, maybe even after several hours (Figure 22-6).

**Signs of injury**   With subdural hematoma, the athlete may be unconscious with dilation of one pupil, usually on the same side as the injury. There may also be signs of headache, dizziness, nausea, or sleepiness.

**Care**   An acute subdural hematoma is a life-threatening situation that requires immediate medical attention. A diagnostic CT scan or magnetic resonance imaging (MRI) is necessary to determine the extent and location of the hemorrhage.

**Figure 22-6**

Subdural hematoma

### Migraine Headaches

**Cause of condition**   Migraine is a disorder characterized by recurrent attacks of severe headache with sudden onset, with or without visual or gastrointestinal problems. The athlete who has a history of repeated minor blows to the head such as those that may occur in soccer or who has sustained a major cerebral injury may, over time, develop migraine headaches. The exact cause is unknown, but it is believed by many to be a vascular disorder.

**Signs of condition**   Flashes of light, blindness in half the field of vision (hemianopia), and paresthesia are thought to be caused by vasoconstriction of intercerebral vessels. Headache is believed to be caused by dilation of scalp arteries. The athlete complains of a severe headache that is diffused throughout the head and often accompanied by nausea and vomiting. There is evidence of a familial predisposition for those athletes who experience migraine headaches after head injury.

**Care**   The best management is prevention. Prophylactic medications are available to help reduce the recurrence of migraines. For severe attacks, administration of a prescription drug called Triptan has a high success rate.

### Scalp Injuries

The scalp can receive lacerations, abrasions, contusions, and hematomas.

**Cause of injury**   The cause of scalp injury is usually blunt or penetrating trauma. A scalp laceration can exist in conjunction with a serious skull or cerebral injury.

**Signs of injury**   The athlete complains of being hit in the head. Bleeding is often extensive, making it difficult to pinpoint the exact site. Matted hair and dirt can also disguise the actual point of injury.

**Care**   The treatment of a scalp laceration poses a special problem because of its general inaccessibility. Wounds that are more than 1/2 inch (1.25 cm) long and 1/8 inch (0.3 cm) deep should be referred to a physician for treatment. In less severe wounds the bleeding should be controlled and an antiseptic applied, followed by the application of a protective coating such as collodion and a sterile gauze pad. A tape adherent is then painted over the skin area to ensure that the tape sticks to the skin.

BIOHAZARD

## ANATOMY OF THE FACE

The facial skin covers primarily subcutaneous bone with very little protective muscle, fascia, or fat. The supraorbital ridges house the frontal sinuses. In general the facial skeleton is composed of dense bony buttresses combined with thin sheets of bone. The middle third of the face consists of the maxillary bone, which supports the nose and nasal passages. The lower aspect of the face consists of the lower jaw or mandible. Besides supporting teeth, the mandible also supports the larynx, trachea, upper airway, and upper digestive tract (refer to Figure 22-1).

## RECOGNITION AND MANAGEMENT OF SPECIFIC FACIAL INJURIES

### Mandible Fracture

**Cause of injury**   Fractures of the lower jaw or mandible (Figure 22-7) occur most often in collision sports. They are second in incidence of all facial fractures. Because it has relatively little padding and sharp contours, the lower jaw is prone to injury from a direct blow. The most frequently fractured area is near the jaw's frontal angle.

**Signs of injury**   The main indications of a fractured mandible are deformity, loss of normal occlusion of the teeth, pain when biting down, bleeding around teeth, and lower lip anesthesia.

**Care**   Fracture of the mandible requires temporary immobilization with an elastic bandage followed by reduction and fixation of the jaw by the physician. Mild repetitive activities can be carried out, such as light weight lifting, swimming, or cycling during recovery. Fixation is from 4 to 6 weeks. Full activity is resumed in 2 to 3 months with appropriate special headgear and customized mouth guard.

**Figure 22-7**

Mandible fracture

### Zygomatic Complex (Cheekbone) Fracture

**Cause of injury**   A fracture of the zygoma represents the third most common facial fracture. The mechanism of injury is a direct blow to the cheekbone.

**Signs of injury**   An obvious deformity occurs in the cheek region, or a bony discrepancy can be felt during palpation. There is usually a nosebleed *(epistaxis),* and the athlete commonly complains of seeing double *(diplopia).* There is also numbness of the cheek.

**Care**   Care usually involves cold application for the control of edema and immediate referral to a physician. Healing takes from 6 to 8 weeks. Proper protective gear must be worn when returning to activity.

### Facial Lacerations

**Cause of injury**   Facial lacerations are common in contact and collision sports. Lacerations about the face are caused by a direct impact to the face with a sharp object or by an indirect compressive force.

**Signs of injury**   The athlete feels pain and there is substantial bleeding and obvious tearing of the epidermis, dermis, and often the subcutaneous layer of skin (Figure 22-8).

**Figure 22-8**

Facial lacerations can be a
medical emergency.

**Care**   Refer to the physician for definitive care, such as suturing.
Coaches should note that in cases of *eyebrow lacerations,* they should not
shave the eyebrow because it may not regrow, or if it does it may do so
in an irregular pattern. Lip, oral, ear, cheek, and nasal lacerations, as with
all facial lacerations, are grossly contaminated and must be carefully
cleaned before suturing can be successful. Infection must be avoided. Systemic antibiotics and tetanus prophylaxis may be necessary.

## DENTAL ANATOMY

The tooth is a composite of mineral salts of which calcium and phospho-
rus are most abundant. The portion protruding from the gum, called the
*crown,* is covered by the hardest substance within the body, the enamel.
The portion that extends into the alveolar bone of the mouth is called the
*root* and is covered by a thin, bony substance known as *cementum.* Underneath the enamel and cementum lies the bulk of the tooth, a hard material known as *dentin.* Within the dentin is a central canal and chamber
containing the *pulp,* which is composed of nerves, lymphatics, and blood
vessels that supply the entire tooth (Figure 22-9).With the use of face
guards and properly fitting mouth guards most dental injuries can be prevented (see Chapter 6).

## PREVENTING DENTAL INJURIES

There is universal agreement within the dental community that all athletes, but particularly those in contact and collision sports, should rou-

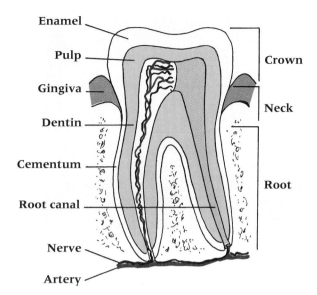

Enamel

Pulp

Gingiva

Dentin

Cementum

Root canal

Nerve

Artery

Crown

Neck

Root

**Figure 22-9**

Normal tooth anatomy

tinely wear mouthguards to prevent injuries to the teeth. Without question the mandatory use of mouthguards by both high school and collegiate football players has significantly reduced the incidence of oral injuries in those sports. However, there is still a high incidence of dental injuries in those sports that do not require mouthguards to be worn.[7,12]

Athletes should practice good dental hygiene that includes regular brushing, rinsing, and flossing. Like everyone else, athletes should have periodically scheduled dental screenings at least once each year to prevent the development of dental caries (cavities) in which there is a gradual decay and degeneration of soft or bony tissue of a tooth. If this decay progresses, the tissue surrounding the tooth can become inflamed and an *abscess* forms from a bacterial infection of the tooth. Poor dental hygiene can also lead to *gingivitis,* which is an inflammation of the gums in which there is swelling, redness, tenderness, and a tendency to bleed easily. Chronic gingivitis can lead to *periodontitis,* in which there is an inflammation and/or a degeneration of the dental periosteum, the surrounding bone, and the cementum; loosening of the teeth; a recession of the gingiva; and infection.[7]

## RECOGNITION AND MANAGEMENT OF SPECIFIC DENTAL INJURIES

### Tooth Fractures

**Cause of injury**   Any impact to the upper or lower jaw or direct trauma can potentially fracture the teeth.[7] There are essentially three types of fractures that can occur to the teeth: an uncomplicated crown fracture, a complicated crown fracture, and a root fracture (Figure 22-10).

**Signs of injury**   In an uncomplicated crown fracture a small portion of the tooth is broken but there is no bleeding from the fracture and the

Tooth fractures:
- uncomplicated crown fracture
- complicatted fracture
- root fracture

**Figure 22-10**

Tooth fractures

A                          B                          C

**Figure 22-10 (cont'd)**

A, Uncomplicated crown
fracture; B, Complicated
crown fracture; C, Root
fracture

pulp chamber is not exposed. In a complicated crown fracture a portion of the tooth is broken and there is bleeding from the fracture. The pulp chamber is exposed and there is a great deal of pain. Because a root fracture occurs below the gum line diagnosis is difficult and may require x-ray. Root fractures account for only 10 to 15 percent of all fractures. The tooth may appear to be in the normal position but there is bleeding from the gum around the tooth and the crown of the tooth may be pushed back or loose. Any impact great enough to cause a fracture of a tooth can also produce a fracture of the mandible or even a concussion.[12]

**Care**   Neither uncomplicated or complicated crown fractures require immediate treatment by a dentist. The fractured piece of tooth can simply be placed in a plastic bag, and if the fractured tooth is not extremely sensitive to air or cold, the athlete can continue to play and see the dentist within 24 to 48 hours after the game. If there is bleeding, a piece of gauze can be placed over the fracture. For the sake of appearance the fractured piece of tooth can either be glued in place or capped using a synthetic composite material.

In the case of a root fracture the athlete may continue to play but should see the dentist as soon as possible after the game. If the tooth is pushed back do not try to force it forward because doing so is likely to make the fracture worse. The dentist will reposition the tooth and apply a brace to be worn for 3 to 4 months. A mouthguard should be worn while competing.

### Tooth Subluxation, Luxation, and Avulsion

**Cause of injury**   The same mechanisms that cause fractures of the teeth may also cause loosening or dislocation of the tooth.[12] Loosening of the tooth can result in concussion or subluxation, luxation, or avulsion.

**Signs of injury**   A tooth may be slightly loosened or totally dislodged. In the case of a concussion or subluxation the tooth is still in its normal place and only slightly loose. There is little if any pain, however, the tooth just feels different. In a luxation there is no fracture but the tooth is very loose and has moved either forward to an extruded position, or backward to an intruded position. In an avulsion, the tooth is knocked completely out of the mouth.

**Care**   For a concussion or subluxation, no immediate treatment is required and the athlete should be referred to a dentist within 48 hours for evaluation only. In a luxation, the tooth should only be moved back into its normal position if it is easy to move. The athlete should be referred to a dentist as soon as possible, especially if it is not possible to reposition the tooth to its normal position. With an avulsion, the coach can safely and easily try to reimplant the tooth. The avulsed tooth can be rinsed off but should never be scraped or scrubbed to get dirt off. If it is not possible to reimplant the tooth, it should be stored in a "Save a Tooth" kit, which contains Hank's Balanced Salt Solution (HBSS), or in milk or saline.[12] The athlete should be referred to the dentist immediately. The sooner the tooth can be reimplanted the better the prognosis.

> An avulsed tooth should be reimplanted immediately.

**BIOHAZARD**

22–4

*Critical Thinking* Exercise

A field hockey player is accidentally hit in the mouth with a stick. One of her front teeth is knocked completely out and she spits the tooth out into her hand.

**?**  What should the coach do in this situation?

## ANATOMY OF THE NOSE

The nose functions to clean, warm, and humidify inhaled air. The external portion of the nose is formed by a combination of bone in the superior portion and fibrocartilage inferiorly that spreads laterally to form the ala. The nasal cavity extends from the nostrils posteriorly to the choane. A nasal septum divides the nasal cavity into right and left chambers.

## RECOGNITION AND MANAGEMENT OF SPECIFIC NASAL INJURIES

### Nasal Fractures and Chondral Separation

**Cause of injury**   A fracture of the nose is one of the most common fractures of the face. The force of the blow to the nose may come either from the side or from  a straight frontal force. A lateral force causes greater deformity than a straight-on blow.

**Signs of injury**   Nasal fractures appear frequently as a separation of the frontal processes of the maxilla, a separation of the lateral cartilages, or a combination of the two (Figure 22-11). In nasal fractures hemorrhage is profuse because of laceration of the mucous lining. Swelling is

**Figure 22-11**

A serious nose fracture may
be a medical emergency.

**Figure 22-12**

Splinting the fractured nose

immediate. Deformity is usually present if the nose has received a lateral blow. Gentle palpation may reveal abnormal mobility and emit a grating sound (crepitus).

**Care**   The coach should control the bleeding and then refer the athlete to a physician for x-ray examination and reduction of the fracture. Simple and uncomplicated fractures of the nose do not hinder and are not unsafe for the athlete, and he or she can return to competition within a few days. Fracture deformity reduction must be performed by a trained person. Adequate protection can be provided through splinting by inserting two pieces of gauze, each 2 inches (5 cm) long and rolled to the size of a pencil into either side of the athlete's nose. Gently but firmly, 4-inch (10 cm) lengths of tape are laid over the gauze rolls (Figure 22-12).

### Deviated Septum

**Cause of injury**   As with fracture, the mechanism of injury to the septum is by compression or lateral trauma.

**Signs of injury**   A careful evaluation of the nose must be made after the trauma. Injury commonly produces bleeding and in some cases a septal hematoma. The athlete complains of nasal pain.

**Care**   At the site where a hematoma may occur, compression is applied. When a hematoma is present, it must be drained immediately through a surgical incision through the nasal septal mucosa. After surgical drainage, a small wick is inserted for continued drainage, and the nose is firmly packed to prevent the hematoma from re-forming. If a hematoma is neglected, an abscess will form, causing bone and cartilage loss and ultimately a difficult deformity to correct.

### Nosebleed (Epistaxis)

**Cause of injury** Nosebleeds in sports are usually the result of direct blows that cause varying degrees of contusion to the septum. *Epistaxis* can be classified as either anterior or posterior. Anterior epistaxis originates from the nasal septum and posterior epistaxis from the lateral wall. Anterior epistaxis is by far the more common and may result from a direct blow, a sinus infection, high humidity, allergies, a foreign body lodged in the nose, or some other serious facial or head injury.[17]

**Signs of injury** Hemorrhages arise most often from the highly vascular anterior aspect of the nasal septum. In most situations the nosebleed presents only a minor problem and stops spontaneously after a short time. However, there are persistent types that require medical attention and possibly cauterization. As always when dealing with blood, universal precautions must be used.

**Care** An athlete with an acute nosebleed should sit upright with a cold compress placed both over the nose and the ipsilateral carotid artery while applying finger pressure to the affected nostril for 5 minutes. It has also been suggested that a piece of rolled-up gauze be placed between the upper lip and gum, thus placing direct pressure on the arteries that supply the nasal mucosa.[17]

**BIOHAZARD**

If this procedure fails to stop the bleeding within 5 minutes, more extensive measures should be taken. With an applicator, paint the hemorrhage point with an astringent or a styptic such as tannic acid or epinephrine hydrochloride solution. The application of gauze or a felt plug provides corking action and encourages blood clotting. If a plug is used, the ends should protrude from the nostrils at least $1/2$ inch to facilitate removal. After bleeding has ceased, the athlete may resume activity but should be reminded not to blow the nose under any circumstances for at least 2 hours after the initial insult.

### ANATOMY OF THE EAR

The ear (Figure 22-13) is responsible for the sense of hearing and equilibrium. It is composed of three parts: the external ear; the middle ear (tympanic membrane) lying just inside the skull; and the internal ear (labyrinth), which is formed in part by the temporal bone of the skull. The middle ear and internal ear are structured to transport auditory impulses to the brain. Aiding the organs of hearing and equalizing pressure between the middle and the internal ear is the eustachian tube, a canal that joins the nose and the middle ear.[15]

Sports injuries to the ear occur most often to the external portion. The external ear is separated into the auricle (pinna) and the external auditory canal (meatus). The auricle, which is shaped like a shell, collects and directs waves of sound into the auditory canal. It is composed of

A

Triangular fossa — 
Concha — 

— Scaphoid fossa
— Helix
— Antihelix
— Lobe

Temporal bone
Malleus (hammer)
Incus (anvil)

Semicircular canals
Stapes (stirrup)
Vestibular nerve
Facial nerve
Cochlea nerve
Cochlea
B
Eustachian tube

Tympanic membrane    Oval window

**Figure 22-13**

Ear anatomy: A, External ear; B, Inner ear

**Figure 22-14**

Cauliflower ear

flexible yellow cartilage, muscles, and fat padding and is covered by a closely adhering, thin layer of skin. Most of the blood vessels and nerves of the auricle turn around its borders, with just a few penetrating the cartilage proper.

## RECOGNITION AND MANAGEMENT OF SPECIFIC INJURIES TO THE EAR

### Auricular Hematoma (cauliflower ear)

**Cause of injury**   Hematoma of the ear is common in boxing, rugby, and wrestling. Hematomas are most common in athletes who do not wear protective headgear. This condition usually occurs from either compression or a shearing injury (single or repeated) to the auricle that causes subcutaneous bleeding into the auricular cartilage.[3]

**Signs of injury**   Trauma may tear the overlying tissue away from the cartilaginous plate, resulting in hemorrhage and fluid accumulation. A hematoma usually forms before the limited circulation can absorb the fluid. If the hematoma goes unattached, a sequence of coagulation, organization, and fibrosis results in a keloid (excessive scar) that appears elevated, rounded, white, nodular, and firm, resembling a cauliflower (Figure 22-14). Often it forms in the region of the helix fossa or concha; once developed, the keloid can be removed only through surgery.[3]

**Care**   To prevent this disfiguring condition, some friction-reducing agent such as petroleum jelly should be applied to the ears of athletes susceptible to this condition. They should also routinely wear ear guards in practice and in competition.

If an ear becomes "hot" because of excessive rubbing or twisting, the immediate application of a cold pack to the affected spot alleviates hemorrhage. Once swelling is present in the ear, special care should be taken to prevent the fluid from solidifying; a cold pack should be placed immediately over the ear and held tightly by an elastic bandage for at least 20 minutes. If the swelling is still present at the end of this time, aspiration by a physician is required.[3] After drainage, pressure is applied to the area to prevent return of the hematoma.

### Rupture of the Tympanic Membrane

**Cause of injury**   Rupture of the tympanic membrane is commonly seen in contact and collision sports, and in water polo and diving.[9] A fall or slap to the unprotected ear or sudden underwater pressure variation can rupture the tympanic membrane.

**Signs of injury**   The athlete complains of a loud pop followed by pain in the ear, nausea, vomiting, and dizziness. The athlete demonstrates hearing loss and a physician can see a visible rupture of the tympanic membrane through an otoscope.

**Care**   Small to moderate perforations of the tympanic membrane usually heal spontaneously in 1 to 2 weeks.[9] Infection can occur and must be continually monitored.

Rupture of the tympanic membrane can cause temporary hearing loss.

### Swimmer's Ear (Otitis Externa)

**Cause of injury**   A common condition in athletes engaged in water sports is *swimmer's ear,* or external otitis. Swimmer's ear is a general term for infection of the ear canal. Contrary to current thought among swimming coaches, swimmer's ear is not usually associated with a fungal infection. Water can become trapped in the ear canal as a result of obstructions created by cysts, bone growths, ear wax plugs, or swelling caused by allergies.[15]

**Signs of injury**   The athlete may complain of itching, discharge, or even a partial hearing loss. The athlete also complains of pain and dizziness.

**Care**   Prevention of ear infection can best be attained by drying the ears thoroughly with a soft towel, using ear drops containing a mild acid (3% boric acid) and alcohol solution before and after each swim, and avoiding situations that can cause ear infections such as overexposure to cold wind or sticking foreign objects into the ear.

When the swimmer displays symptoms of external otitis, immediate referral to a physician must be made. Tympanic membrane rupture should be ruled out. Antibiotics may be used in athletes with a mild ear infection.[15] In the event of a perforated ear drum, custom-made ear plugs must be used.

### Middle Ear Infection (Otitis Media)

**Cause of injury**   Otitis media is an accumulation of fluid in the middle ear caused by local and systemic inflammation and infection.

**Signs of injury**   There usually is intense pain in the ear, fluid draining from the ear canal, and a transient loss of hearing. In addition, the systemic infection may also cause fever, headache, irritability, loss of appetite, and nausea.[15]

**Care**   A physician may choose to draw a small amount of fluid from the middle ear to determine the most appropriate antibiotic therapy.

Analgesics can be used to help reduce pain. The problem generally begins to resolve within 24 hours, although pain may last for 72 hours.

### Impacted Cerumen

**Cause of condition**   *Cerumen* or ear wax is secreted by glands in the outer portion of the ear canal. Occasionally an excessive amount of ear wax may accumulate, clogging the ear canal.

**Signs of condition**   When cerumen becomes impacted there is some degree of hearing loss that is usually muffled. However, there generally is little or no pain because no infection is involved.[15]

**Care**   Initially an attempt can be made to remove excess cerumen by irrigating the ear canal with warm water. The athlete should not attempt to remove the cerumen with a cotton tip applicator because that may increase the degree of impaction. If irrigation fails, the impacted cerumen must be physically removed by a physician using a curette.

## ANATOMY OF THE EYE

The eye has many anatomical protective features. It is firmly retained within an oval socket formed by the bones of the head. A cushion of soft fatty tissue surrounds it, and a thin skin flap (the eyelid), which functions by reflex action, covers the eye for protection. Foreign particles are prevented from entering the eye by the lashes and eyebrows, which act as a filtering system. A soft mucous lining that covers the inner conjunctiva transports and spreads tears, which are secreted by many accessory lacrimal glands. A larger lubricating organ is located above the eye and secretes quantities of fluid through the lacrimal duct to help wash away foreign particles. The eye proper is well protected by the sclera, a tough white outer layer possessing a transparent center portion called the *cornea*.

The cornea covers the pupil, which is the central opening of the eye. Light passes through the cornea, then through the anterior chamber past the iris to the lens, and finally through the vitreous body, all of which function collectively to focus an image on the retina that is detected by the optic nerve (Figure 22-15).

## RECOGNITION AND MANAGEMENT OF SPECIFIC EYE INJURIES

### Orbital Hematoma (Black Eye)

**Cause of injury**   Although well protected, the eye may be bruised during sports activity. The severity of eye injuries varies from a mild bruise to an extremely serious condition affecting vision to the fracturing of the orbital cavity. Fortunately, most of the eye injuries sustained in sports are mild. A blow to the eye may initially injure the surrounding tissue and produce capillary bleeding into the tissue spaces. If the hemorrhage goes unchecked, the result may be a classic "black eye."

**Signs of injury**   The signs of a more serious contusion may be displayed as a subconjunctival hemorrhage or as faulty vision.

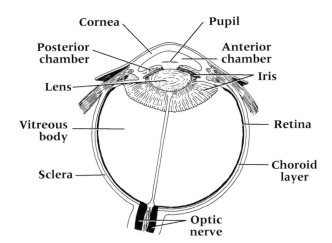

**Figure 22-15**

Eye anatomy

**Care**   Care of an eye contusion requires cold application for at least half an hour, plus a 24-hour rest period if the athlete has distorted vision. Under no circumstances should an athlete blow the nose after an acute eye injury. To do so might increase hemorrhaging.

### Orbital Fractures

**Cause of injury**   A fracture of the bony framework of the orbit surrounding the eye can occur when a blow to the eyeball forces it backwards, compressing the orbital fat until a blow-out or rupture occurs to the floor of the orbit. Both fat and the inferior extraocular muscles can bulge through this fracture.[11]

**Signs of injury**   The athlete with a fracture of the orbit often exhibits *diplopia* (double vision), restricted movement of the eye, a downward displacement of the eye, and pain accompanied by soft tissue swelling and hemorrhage. There may be numbness associated with injury to the infraorbital nerve on the floor of the orbit. An x-ray must be taken to confirm the fracture.

**Care**   A physician should administer antibiotics prophylactically to decrease the likelihood of infection. A fracture in the orbital floor allows communication with the maxillary sinus, which may contain potentially infectious bacteria. Most orbital fractures are treated surgically although some physicians prefer to wait and see if the symptoms resolve on their own.

### Foreign Body in the Eye

**Cause of injury**   Foreign bodies in the eye are a frequent occurrence in sports and are potentially dangerous.[11]

**Signs of injury**   A foreign object produces considerable pain and disability. No attempt should be made to remove the body by rubbing or to remove it with the fingers.

**Care**   Have the athlete close the eye until the initial pain has subsided, and then attempt to determine if the object is in the vicinity of the

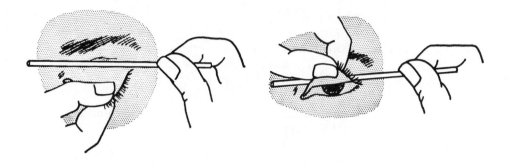

**Figure 22-16**

Removing a foreign object from the eye

upper or lower lid. Foreign bodies in the lower lid are relatively easy to remove by depressing the tissue and then wiping it with a sterile cotton applicator. Foreign bodies in the area of the upper lid are usually much more difficult to localize. Gently pull the upper eyelid over the lower lid while the subject looks downward. This causes tears to be produced, which may flush the object down onto the lower lid. If this method is unsuccessful, gently pull the eyelid down and place an applicator stick crosswise at its base; have the athlete look down; then grasp the lashes and turn the lid back over the stick. Holding the lid and the stick in place with one hand, use the sterile cotton swab to lift out the foreign body (Figure 22-16). After the foreign particle is removed, the affected eye should be washed with saline solution. Often after removal of the foreign body there is residual soreness, which may be alleviated by the application of petroleum jelly or some other mild ointment. If there is extreme difficulty in removing the foreign body or if it has become embedded in the eye itself, the eye should be closed and "patched" with a gauze pad, which is held in place by strips of tape. The athlete is referred to a physician as soon as possible.

### Corneal Abrasions

**Cause of injury**   An athlete who gets a foreign object in his or her eye usually tries to rub it away. In doing so, the cornea can become abraded.[11]

**Signs of injury**   The athlete complains of severe pain and watering of the eye, photophobia, and spasm of the orbicular muscle of the eyelid.

**Care**   The eye should be patched, and the athlete should be sent to a physician. Antibiotic ointment is applied and a semipressure patch placed over the closed eyelid.

### Hyphema

**Cause of injury**   A blunt blow to the anterior aspect of the eye can produce a *hyphema,* which is a collection of blood within the anterior chamber.[14] This injury is often caused by being struck in the eye with a racquetball or squash ball when not wearing appropriate protective eyewear.

**Signs of injury**   Initially there is a reddish tinge in the anterior chamber and within the first 2 hours the blood settles inferiorly or may fill the entire chamber. The blood may turn pea green. Vision is partially or completely blocked. The coach must be aware that a hyphema is a major eye injury that can lead to serious problems of the lens, choroid, or retina.

**Care**   Athletes with a hyphema should be immediately referred to a physician. Conventional treatment involves hospitalization and bed rest with the head elevated 30 to 45 degrees, patching of both eyes, sedation, and medication to reduce pressure in the anterior chamber. The initial hemorrhage resorbs in a few days, although occasionally there is rebleeding. If not managed properly, irreversible visual damage can occur.

### Retinal Detachment

**Cause of injury**   A blow to the athlete's eye can partially or completely separate the retina from its underlying attachment. Retinal detachment is more common among athletes who have myopia (nearsightedness).[8]

**Signs of injury**   Detachment is painless; however, early signs include seeing specks floating before the eye, flashes of light, or blurred vision. As the detachment progresses, the athlete complains of a "curtain" falling over the field of vision. Any athlete with symptoms of detachment must be immediately referred to an ophthalmologist (Figure 22-17).

**Care**   Initial treatment is bed rest with patches on both eyes. The athlete should immediately be referred to an ophthalmologist to determine if surgery is required.

**Figure 22-17**

A blow to the eye can cause the retina to become detached.

## Acute Conjunctivitis

**Cause of injury**    The conjunctiva is the tissue that lines the back of the eyelid, moves into the space between the eyelid and eye globe, and spreads up over the sclera to the corena.[15] Acute conjunctivitis is usually caused by various bacteria or allergens. It may begin with conjunctival irritation from wind, dust, smoke, or air pollution. It may also be associated with the common cold or other upper respiratory conditions.

**Signs of injury**    The athlete complains of eyelid swelling, sometimes with a purulent discharge. Itching is associated with allergy. Eyes may burn or itch.

**Care**    Acute conjunctivitis can be highly infectious. The athlete should be referred to a physician for treatment.

## RECOGNITION AND MANAGEMENT OF INJURIES TO THE THROAT

### Contusions

**Cause of injury**    Blows to the throat do not occur frequently in sports, but occasionally an athlete may receive a kick or blow to the throat. One type of trauma is known as "clotheslining," in which the athlete is struck in the throat region. Such a force can conceivably injure the carotid artery, causing a clot to form that occludes the blood flow to the brain. This same clot can become dislodged and migrate to the brain. In either case, serious brain injury may result.

**Signs of injury**    Immediately after throat trauma the athlete may experience severe pain and spasmodic coughing, speak with a hoarse voice, and complain of difficulty in swallowing. Fracture of throat cartilages of the larynx is rare, but it is possible and may be indicated by an inability to breathe and expectoration of frothy blood.[16] Cyanosis may be present. Throat contusions are extremely uncomfortable and are often frightening to the athlete.

**Care**    The most immediate concern is the integrity of the airway. If the athlete is experiencing difficulty in breathing he or she should be sent to an emergency care facility immediately. In most situations cold may be applied intermittently to control superficial hemorrhage and swelling, and after a 24-hour rest period moist hot packs may be applied. For the most severe neck contusions, stabilization with a well-padded collar is beneficial.

## SUMMARY

• An athlete who receives either a direct blow to the head or body contact that causes the head to snap forward, backward, or rotate to the side must be carefully evaluated for injury to the brain. Injuries to the brain may or may not result in unconsciousness; disorientation or amnesia; motor, coordination, or balance deficits; and cognitive deficits.

• It is important to realize that in the athletic population, the majority of concussions do not involve loss of consciousness.

- Concussions usually occur as a result of a direct impact or through a combination of rotational acceleration and deceleration forces.

- A variety of classification systems have been proposed for determining severity of concussion. To date, none of these classification systems has been universally endorsed and thus debate continues.

- Returning an athlete to competition following concussion often creates a difficult dilemma for the sports medicine team. There must be ongoing concern about second impact syndrome and epidural and subdural hematomas.

- Injuries to the face can involve fractures of the mandible, maxilla, or zygoma, dislocations of the mandible, and facial lacerations.

- Any impact to the upper or lower jaw or direct trauma can cause one of three types of fractures to the teeth: an uncomplicated crown fracture, a complicated crown fracture, and a root fracture. A tooth may also be subluxated, luxated, or avulsed. The coach should be aware of when to refer an athlete for dental care.

- Most injuries to the ear involve the auricle; cauliflower ear is the most common injury. Rupture of the tympanic membrane, swimmer's ear, and middle ear infections are common in the athletic population.

- For the most part, injuries to the eye should be treated by physicians who are specifically trained. Orbital fractures, a foreign body in the eye, a hyphema, and retinal detachments are all considered serious injuries to the eye.

- The most serious consequence of a throat contusion is airway interference.

---

*Solutions to Critical Thinking* Exercises

**22-1** The coach should ask him or her to count backwards from 100 by 7s and to name the months in reverse order. Both of these tests assess cognitive function.

**22-2** The athlete should be out of play for at least 1 month. After this period he or she may return to play if asymptomatic for 1 week. The physician may consider terminating the athlete for the rest of the season.

**22-3** Absolutely not. Whenever an athlete suffers a loss of consciousness, they are automatically finished for that day and should be cleared by a physician before being allowed to return to play.

**22.4** The coach should take the tooth and without trying to clean it off attempt to reimplant the tooth. The athlete should then be immediately referred to a dentist.

## REVIEW QUESTIONS AND CLASS ACTIVITIES

1. What is the difference between the terms *concussion* and *mild head injury?*
2. Identify a classification system for determining grades of concussion.
3. How is second impact syndrome related to concussion?
4. What immediate care procedures should be performed for athletes with facial lacerations?

5. Describe the immediate care procedures that should be performed when a tooth is fractured and when it is dislocated.
6. Describe the procedures that should be performed for an athlete with a nosebleed.
7. How can cauliflower ear be prevented?
8. How should a foreign body in the eye be treated?

 **Dynamic Human CD**

For more information on skeletal anatomy of the thorax and abdomen click on:

- Skeletal
- Anatomy
- Gross anatomy
- Skull
- Then, 3D Viewer: cranial

To take a closer look at the muscles that are involved in thorax and abdomen movement click on:

- Muscular
- Anatomy
- Body regions
- Head and face

### REFERENCES

1. Cantu RC: Second impact syndrome. In Cantu RC: *Clin Sports Med* 17(1):37, 1998.
2. Curtis SM: Disorders of brain function. In Porth CM, editor: *Pathophysiology,* ed 4, Philadelphia, 1994, Lippincott.
3. Davidson TM, Neuman TR: Managing ear trauma, *Physician Sportsmed* 22(7):27, 1994.
4. Guskiewicz K, Perrin D, Gansneader B: Effect of mild head injury on postural stability in athletes, *J Ath Train* 31(4):300, 1996.
5. Jordan BD: Management of concussion in sports, *Neurology* 53(4):892, 1999.
6. Kelly JP: Traumatic brain injury and concussion in sports, *JAMA* 282(10):989, 1999.
7. Kumamoto DP et al: Oral trauma, *Physician Sportsmed* 23(5):53, 1995.
8. Laio J, Zagelbaum BM: Eye injuries in sports, *Ath Ther Today* 4(5):36, 1999.
9. Lenker C: Traumatic tympanic membrane perforation in a collegiate football player, *Ath Ther Today* 5(1):43, 2000.
10. Lindley TR: Concussion management on the field: the recognition and treatment of head injuries in athletes, *Rehab management* 13(3):20, 2000.
11. Pashby RC, Pashby TJ: Ocular injuries. In Torg JS, Shephard RJ, editors: *Current therapy in sports medicine.* St Louis, 1995, Mosby.
12. Roberts WO: Field care of the injured tooth, *Physician Sportsmed* 28(1):101, 2000.
13. Sherman AL, Young JL: Musculoskeletal rehabilitation and sports medicine. 1. Head and spine injuries, *Arch Phys Med Rehab* 80(5 suppl 1):540, 1999.

14. Stilger VG, Alt JM, Robinson TW: Traumatic hyphema in an intercollegiate baseball player: a case report, *J Ath Train* 34(1):25, 1999.

15. *Tabers cyclopedic medical dictionary,* Philadelphia, 1997, FA Davis.

16. Torg JS: Emergency management of head and cervical spine injuries. In Torg JS, Shepard RJ, editors: *Current therapy in sports medicine,* St Louis, 1995, Mosby.

17. Weir J: Effective management of epistaxis in athletes, *J Ath Train* 32(3):254, 1997.

18. Wojtys EM et al: Concussion in sports, *Am J Sports Med* 27(5):676, 1999.

## ANNOTATED BIBLIOGRAPHY

Cantu RC: Neurologic athletic head and neck injuries, *Clin Sports Med,* 17(1):37, 1998.

*A recent text that looks at head and neck trauma that occurs specifically in the athletic population.*

Currie D, Ritchie E, Scott S: *The management of head injuries,* London, 2000, Oxford University Press.

*Chapters cover initial assessment, resuscitation, neurological deterioration, scalp and skull injuries, cervical spine injuries, children's injuries, and more.*

National Athletic Trainers Association Research and Education Foundation: *Proceedings: Mild brain injury in sports,* Washington, DC, 1994.

*A collection of papers presented at a conference dealing with mild brain injuries. Provides a concise summary of information on this topic.*

## WEBSITES

American Academy of Ophthalmology: http://www.master@aao.org and http://www.nbc.com

American Academy of Otolaryngology Head and Neck Surgery: http://www.entnet.org/weblink.html

American Dental Association Online: http://www.ada.org/

ADA ONLINE, the official website of the American Dental Association

SPORTS DENTISTRY ON LINE: http://www.sportsdentistry.com/

## Chapter 23

# Additional Health Concerns

*When you finish this chapter you will be able to:*

- Explain the causes, prevention, and care of the most common skin infections in sports.
- Describe respiratory tract illnesses common to athletes.
- Identify disorders of the gastrointestinal tract.
- Describe how to avoid problems with the diabetic athlete.
- Describe the dangers that hypertension presents to an athlete.
- Describe the adverse effects that various anemias have on the athlete.
- Explain what a coach should do with an athlete who is having a grand mal seizure.
- Identify contagious viral diseases that may be seen in athletes.
- Explain the concerns of the female athlete in terms of menstruation, osteoporosis, and reproduction.
- Explain the many concerns inherent in medical and nonmedical drug use among athletes.
- Identify specific sexually transmitted infections.

I n addition to the injuries that have been discussed in previous chapters, there are a variety of additional health-related conditions that can potentially affect the athlete. Like everyone else, athletes inevitably become ill. When illnesses occur, it becomes incumbent on the coach to recognize these conditions and to follow up with appropriate care. With the illnesses and conditions discussed in this chapter, appropriate care often means referring the athlete to a physician to provide medical care that is beyond the scope of the coach and, in many instances, beyond that of the athletic trainer. The information provided in this chapter serves as a reference for the coach in making appropriate decisions regarding care of the sick athlete.

## SKIN INFECTIONS

The skin is the largest organ of the human body. It is composed of three layers—epidermis, dermis, and subcutis. The most common skin infections in sports are caused by viruses, bacteria, and fungi.[15] Focus Box 23-1 lists the most common skin infections.

### Viral Infections

A virus is the smallest of the microorganisms that can live only inside a cell. When the virus enters a cell it may immediately trigger a disease (influenza) or it can remain dormant for years (herpes). A virus can damage

Herpes is a common virus that attacks the skin of athletes.

---

23-1   *Focus Box*

---

**Common Viral, Bacterial, and Fungal Skin Infections Found in Athletes**

*Viral infections*
   herpes simplex type 1—cold sore, fever blister
   herpes simplex type 2—genital herpes
   herpes gladiatorum (back or shoulders)
   herpes zoster
*Bacterial infections*
   staphylococcus
      boils
   streptococcus
      impetigo
      infected hair follicles
      infected sweat glands
*Fungal infections*
   ringworm (tinea)
      tinea capitis (head)
      tinea corporis (body)
      tinea unguium (toenails and fingernails)
      tinea cruris (jock rash)
      tinea pedis (athlete's foot)

---

the host cell by blocking its normal function and using the metabolism of the host cell for its own reproduction. Eventually the virus destroys the host cell and progressively invades other cells.

Viral infections most likely to affect the skin are herpes simplex and herpes zoster.

### Herpes

**Cause of condition**    Herpes simplex is a viral infection that results in a skin eruption of vesicles that tend to recur in the same place, usually at sites at which mucous membranes join the skin. Herpes simplex is further classified as either type 1 or type 2. Type 1 occurs as a cold sore or fever blister around the lips and type 2 usually occurs around the genitals and is classified as a sexually transmitted infection (Figure 23-1). Herpes simplex that appears on the back or shoulders is called *herpes gladiatorum* and occurs most often in wrestlers.

Herpes zoster appears in a specific pattern on the body in an area that is innervated by a specific nerve root. It may appear on the face or anywhere on the trunk. Herpes zoster is the reappearance of the chicken pox virus that has remained dormant for many years. It is most likely to appear when the immune system is compromised.

**Symptoms of condition**    Athletes about to experience an outbreak of herpes usually feel a tingling, itching soreness immediately before a small area of redness appears. The athlete also reports feeling ill, particularly

**Figure 23-1**

Herpes simplex type 1

with first episode outbreaks. These symptoms are followed by the appearance of painful, fluid-filled vesicles that take on a crusty appearance. These vesicles usually heal in about 10 days.

**Care**   It is important to take universal precautions when dealing with the herpes virus. Herpes may spread by contact with the fluid inside the vesicles. Outbreaks of herpes must run their course. Acyclovir, an over-the-counter medication taken orally and applied topically, has been effective in treating the symptoms. However, athletes must realize that the virus is not destroyed and that the herpes will probably reappear in the same area.

### Bacterial Infections

**Cause of condition**   Bacteria are one-celled plantlike microorganisms that are capable of multiplying in an environment that supports their reproduction. Bacteria that cause disease are called *pathogens*. Millions of nonpathogenic bacteria normally live on the skin and mucous membranes of the body. Development of a disease involves entry of the bacterial pathogen into a host, growth of bacteria and production of toxic substances, and the response of the host to fight that infection. Many different types of bacterial pathogens can produce infection in the body. The two types of bacteria most likely to infect the skin are *streptococcus* (strep) and *staphyloccus* (staph).[15] Impetigo contagiosa is a common skin disease, primarily observed in children, with the greatest number of cases occurring in late summer and early fall. It is caused by streptococci and spreads rapidly when athletes are in close contact with one another. It is characterized by the eruption of small vesicles that form into pustules and later yellow crustations.

**Symptoms of condition**   The symptoms of localized infection are similar to the signs of inflammation, including tenderness, warmth, redness, and swelling. Pus may form in an infected area from either staph or strep.

**Care**   Bacterial infections should be treated with specific antibiotic medications that inhibit the growth and proliferation of a particular bacterium. The area should also be treated with warm compresses. If an open, pus-filled lesion develops, it should be drained. Every precaution

**Figure 23-2**

Tinea of the groin

should be taken to minimize the spread of infection and transmission to another person.

## Fungal Infections

**Cause of condition**    The most common fungal infection found in athletes is *ringworm*. Ringworm fungi are the cause of most skin, nail, and hair fungal infections. Ringworm can be found all over the body and is more appropriately referred to by the term *tinea* plus the Latin term for whatever body part is affected. The two most common sites for ringworm are in the groin (tinea cruris) and in the foot (tinea pedis).[9]

**Symptoms of tinea of the groin (tinea cruris)**    Tinea of the groin (tinea cruris), more commonly called "jock rash," appears as a bilateral and often symmetrical brownish or reddish lesion resembling the outline of a butterfly in the groin area (Figure 23-2).

The athlete complains of mild to moderate itching, which can lead to scratching and the possibility of a secondary bacterial infection.

**Care**    Coaches must be able to identify lesions of tinea cruris and treat them accordingly. Conditions of this type must be treated until cured (Figure 23-3). Infection not responding to normal management must be referred to the team physician. Most ringworm infections respond to the many nonprescription medications that are available as aerosol sprays, liquids, powders, or ointments. Medications that are irritating or tend to mask the symptoms of a groin infection must be avoided.

**Symptoms of athlete's foot (tinea pedis)**    The foot is the area of the body most commonly infected by dermatophytes, usually by tinea pedis, or athlete's foot. The fungus is usually found in the space between the

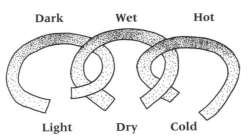

Dark    Wet    Hot

Light    Dry    Cold

**Figure 23–3**

When managing a fungal infection, it is essential to break the chain of infection in one or more ways: Dark-light, wet-dry, hot-cold.

**Figure 23–4**

Athlete's foot (tinea pedis)

third and fourth digits and in the plantar surface of the arch. The same organism attacks toenails. This fungus causes scaling and thickening of the soles. The athlete wearing shoes that are enclosed sweats, encouraging fungal growth. However, the likelihood of getting athlete's foot is based mainly on the athlete's individual susceptibility. Other conditions that may be thought to be athlete's foot include a dermatitis caused by allergy or an eczema-type skin infection.

Athlete's foot can reveal itself in many ways but appears most often as an extreme itching on the soles of the feet and between and on top of the toes. It appears as a rash, with small pimples or minute blisters that break and exude a yellowish serum (Figure 23-4). Scratching because of itchiness can cause the tissue to become inflamed and infected, manifesting a red, white, or gray scaling of the affected area.[2]

**Care**   Griseofulvin is the most effective medication for management of tinea pedis. Of major importance is good foot hygiene. Topical medications used for tinea corporis can be beneficial (Focus Box 23-2).[2]

## RESPIRATORY CONDITIONS

The respiratory tract is an organ system through which various communicable diseases can be transmitted.[16] It is commonly the port of entry for acute infectious diseases that are spread from person to person or by direct contact. Some of the more prevalent conditions affecting athletes are the common cold, sore throat, asthma, hay fever, and air pollution.

### The Common Cold

**Cause of condition**   Upper respiratory tract infections, especially colds and associated conditions, are common in the sports program and can play havoc with entire teams. The common cold is attributed to a filterable virus, which produces an infection of the upper respiratory tract

23-2   *Focus Box*

**Basic Care of Athlete's Foot**

- Keep the feet as dry as possible through frequent use of talcum powder.
- Wear clean white socks to avoid reinfection, changing them daily.
- Use a standard fungicide for specific medication. Over-the-counter medications such as Desenex and Tinactin are useful in the early stages of the infection. For stubborn cases see the team physician; a dermatologist may need to make a culture from foot scrapings to determine the best combatant to be used.

The best cure for athlete's foot is prevention. To keep the condition from spreading to other athletes, the following steps should be faithfully followed by individuals in the sports program:

- Powder the feet daily.
- Dry the feet thoroughly, especially between and under the toes, after every shower.
- Keep sports shoes and street shoes dry by dusting them with powder daily.
- Wear clean sports socks and street socks daily.
- Clean and disinfect the shower and dressing rooms daily.

of a susceptible individual.[16] The susceptible person is believed to be one who has, singly or in combination, any of the following characteristics:

- Physical debilitation from overwork or lack of sleep
- Chronic inflammation from a local infection
- Inflammation of the nasal mucosa from an allergy
- Inflammation of the nasal mucosa from breathing foreign substances such as dust
- Sensitivity to stress

**Symptoms of condition**   The onset of the common cold is usually rapid; symptoms vary among individuals. The typical effects are a general feeling of **malaise** with an accompanying headache, sneezing, and nasal discharge. Some individuals may register a fever of 100° to 102° F (38° to 39° C) and have chills. Various aches and pains may also accompany the symptoms. The nasal discharge starts as a watery secretion and gradually becomes thick and discolored from the inflammation.[16]

**Care**   Care of the cold is usually symptomatic, with emphasis on isolation, bed rest, and light eating. Medications include aspirin for relieving general discomfort, rhinitis tablets for drying the secreting mucosa, and nasal drops to relieve nasal congestion. If a cough is present, various syrups may be given to afford relief. The athlete should avoid intense training while experiencing a severe respiratory infection. Intense training can suppress the immune system.[16]

**malaise** (muh **laze**)
Discomfort and uneasiness
caused by an illness.

## Sinusitis

**Cause of condition**    Sinusitis is an inflammation of the nasal sinuses. Sinusitis can stem from an upper respiratory infection caused by a variety of bacteria. As a result, nasal mucous membranes swell and block the sinuses. A painful pressure occurs from an accumulation of mucus.

**Symptoms of condition**    The skin area over the sinus may be swollen and painful to the touch. The athlete may experience a headache and a feeling of being out of sorts.

**Care**    If an infection is present, antibiotics may be warranted. Nasal vasoconstrictors may be helpful in nasal drainage.

## Sore Throat (Pharyngitis)

**Cause of condition**    A sore throat, or pharyngitis, usually is the result of postnasal drip associated with a common cold or sinusitis. It may also be an indication of a more serious condition, including either viral or bacterial infection.

**Symptoms of condition**    Frequently the condition starts as a dryness in the throat and progresses to soreness with pain and swelling. It is sometimes accompanied by a headache, a fever of 101° to 102° F (38° to 39° C), chills, coughing, and a general feeling of fatigue. On examination the throat may appear dark red and swollen, and mucous membranes may be coated.

**Care**    In most cases bed rest is considered the best treatment, combined with symptomatic medications such as aspirin and a hot saltwater gargle. Antibiotics may be prescribed by a physician if other measures are inadequate.

## Influenza

**Cause of condition**    Influenza, or the flu, is one of the most persistent and debilitating diseases. It usually occurs in various forms as an annual epidemic, causing severe illness among the populace.[19]

Influenza is caused by a virus that enters the tissue's cell through its genetic material. Within the tissue, the virus multiplies and is released from the cell by a budding process and is spread throughout the body. Not all athletes need influenza vaccines; however, athletes engaging in winter sports, basketball, wrestling, and swimming may require them.

**Symptoms of condition**    The athlete with the flu has the following symptoms: fever, cough, headache, malaise, and inflamed respiratory mucous membranes with coryza. It should be noted that certain viruses can increase the body's core temperature. Flu generally has an incubation period of 48 hours and comes on suddenly, accompanied by chills and a fever of 102° to 103° F (39° to 39.5° C), which develops over a 24-hour period. The athlete complains of a headache and general aches and pains—mainly in the back and legs. The headache increases in intensity, along with photophobia and aching at the back of the skull. There is of-

ten sore throat, burning in the chest, and in the beginning, a nonpro-
ductive cough, which later may develop into bronchitis. The skin is
flushed, and the eyes are inflamed and watery. The acute stage of the disease usually lasts up to 5 days. Weakness, sweating, and fatigue may persist for many days.

**Care**   Flu prevention includes staying away from infected persons,
maintaining good resistance through healthy living, and annual vaccines.
If the flu is uncomplicated, its management consists of bed rest. During
the acute stage, the temperature often returns to normal. Symptomatic
care such as aspirin, steam inhalation, cough medicines, and gargles may
be given.[19]

## Seasonal Allergies (Rhinitis)

**Cause of condition**   Hay fever is an acute seasonal allergic condition
that results from airborne pollens. Hay fever can occur during the spring
as a reaction to tree pollens such as oak, elm, maple, alder, birch, and cot-
tonwood. During the summer, grass and weed pollens can be the culprits.
In the fall, ragweed pollen is the prevalent cause. Airborne fungal spores
also have been known to cause hay fever.[5]

**Symptoms of condition**   In the early stages, the athlete's eyes,
throat, mouth, and nose begin to itch, followed by watering of the eyes,
sneezing, and a clear, watery, nasal discharge. The athlete may complain
of a sinus-type headache, emotional irritability, difficulty in sleeping, red
and swollen eyes and nasal mucous membranes, and a wheezing cough.
It should be noted that other common adverse allergic conditions are
asthma, anaphylaxis, urticaria, angioedema, and **rhinitis**.[22]

**Care**   Most athletes obtain relief from hay fever through over-the-
counter oral antihistamines. To avoid the problem of sedation stemming
from these drugs, the athlete may ingest a decongestant during the day
and a long-acting antihistamine before going to bed.

## Acute Bronchitis

**Cause of condition**   Bronchitis is an inflammation of the mucous
membranes of the bronchial tubes. It occurs in both acute and chronic
forms. Bronchitis in an athlete is more likely to be in the acute form.
Acute bronchitis usually occurs as an infectious winter disease that follows a common cold or other viral infection of the upper respiratory region. Secondary to this inflammation is a bacterial infection that may follow overexposure to air pollution. Fatigue, malnutrition, and/or chills
could be predisposing factors.

**Symptoms of condition**   The symptoms of an athlete with acute
bronchitis usually start with an upper respiratory tract infection, nasal inflammation and profuse discharge, slight fever, sore throat, and back and
muscle pains. A cough signals the beginning of bronchitis. In the beginning, the cough is dry, but in a few hours or days, a clear mucous secretion begins, becoming yellowish, indicating an infection. In most cases,

---

23–2

***Critical Thinking*** Exercise

A swimmer complains of fever,
cough, headache, malaise,
aching in the back and neck,
and a sore throat.

**?**  What is probably wrong
with this athlete, and how can it
be managed?

---

**rhinitis** (rye **nye** tis)
Inflammation of the nasal
mucous lining.

the fever lasts 3 to 5 days, and the cough lasts 2 to 3 weeks or longer. The athlete may wheeze and rale when auscultation of the chest is performed. Pneumonia can complicate bronchitis.

**Care**   To avoid bronchitis, an athlete should not sleep in an area that is extremely cold or exercise in extremely cold air without wearing a face mask to warm inhaled air. Management of acute bronchitis involves rest until fever subsides, drinking three to four glasses of water per day, and ingesting an antifever medication, a cough suppressor, and using an antibiotic (when severe lung infection is present) daily.

### Bronchial Asthma

**Cause of condition**   As one of the most common respiratory diseases, bronchial asthma can be produced from a number of stressors, such as a viral respiratory tract infection, emotional upset, changes in barometric pressure or temperature, exercise, inhalation of a noxious odor, or exposure to a specific allergen.[13]

**Symptoms of condition**   Bronchial asthma is characterized by a spasm of the bronchial smooth muscles, edema, and inflammation of the mucous lining. In addition to asthma's narrowing of the airway, copious amounts of mucus are produced. Difficulty in breathing may cause the athlete to hyperventilate, resulting in dizziness. The attack may begin with coughing, wheezing, shortness of breath, and fatigue (Focus Box 23-3).

**Care**   Prevention should include efforts to identify and control the causative factors. Acute attacks can be managed by using physician-prescribed medications administered through inhalers. Relief from an inhaler usually occurs in a matter of minutes. If breathing difficulty persists, the athlete should be taken to an emergency care facility.

### Exercise-Induced Asthma (EIA)

**Cause of condition**   Exercise-induced asthma (EIA) is also known as exercise-induced bronchial obstruction. It is a disease that occurs almost exclusively in asthmatic persons. An asthmatic attack can be stimulated by exercise in some individuals and can be provoked in others, only on rare occasions, during moderate exercise. The exact cause of EIA is not clear. Loss of heat and water causes the greatest loss of airway reactivity. Eating certain foods such as shrimp, celery, and peanuts can cause EIA. Sinusitis can also trigger an attack in an individual with chronic asthma.[24]

**Symptoms of condition**   The athlete with EIA may show signs of swelling of the face, swelling of the palms and soles of the feet, chest tightness, shortness of breath, coughing, nausea, hypertension, diarrhea, fatigue, itching, respiratory stridor (high-pitched noise on respiration), headaches, and redness of the skin.[24]

**Care**   Long, continuous running causes the most severe bronchospasm. Swimming is the least bronchospasm producing, which may be because of the moist, warm air environment. A regular exercise program can benefit asthmatics and nonasthmatics. Fewer symptoms occur

The athlete undergoing a sudden asthma attack should:
• Be relaxed and reassured
• Use a previously specified medication
• Drink water
• Perform controlled breathing
• Be removed from what might be triggering the attack

( 23-3 ) **Focus Box**

**Management of the Acute Asthmatic Attack**

Athletes who have a history of asthma usually know how to care for
themselves when an attack occurs. However, the athletic trainer must be
aware of what to look for and what to do if called on.

*Early symptoms and signs*

- Anxious appearance
- Sweating and paleness
- Flared nostrils
- Breathing with pursed lips
- Fast breathing
- Vomiting
- Hunched-over body posture
- Physical fatigue unrelated to activity
- Indentation in the notch below the Adam's apple
- Sinking in of rib spaces as the athlete inhales
- Coughing for no apparent reason
- Excess throat clearing
- Irregular, labored breathing or wheezing

*Actions to take*

- Attempt to relax and reassure the athlete.
- If medication has been cleared by the team physician, have the athlete
  use it.
- Encourage the athlete to drink water.
- Have the athlete perform controlled breathing along with relaxation ex-
  ercises.
- If an environmental factor triggering the attack is known, remove it or
  the athlete from the area.
- If these procedures do not help, immediate medical attention may be
  necessary.

with short, intense work followed by rest than occur with sustained exercise. There should be a gradual warm-up and cooldown. The duration
of exercise should build slowly to 30 to 40 minutes four or five times a
week. Exercise intensity and loading also should be graduated slowly. An
example is 10 to 30 seconds of work followed by 30 to 90 seconds of rest.
Many athletes with chronic asthma and/or EIA use an inhaled bronchodilator. Metered-dose inhalers are preferred for administration. It has
also been found that prophylactic use of the bronchodilator 15 minutes
before exercise delays the symptoms by 2 to 4 hours.[24] Asthmatic athletes
who receive medication for their condition should make sure that what
they take is legal for competition.

A balanced diet is as
important as brushing the
teeth in preventing gum
disease.

# GASTROINTESTINAL DISORDERS

Like any other individual, the athlete may develop various complaints associated with the digestive system. The athlete may display various disorders of the gastrointestinal tract as a result of poor eating habits or the stress related to competition. The responsibility of the coach in such cases is to recognize the more severe conditions so that early referrals to a physician can be made.

## Indigestion

**Cause of condition**   Indigestion (dyspepsia) can be caused by any number of conditions, including food idiosyncrasies, emotional stress before competition, esophageal and stomach spasms, and/or inflammation of the mucous lining of the esophagus and stomach.

**Symptoms of condition**   Indigestion can cause sour stomach, nausea, and flatulence (gas).

**Care**   Care of acute dyspepsia involves the elimination of irritating foods from the diet, development of regular eating habits, and avoidance of anxieties that may lead to gastric distress.

## Vomiting

**Cause of condition**   Vomiting results from some type of irritation, most often in the stomach, that stimulates the vomiting center in the brain to cause a series of forceful contractions of the diaphragm and abdominal muscles, compressing the stomach and forcefully expelling the contents.

**Care**   Antinausea medications should be administered. Fluids to prevent dehydration should be administered by mouth if possible. If vomiting persists, fluids and electrolytes must be administered intravenously.

## Diarrhea

Indigestion, vomiting,
diarrhea, and constipation
are common problems in the
athlete.

**Cause of condition**   Diarrhea can be caused by problems in diet, inflammation of the intestinal lining, gastrointestinal infection, ingestion of certain drugs, and psychogenic factors.

**Symptoms of condition**   Diarrhea is characterized by abdominal cramps, nausea, and possibly vomiting coupled with frequent elimination of stools. Extreme weakness caused by fluid dehydration is usually present. The cause of diarrhea is often difficult to establish.

**Care**   Less severe cases can be cared for by omitting foods that cause irritation, eating bland food until symptoms have ceased, and using over-the-counter medications to control intestinal activity.

## Constipation

**Cause of condition**   Constipation can be caused by insufficient moisture in the feces, causing it to be hard and dry, lack of sufficient roughage and bulk in the diet, poor bowel habits, nervousness and anxiety, or overuse of laxatives and enemas.

**Symptoms of condition**   There is occasional intense cramping and pain in the lower abdomen, with difficulty eliminating hard-packed stools.

**Care**   Athletes can eliminate constipation by eating cereals, fruits, vegetables, and fats that stimulate bowel movement. Laxatives or enemas should be avoided unless their use has been prescribed by a physician.

### Food Poisoning

**Cause of condition**   Food poisoning (gastroenteritis), which may range from mild to severe, results from infectious organisms (bacteria) that enter the body in either food or drink. Foods become contaminated by improper food refrigeration or from an infected food handler.

**Symptoms of condition**   Infection results in nausea, vomiting, cramps, and diarrhea that usually subside in 3 to 6 hours.

**Care**   Management requires rapid replacement of lost fluids and electrolytes, which in severe cases may need to be replaced intravenously. If tolerated, light fluids or foods such as clear, strained broth, bouillon, or bland cereals may be given.

### Gastrointestinal Bleeding

**Cause of condition**   Gastrointestinal bleeding that is reflected in bloody stools can be caused by gastritis, iron-deficiency anemia, ingestion of aspirin or other antiinflammatory agents, colitis, or even stress and bowel irritation. Distance runners often have blood in their stools during and following a race.

**Care**   Athletes with gastrointestinal bleeding must be referred immediately to a physician.

## OTHER CONDITIONS THAT CAN AFFECT THE ATHLETE

### Infectious Mononucleosis

**Cause of condition**   Infectious mononucleosis is an acute viral disease that affects mainly young adults and children. It has major significance to athletes because it can produce severe fatigue and raise the risk of spleen rupture.[20] Incubation is 4 to 6 weeks. The virus is carried in the throat and transmitted to another person by saliva. It has been called the "kissing disease."[20]

**Symptoms of condition**   The disease usually starts with a 3- to 5-day period of headache, fatigue, loss of appetite, and general muscle ache. From the fifth to the fifteenth day, there is fever, swollen lymph glands, and a sore throat.[20] By the second week, 50 to 70 percent of those infected have an enlarged spleen, 10 to 15 percent have jaundice, and 5 to 15 percent have a skin rash, a pinkish flush to the cheeks, and puffy eyelids.[20]

**Care**   Care of mononucleosis is supportive and symptomatic. In many cases the athlete with this disease may resume easy training in 3 weeks after the onset of illness if: (1) the spleen is not markedly enlarged or painful; (2) the athlete is without a fever; (3) liver function tests are normal; and (4) the sore throat and any other complications have been resolved.

## Anemia in Athletes

### Iron-Deficiency Anemia

**Cause of condition**    Iron deficiency is the most common form of true anemia among athletes.[3] It occurs as the result of low levels of **hemoglobin** (the oxygen-carrying molecules in blood) and also of red blood cells (hematocrit). For men, iron deficiency is usually caused by blood loss in the gastrointestinal tract. For women, the most common causes are menstruation and not taking in enough iron in the diet. Athletes who are vegetarians might lack iron.

**Symptoms of condition**    In the first stages of iron deficiency, the athlete's performance begins to decline. The athlete may complain of feeling tired and lethargic. During training there may also be complaints of muscle fatigue and nausea. Athletes with mild iron-deficiency anemia may display some mild impairment in their maximum performance.

**Care**    The athlete with symptoms of anemia should be sent to a physician for blood work to determine the level of hemoglobin and the hematocrit. It is important to differentiate anemia from mononucleosis because symptoms are similar. Some ways that athletes can manage iron deficiency are: (1) follow a proper diet, including more red meat or dark chicken; (2) avoid coffee or tea, which hamper iron absorption from grains; (3) ingest vitamin C sources, which enhance iron absorption; and (4) take an iron supplement.

### Sickle-Cell Anemia

**Cause of condition**    Sickle-cell anemia is a chronic hereditary anemia. The red blood cell with an abnormal sickle shape has less potential for transporting oxygen and is more fragile than normal cells. A sickle cell's life span is 15 to 25 days, compared to the 120-day life span of a normal red cell; this short life of the sickle cell can produce severe anemia in individuals with acute sickle-cell anemia. Approximately 35 percent of the black population in the United States has this condition; 8 to 13 percent are not anemic but carry this trait in their genes (sicklemia).[7] The person with the sickle-cell trait may participate in sports and never encounter problems until symptoms are brought on by some unusual circumstance.[7]

**Symptoms of condition**    An athlete may never experience any complications from having the sickle-cell trait. However, a sickle-cell crisis can be brought on by exposure to high altitudes or by elevated body temperature. Crisis symptoms include fever, severe fatigue, skin pallor, muscle weakness, and severe pain in the limbs and abdomen. Abdominal pain in the right upper quadrant is somewhat common. The athlete may also experience headache and convulsions.[7]

**Care**    Treatment of a sickle-cell crisis is usually symptomatic. The physician may elect to give anticoagulants and analgesics for pain.

---

**hemoglobin**
Molecules that carry oxygen in blood.

## Diabetes Mellitus

**Cause of condition**    Diabetes mellitus is a complex hereditary or developmental disease involving some imbalance between blood sugar and the hormone insulin, which is produced by the pancreas. Decreased effectiveness of insulin or an insufficient amount is responsible for most cases of diabetes. Until recently diabetics were usually discouraged from or forbidden competitive sports participation. Today an ever-increasing number of diabetics are active sports participants, functioning effectively in almost all sports. Because the key to the control of diabetes is the control of blood sugar, the insulin-dependent athlete must constantly juggle food intake, insulin, and exercise to maintain blood sugar in its proper range if he or she is to perform at maximum levels. Diet, exercise, and insulin are the major factors in the everyday lifestyle of the diabetic athlete, who out of necessity must develop an ordered and specific living pattern to cope with the demands of daily existence and strenuous physical activity.[4]

Diabetic athletes engaging in vigorous physical activity should eat before exercising and, if the exercise is protracted, should have hourly glucose supplementation. As a rule the insulin dosage is not changed, but food intake is increased. The response of diabetics varies among individuals and depends on many variables. Although there are some hazards, with proper medical evaluation and planning by a consultant in metabolic diseases, diabetics can feel free to engage in most physical activities.[4]

Problems in the diabetic athlete result either in insulin shock, in which there is too little blood sugar relative to insulin, or in diabetic coma, in which there is too much blood sugar and not enough insulin. Those who work with athletes who have diabetes mellitus must be aware of the major symptoms of diabetic coma and insulin shock and of the proper actions to take when either one occurs.[4]

**Symptoms of insulin shock**    Insulin shock occurs when there is too little blood sugar, resulting in hypoglycemia and shock. It is characterized by physical weakness, moist and pale skin, drooping eyelids, and normal or shallow respirations.

**Care for insulin shock**    The diabetic athlete who either forgets to eat or who engages in intense exercise and metabolizes large amounts of glycogen is more likely to experience insulin shock. To avoid this problem, the athlete must adhere to a carefully planned diet that includes a snack before exercise. The snack should contain a combination of a complex carbohydrate and a protein, for example, cheese and crackers. Activities that last for more than 30 to 40 minutes should be accompanied by snacks and simple carbohydrates. Some diabetics carry with them a lump of sugar or have candy or orange juice readily available in the event that an insulin reaction seems imminent.[4]

Key questions to ask a diabetic athlete are:

- Have you eaten today and when?
- Have you taken your insulin today and when?

**Symptoms of diabetic coma**  The signs of a diabetic coma include labored breathing or gasping for air, fruity-smelling breath (caused by acetone), nausea and vomiting, extreme thirst, dry mucous lining of the mouth, flushed skin, and mental confusion or unconsciousness followed by coma.

**Care for diabetic coma**  Because the diabetic coma threatens life, early detection is essential.  The only way to correct the insulin–blood sugar imbalance of a diabetic coma is to inject insulin. An injection of insulin into the athlete normally prevents coma. If the athlete does not respond within minutes following injection, emergency care is needed.

## Epilepsy

Individuals who have major daily or weekly seizures may be prohibited from collision sports.

**Cause of condition**  Epilepsy is not a disease but is a symptom manifested by a large number of underlying disorders. For some types of epilepsy there is a genetic predisposition and a low threshold to having seizures. In others, altered brain metabolism or a history of injury may be the cause.

Each person with epilepsy must be considered individually as to whether he or she should engage in competitive sports. The general recommendation is that an individual who has daily or even weekly major seizures should not participate in collision sports. This prohibition is not because a hit in the head necessarily triggers a seizure, but because unconsciousness during participation could result in a serious injury. If the seizures are properly controlled by medication or only occur during sleep, little if any sports restriction should be imposed except for scuba diving, swimming alone, or participation in activities at some height.[23]

**Symptoms of condition**  Epilepsy is defined as "a recurrent disorder of cerebral function characterized by a sudden, brief attack of altered consciousness, motor activity, sensory phenomena, or inappropriate behavior." A seizure can range from extremely brief episodes (petit mal seizures) to major episodes (grand mal seizures), unconsciousness, and tonic-clonic muscle contractions.[23]

**Care**  The athlete commonly takes an anticonvulsant medication that is specific for the type and degree of seizures that occur. On occasion an athlete may experience some undesirable side effects from drug therapy, such as drowsiness, restlessness, nystagmus, nausea, vomiting, problems with balance, skin rash, or other adverse reactions.[23]

When an athlete with epilepsy becomes aware of an impending seizure, he or she should immediately sit or lie down to avoid injury. When a seizure occurs without warning, the following steps should be taken by the coach:

- Be emotionally composed.
- If possible, cushion the athlete's fall.
- Keep the athlete away from surrounding objects that may cause injury.
- Loosen restricting clothing.

| **TABLE 23-1** Age and blood pressure limits | |
| --- | --- |
| **Age** | **Upper Blood Pressure Limits at Rest\*** |
| <10 | 120/75 mm Hg |
| 10–12 | 125/80 mm Hg |
| 13–15 | 135/85 mm Hg |
| 16–18 | 140/90 mm Hg |
| >18 | 140/90 mm Hg |

\*If the upper limits of blood pressure are exceeded during three measurements, the athlete may have hypertension.

- Do not try to force anything between the athlete's teeth.
- Allow the athlete to awaken normally after the seizure.

## Hypertension (High Blood Pressure)

**Cause of condition**   Excessive pressure applied against the arterial wall while the blood circulates is known as hypertension, or high blood pressure (HBP). A normal, average pressure is 120/80 mm Hg. HBP is 140/90 mm Hg and over (Table 23-1.)

Hypertension is classified as primary, or essential, and secondary. Primary hypertension accounts for 90 percent of all cases and has no disease associated with it.[12] Secondary hypertension is related to a specific underlying cause such as a kidney disorder, overactive adrenal glands (increased blood volume), hormone-producing tumor, narrowing of the aorta, pregnancy, or medications (oral contraceptives, cold remedies, etc.). The presence of prolonged HBP increases the chances of coronary artery disease, congestive heart failure, or stroke.[12]

**Symptoms of condition**   Primary hypertension is usually asymptomatic until complications occur. Uncomplicated HBP may cause dizziness, a flushed face, headache, fatigue, epistaxis, and nervousness.

**Care**   The existence of HBP is not established until many pressure readings have been taken at various times. A thorough physical examination must be conducted to ascertain the type of hypertension. Primary hypertension can be controlled with life changes such as weight loss, salt restriction, and aerobic exercise. In secondary hypertension, when the underlying condition is cured, the blood pressure commonly returns to normal. Athletes with HBP should avoid isometrics and resistive exercise against very heavy weight.[12]

## Common Contagious Viral Diseases

It is not within the scope of this text to describe in detail all the various infectious diseases to which athletes may be prone. However, on occasion the athlete may exhibit recognizable manifestations of such a disease; a coach should be aware of certain signs that might indicate a contagious viral disease (Table 23-2). When indications of a contagious

**TABLE 23-2** Some infectious viral diseases

| Disease | Sites Involved | Signs of Conditions | Care | Prevention |
|---|---|---|---|---|
| Measles (rubeola) | Skin, respiratory tract, and conjunctivae | Appearance—like common cold with fever, cough, conjunctivitis, photophobia, and spots in throat, followed by skin rash | Bed rest and use of smoked glasses; symptomatic | Vaccine available |
| German measles (rubella) | Skin, respiratory tract, and conjunctivae | Cold symptoms, skin rash, and swollen lymph nodes behind ear | Symptomatic | Vaccine available; gamma globulin given in postexposure situations |
| Chicken pox (varicella) | Trunk; then face, neck, and limbs | Mild cold symptoms followed by appearance of vesicles | Symptomatic | Vaccine available, including zoster immune globulin (ZIG) or varicell-zoster immune globulin (VZIG) |
| Mumps (epidemic parotiditis) | Salivary glands | Headache, drowsiness, fever, abdominal pain, pain during chewing and swallowing, swelling of neck under jaw | Symptomatic | Temporary immunization by virus vaccine |
| Influenza (flu) | Respiratory tract | Aching of low back, generalized aching, chills, headache, fever, and bronchitis | Symptomatic | Moderate temporary protection from polyvalent influenza virus |
| Cold (coryza) | Respiratory tract | Mild fever, headache, chills, and nasal discharge | Symptomatic | Possible help from vitamins and/or cold vaccine; avoid exposure |
| Infectious mononucleosis | Trunk | Sore throat, fever, skin rash, general aching, and swelling of lymph glands | Symptomatic | None; avoid extreme fatigue |

disease are present, the coach must refer the athlete to a physician without delay.

## SUBSTANCE ABUSE AMONG ATHLETES

There is increasing concern about the number of athletes engaging in substance abuse (Focus Box 23-4). Some do so in an attempt to improve performance, whereas others engage in it as a recreational pursuit. Much material has been written and discussed about the use of performance-enhancing drugs among Olympic athletes and about the widespread use of street drugs by high school, collegiate, and professional athletes. **Clearly, substance abuse has no place in the athletic population.**[10]

### Performance-Enhancing Drugs

In sports medicine, the administration of a drug that is designed to improve the competitor's performance is known as **doping.** The Interna-

**doping**
The administration of a drug that is designed to improve the competitor's performance.

(23-4)  *Focus Box*

**Identifying the Substance Abuser**

The following are signs of drug abuse:

1. Sudden personality changes
2. Severe mood swings
3. Changing peer groups
4. Decreased interest in extracurricular and leisure activities
5. Worsening grades
6. Disregard for household chores and curfews
7. Feeling of depression most of the time
8. Breakdown in personal hygiene habits
9. Increased sleep and decreased eating
10. Clothes and skin smell of alcohol or marijuana
11. Sudden weight loss
12. Lying, cheating, stealing, etc.
13. Arrests for drunk driving or for possessing illegal substances
14. Truancies from school
15. Frequent job changes or loss
16. Defensiveness at the mention of drugs or alcohol
17. Increased isolation (spends time in room)
18. Family relationship deteriorates
19. Drug paraphernalia (needles, empty bottles, etc.) found
20. Others make observations about negative behavior
21. Signs of intoxication
22. Constantly misses appointments
23. Falls asleep in class or at work
24. Has financial problems
25. Misses assignments or deadlines
26. Diminished productivity

tional Olympic Committee (IOC) defines doping as "the administration or use of substances in any form alien to the body or of physiological substances in abnormal amounts and with abnormal methods by healthy persons with the exclusive aim of attaining an artificial and unfair increase in performance in sports."

### Stimulants

The intention of the athlete when he or she ingests a stimulant may be to increase alertness, to reduce fatigue, or in some instances, to increase competitiveness; ingestion can produce hostility. Some athletes respond to stimulants with a loss of judgment that may lead to personal injury or injury to others.[10]

**Amphetamines** Amphetamines, caffeine and cocaine are the stimulant drugs most commonly used in sports. (Cocaine is discussed in the section on recreational drug abuse.) Amphetamines present an extremely difficult problem in sports because they are commonly found in cold remedies, nasal and ophthalmic decongestants, and most asthma preparations. The IOC has approved some substances to be used by asthmatics who develop exercise-induced bronchospasms. Before an athlete engages in Olympic competition, his or her team physician must notify the IOC Medical Subcommission in writing concerning drug usage.

Amphetamines are extremely powerful and dangerous drugs. They may be injected, inhaled, or taken as tablets. Amphetamines are among the most abused of the drugs used for enhancing sports performance. In ordinary doses, amphetamines can produce an increased sense of well-being and heightened mental activity—until fatigue sets in (from lack of sleep), accompanied by nervousness, insomnia, and anorexia. In high doses, amphetamines reduce mental activity and impair performance of complicated motor skills. The athlete's behavior may become irrational. The chronic user may get hung up, or in other words, become stuck, in a repetitive behavioral sequence. This behavior may last for hours, becoming increasingly more irrational. The long-term, or even short-term, use of amphetamines can lead to amphetamine psychosis, manifested by auditory and visual hallucinations and paranoid delusions. Physiologically, high doses of amphetamines can cause abnormal pupillary dilation, increased blood pressure, and hyperthermia.

Athletes believe that amphetamines improve sports performance by promoting quickness and endurance, delaying fatigue, and increasing confidence, thereby causing increased aggressiveness. Studies indicate that there is no improvement in performance, but there is an increased risk of injury, exhaustion, and circulation collapse.

**Caffeine** Caffeine is found in coffee, tea, cocoa, and cola, and is readily absorbed into the body (Table 23-3). It is a central nervous system stimulant and diuretic and also stimulates gastric secretion. One cup of coffee can contain from 100 to 150 mg of caffeine. In moderation, caf-

**TABLE 23-3** Examples of caffeine-containing products

| Product | Dose |
| --- | --- |
| Coffee (1 cup) | 100 mg |
| Diet Coke (12 oz) | 45.6 mg |
| Diet Pepsi (12 oz) | 36.0 mg |
| No-Doz (1) | 100.0 mg |
| Anacin (1) | 32.0 mg |
| Excedrin (1) | 65.0 mg |
| Midol (1) | 32.4 mg |

feine results in wakefulness and mental alertness. In larger amounts and in individuals who ingest caffeine daily, it raises blood pressure, and decreases and then increases the heart rate. It affects coordination, sleep, mood, behavior, and thinking processes. In terms of exercise and sports performance, caffeine is controversial. Like amphetamines, caffeine can affect some athletes by acting as an ergogenic aid during prolonged exercise. A habitual user of caffeine who suddenly stops may experience withdrawal, including headache, drowsiness, lethargy, rhinorrhea, irritability, nervousness, depression, and loss of interest in work. Caffeine also acts as a diuretic when hydration may be important.

### Narcotic Analgesic Drugs

Narcotic analgesic drugs are derived directly or indirectly from opium. Morphine and codeine (methylmorphine) are examples of substances made from opium. Narcotic analgesics are used for the management of moderate-to-severe pain. They have been banned by the IOC because of the high risk of physical and psychological dependency and because of many other problems stemming from their use. Slight-to-moderate pain can be effectively dealt with by drugs other than narcotics.

### Beta Blockers

In sports, beta blockers have been used by athletes who require steadiness, whose signs of nervousness must be in control while engaging in sports such as target shooting, sailing, archery, fencing, ski jumping, and luge. Beta blockers relax the blood vessels. This relaxation, in turn, slows heart rate and decreases cardiac output. Therapeutically, beta blockers are used for a variety of cardiac diseases and for treating hypertension.

### Diuretics

Diuretics are used for a variety of cardiovascular and respiratory conditions (e.g., hypertension) in which elimination of fluids from tissues is necessary. Sports participants have misused diuretics mainly in two ways: to reduce body weight quickly or to decrease a drug's concentration in the urine (increasing its excretion to avoid the detection of drug misuse). In both cases, there are ethical and health grounds for banning certain classes of diuretics from use during Olympic competition.

### Anabolic Steroids and Human Growth Hormone

Two substances related to the increase of muscle build, strength, power, and growth are anabolic steroids and human growth hormone (HGH).

**Anabolic steroids**   Androgenic hormones are products of the male testes. Of these hormones, testosterone is the principal one; it possesses the ability to function androgenically (to stimulate male characteristics) and anabolically (through improved protein assimilation, increase muscle mass and weight, general growth, bone maturation, and virility).[21] When prescribed by a physician to improve certain physiological conditions,

**Examples of Deleterious Effects of Anabolic Steroids**

- *Teens*—presmature closure of long bones, acne, hirsutism, voice deepening, enlarged mammary glands (gynecomastia) of the male
- *Men*—male-pattern baldness, acne, voice deepening, mood swings, aggressive behavior, decreased high-density lipoprotein, increased cholesterol, reduction in size of testicle, reduced testosterone production, changes in libido
- *Women*—female-pattern baldness, acne, voice deepening (irreversible), increased facial hair, enlarged clitoris (irreversible), increased libido, menstrual irregularities, increased aggression, decreased body fat, increased appetite, decreased breast size
- *Abuse*—may lead to liver tumors and cancer, heart disease, and hypertension

these drugs have value. In 1984, the American College of Sports Medicine (ACSM) reported that anabolic androgenic steroids taken with an adequate diet could contribute to an increase in body weight and, with a heavy resistance program, to a significant gain in strength. However, in sports, anabolic steroids constitute a major threat to the health of the athlete (Focus Box 23-5). Anabolic steroids present an ethical dilemma for the sports world. It is estimated that more than a million young male and female athletes are taking them, with most being purchased through the black market. It is estimated that 6.5 percent of male and 1.4 percent of female high school students take or have taken anabolic steroids. Also an estimated 2 to 20 percent of male intercollegiate athletes take anabolic steroids.

If these drugs are given to the prepubertal boy, a most certain hazard is a decrease in his ultimate height because of the cessation of long bone growth. Acne, hirsutism, a deepening of the voice in the prepubescent boy, and in some cases, a swelling of the breasts, called *gynecomastia*, are among other androgen effects. The ingestion of steroids by females can result in **hirsutism** and in a deepening of the voice because of vocal cord alteration. When the dosage is halted, the hirsutism may cease, but the change in the vocal cords is irreversible. As the duration and dosage increase, the possibility of producing androgen effects also increases. Because self-administered overdosage seems to be the pattern of those who use steroids, the preceding statement is most significant. Abuse of these drugs may also lead to cancer of the liver and prostate glands and to heart disease.[21]

Anabolic steroids are most abused in sports that involve strength. Power lifting, the throwing events in track and field, and American football are some of the sports in which the use of anabolic steroids is a serious problem. Because female athletes are developing the attitude of "win

**hirsutism (her** soot ism)
Excessive hair growth
and/or the presence of hair
in unusual places.

at all costs," their abuse of anabolic steroids is also becoming a major health concern.

**Human growth hormone**   Human growth hormone (HGH) is a hormone produced by the pituitary gland. It is released into circulation in a pulsating manner. This release can vary with a person's age and developmental period. A lack of HGH can result in dwarfism. In the past, HGH was in limited supply because it was extracted from cadavers. Now, however, it can be made synthetically and is more available.[18]

Experiments indicate that HGH can increase muscle mass, skin thickness, connective tissues in muscle, and organ weight and can produce lax muscles and ligaments during rapid growth phases. It also increases body length and weight and decreases body fat percentage.

The use of HGH by athletes throughout the world is on the increase because it is more difficult to detect in urine than anabolic steroids are. There is currently a lack of concrete information about the effects of HGH on the athlete who does not have a growth problem. It is known that an overabundance of HGH in the body can lead to premature closure of long-bone growth sites or, conversely, can cause acromegaly, a condition that produces elongation and enlargement of bones of the extremities and thickening of bones and soft tissues of the face. Also associated with acromegaly is diabetes mellitus, cardiovascular disease, goiter, menstrual disorders, decreased sexual desire, and impotence. It decreases the life span by up to 20 years. Like anabolic steroids, HGH presents a serious problem for the sports world. At this time there is no proof that an increase of HGH combined with weight training contributes to strength and muscle hypertrophy.

### Androstenedione

Androstenedione is a relatively weak androgen that is produced primarily in the testes and in lesser amounts by the adrenal cortex and ovaries.[21] It has been used in humans to increase testosterone in men and particularly women, however, the effect lasted only for a few hours. Currently, the FDA classifies commercially produced androstenedione as a dietary supplement. To date, there is no scientific base of research to support or deny the efficacy or safety of using this ergogenic aid.

### Creatine Supplementation

Creatine is a naturally occurring organic compound synthesized by the kidneys, liver, and pancreas. Creatine can also be obtained from the ingestion of meat and fish, which contain approximately 5 g/kg. Creatine has an integral role in energy metabolism. The positive physiological effects of creatine include increasing the intensity in a workout; prolonging maximal effort and improving exercise recovery time during maximal intensity activities; stimulating protein synthesis; decreasing total cholesterol; decreasing total triglycerides; and increasing fat-free mass. Side effects of creatine supplementation include weight gain and occasional muscle cramping, however, there are apparently no other

Recognition and
Management of Specific
Injuries and Conditions

23–3

*Critical Thinking* Exercise

A high school shot putter has read about the effects of creatine in a trade magazine and is excited about trying this supplement. He comes to the coach to ask about the benefits of using creatine.

**?** How should the coach respond?

Not only is the use of blood reinjection in competition unethical, but when conducted by nonmedical personnel, it could prove dangerous.

known long-term side effects. It has been suggested that oral supplementation with creatine may enhance muscular performance during high-intensity resistance exercise.[14]

### Other Drugs Subject to IOC Restriction

The IOC indicates that although it does not expressly prohibit alcohol, blood alcohol levels may be determined at the request of the committee. Local anesthetics that are injected (excluding cocaine) are permitted. Corticosteroids have been abused because of their ability to produce euphoria and certain side effects. They are, therefore, banned during the Olympic Games except for topical use or for inhalation therapy and intraarticular injections.

### Blood Reinjection (Blood Doping, Blood Packing, and Blood Boosting)

Endurance, acclimatization, and altitude make increased metabolic demands on the body, which responds by increasing blood volume and red blood cells to meet the increased aerobic demands.[1]

Recently researchers have replicated these physiological responses by removing 900 ml of blood, storing it, and reinfusing it after 6 weeks. The reason for waiting at least 6 weeks before reinfusion is it takes that long for the athlete's body to reestablish a normal hemoglobin and red blood cell concentration. Using this method, endurance performance has been significantly improved. From the standpoint of scientific research, such experimentation has merit and is of interest. However, not only is use of such methods in competition unethical, but when conducted by nonmedical personnel, it could prove to be dangerous, especially when a matched donor is used.

There are serious risks with transfusing blood and related blood products. The risks include allergic reactions, kidney damage (if the wrong type of blood is used), fever, jaundice, the possibility of transmitting infectious diseases (viral hepatitis or HIV), or blood overload, resulting in circulatory and metabolic shock.

### Recreational Drug Abuse

Just as it has become a part of the general world, recreational drug use has become a part of the world of sports. Reasons for using these substances may include desire to experiment, to temporarily escape from problems, or to just be part of a group (peer pressure). For some, recreational drug use leads to abuse and dependence. There are two general aspects of dependence: psychological and physical. Psychological dependence is the drive to repeat the ingestion of a drug to produce pleasure or to avoid discomfort. Physical dependence is the state of drug adaptation that manifests itself as the development of tolerance and, when the drug is removed, causes a withdrawal syndrome. Tolerance of a drug is the need to increase the dosage to create the effect that was obtained previously by smaller amounts. The withdrawal syndrome consists of an unpleasant physiological reaction when the drug is abruptly stopped. Some drugs that are abused by the athlete overlap with those thought to enhance performance. Examples include amphetamines and cocaine. Tobacco (nicotine), alcohol, cocaine, and marijuana are the most abused recreational drugs. The coach might also come in contact with abuse by athletes of barbiturates, nonbarbiturate sedatives, psychotomimetic drugs, or different inhalants.

### Tobacco

A number of current problems are related to tobacco and sports. They can be divided into two headings: cigarette smoking and the use of smokeless tobacco.

**Cigarette smoking**    On the basis of various investigations into the relationship between smoking and performance, the following conclusions can be drawn:

- Individuals vary in sensitivity to tobacco, and relatively high sensitivity may seriously affect performance. Because more than one-third of men studied indicate tobacco sensitivity, it may be wise to prohibit smoking by athletes.
- Tobacco smoke has been associated with as many as 4,700 different chemicals, many of which are toxic.
- As few as ten inhalations of cigarette smoke cause an average maximum decrease in airway conductance of 50 percent. This decrease occurs as well in nonsmokers who inhale secondhand smoke.
- Smoking reduces the oxygen-carrying capacity of the blood. A smoker's blood carries five to ten times more carbon monoxide than normal; thus the red blood cells are prevented from picking up sufficient oxygen to meet the demands of the body's tissues. The carbon monoxide also tends to make arterial walls more permeable to fatty substances, a factor in atherosclerosis.
- Smoking aggravates and accelerates the heart muscle cells through overstimulation of the sympathetic nervous system.
- Total lung capacity and maximum breathing capacity are significantly decreased in heavy smokers; this is important to the athlete because both changes impair the capacity to take in oxygen and make it readily available for body use.
- Smoking decreases pulmonary diffusing capacity.
- After smoking, an accelerated thrombolic tendency is evidenced.
- Smoking is a carcinogenic factor in lung cancer and is a contributing factor to heart disease.

The addictive chemical of tobacco is nicotine, which is one of the most toxic drugs. When ingested, nicotine causes blood pressure elevation, increased bowel activity, and an antidiuretic action. Moderate tolerance and physical dependence occur. It also has been noted that passive inhalation of cigarette smoke can reduce maximum aerobic power and endurance capacity.

**Use of smokeless tobacco**   It is estimated that 36 percent of athletes use smokeless tobacco, which comes in three forms: loose-leaf, moist or dry powder (snuff), and compressed. The tobacco is placed between the cheek and the gum, where it is sucked and chewed. Aesthetically, this is an unsavory habit during which an athlete is continually spitting into a container. Besides the unpleasant appearance, the use of smokeless tobacco poses an extremely serious health risk. Smokeless tobacco causes bad breath, stained teeth, tooth sensitivity to heat and cold, cavities, gum recession, tooth bone loss, leukoplakia, and oral and throat cancer. Aggressive oral and throat cancer and periodontal destruction (with tooth loss) have been associated with this habit. The major substance injested is nitrosonornicotine, which is the drug responsible for this habit's addictiveness. This chemical makes smokeless tobacco a more addictive habit than smoking is. Smokeless tobacco increases heart rate but does not affect reaction time, movement time, or total response time among athletes or nonathletes.

Coaches, athletic trainers, and professional athletes themselves must avoid the use of smokeless tobacco to present a positive role model.

### Alcohol

Alcohol consumption, at any time or in any amount, does not improve mental or physical abilities and should be avoided by athletes.

Alcohol is the number one abused drug in the United States. Alcohol is absorbed directly into the bloodstream through the small intestine. It accumulates in the blood because alcohol absorption is faster than its oxidation. It acts as a central nervous system depressant, producing sedation and tranquility. Characteristically, alcohol consumption, at any time and in any amount, does not improve mental or physical abilities and should be completely avoided by athletes. Alcohol consumption on a large scale can lead to a moderate degree of tolerance. Alcohol has no place in sports participation.[6]

### Cocaine

Cocaine, sometimes called "coke," "snow," "toot," "happy dust," and "white girl," is a powerful central nervous system stimulant and a local anesthetic and vasoconstrictor. Besides being a banned performance enhancer, cocaine is one of the most abused recreational drugs. It can be inhaled, smoked, or injected (intravenously, subcutaneously, or intramuscularly).

In high doses cocaine, which is found in the leaves of the coca bush, causes a sense of excitement and euphoria. On occasion it also produces hallucinations. When applied locally to the skin, cocaine acts as an anesthetic; however, when taken into the body through inhalation, snorting, or injection, it acts on the central nervous system.

**Crack**   Crack, a highly purified form of cocaine, is smoked and is known to produce a virtually instantaneous high. Habitual use of cocaine does not lead to physical tolerance or dependence but does cause psychological dependence and addiction. When cocaine is used recreationally, the athlete feels alert, self-satisfied, and powerful. Heavy usage can produce paranoid delusions and violent behavior. Overuse can lead to overstimulation of the sympathetic nervous system and can cause tachycardia, hypertension, extra heartbeats, coronary vasoconstriction, strokes, pulmonary edema, aortic rupture, and sudden death.

### Marijuana

Marijuana is another one of the most abused drugs in Western society. It is more commonly called "grass," "weed," "pot," "dope," or "hemp." The marijuana cigarette is called a "joint," "j," "number," "reefer," or "root." Marijuana is not a harmless drug. The components of marijuana smoke are similar to those of tobacco smoke and the same cellular changes are observed in the user.

Continued use leads to respiratory diseases such as asthma and bronchitis and to a decrease in vital capacity of 15 to 40 percent (certainly detrimental to physical performance). Among other deleterious effects are lowered sperm counts and testosterone levels. Evidence of interference with the functioning of the immune system and cellular metabolism has also been found. The most consistent sign of this interference is an increase in pulse rate, which averages close to 20 percent higher during exercise and is a definite factor in limiting performance. Some decrease in leg, hand, and finger strength has been found at higher dosages. Like tobacco, marijuana must be considered carcinogenic.

Psychological effects such as a diminution of self-awareness and judgment, a slowdown of thinking, and a shorter attention span appear early in the use of the drug. Postmortem examinations of habitual users reveal not only cerebral atrophy but alterations of anatomical structures, which suggest irreversible brain damage. Marijuana also contains unique substances (cannabinoids) that are stored, in much the same manner as are fat cells, throughout the body and in the brain tissues for weeks and even months. These stored quantities result in a cumulative deleterious effect on the habitual user.

A drug such as marijuana has no place in sports. Claims for its use are unsubstantiated, and the harmful effects, both immediate and long-term, are too significant to permit indulgence at any time.

## MENSTRUAL IRREGULARITIES AND THE FEMALE REPRODUCTIVE SYSTEM

During the prepubertal period, girls are the equal of, and are often superior to, boys of the same age in activities requiring speed, strength, and endurance. The difference between males and females is not readily apparent until after puberty. At puberty males begin to exhibit a slow, gradual increase in strength, speed, and endurance.

Menarche, the onset of the menses, normally occurs between the tenth and the seventeenth year, and the majority of girls enter it between

During the prepubertal period, girls are the equal of, and are often superior to, boys of the same age in activities requiring speed, strength, and endurance.

Recognition and
Management of Specific
Injuries and Conditions

The onset of menarche may
be delayed by strenuous
training and competition.

13 and 15 years of age. There is some indication that strenuous training and competition may delay the onset of menarche. The greatest delay is related to higher caliber competition. The late-maturing girl commonly has longer legs, narrower hips, and less adiposity and body weight for her height, all of which are more conducive to sports.[11]

As interest and participation in girls' and women's sports grow, the various myths that have surrounded female participation and the effects of participation on menarche, menstruation, and childbirth are gradually being dispelled. The effects of sustained and strenuous training and competition on the menstrual cycle and the effects of menstruation on performance, however, still cannot be fully explained.

## Menstrual Irregularities

> **amenorrhea**
> (amen oh **ree** ah)
> Absence or suppression of
> menstruation.

Menarche may be delayed in highly physically active women. **Amenorrhea** (absence of menses) and *oligomenorrhea* (diminished flow) have been common in professional female ballet dancers, gymnasts, and long-distance runners.[8] Runners who decrease training, because of an injury for example, often report a return of regular menses. Weight gain together with less intense exercise also is reported to reverse amenorrhea and oligomenorrhea. Because these irregularities may or may not be normal aspects of thinness and hard physical training, it is advisable that a physician be consulted. To date, there is no indication that these conditions adversely affect reproduction. Almost any type of menstrual disorder can be caused by overly stressful and demanding sports activity—amenorrhea, dysmenorrhea, menorrhagia (excessive menstruation), oligomenorrhea, polymenorrhea (abnormal frequent menstruation), irregular periods, or any combination of these.[11]

### Dysmenorrhea

Women who have moderate-to-severe dysmenorrhea require examination by a physician.

Dysmenorrhea (painful menstruation) apparently is prevalent among more active women; however, it is inconclusive whether specific sports participation can alleviate or produce dysmenorrhea. For women with moderate-to-severe dysmenorrhea, gynecological consultation is warranted to rule out a pathological condition.

Dysmenorrhea is caused by ischemia (a lack of normal blood flow to the pelvic organs) or by a possible hormonal imbalance. This syndrome, which is identified by cramps, nausea, lower abdominal pain, headache, and, on occasion, emotional lability, is the most common menstrual disorder. Physicians usually prescribe mild-to-vigorous exercises that help ameliorate dysmenorrhea. Physicians also generally advise a continuance of the usual sports participation during the menstrual period, provided the performance level of the individual does not drop below her customary level of ability. Among athletes, swimmers have the highest incidence of dysmenorrhea; it occurs most often, quite probably, as the result of strenuous sports participation during the menses. Generally, oligomenorrhea, amenorrhea, and irregular or scanty flow are more common in sports that require strenuous exertion over a long period. A

23–4

*Critical Thinking* Exercise

A female athlete has been
diagnosed as having both an
eating disorder and
amenorrhea.

? Why may these two medical
disorders eventually be
associated with osteoporosis?

great deal of variability exists among female athletes with regard to the menstrual pattern and its effect on physical performance. Each individual must learn to make adjustments to her lifestyle that permit her sto function effectively and efficiently with a minimum of discomfort or restriction.

## The Female Athletic Triad

A young female athlete, driven to excel in her chosen sport and pressured to fit a specific athletic image to reach her goals, is at risk for the development of the *female athletic triad*. It is a combination of three medical disorders including disordered eating, amenorrhea, and osteoporosis, a bone disease marked by softening and decreased density.[17] Focus Box 23-6 identifies lifestyle habits that may place a woman at risk for female athletic triad.

Disordered eating can include any combination of anorexia, bulimia, and/or excessive exercise. It can lead to malnutrition, which obviously has a negative impact on the ability of the female to perform athletically. In addition, chronic fatigue, compromise of the immune system, and often depression have been associated with disordered eating. Certainly disordered eating can lead to serious illness and even death.[17]

Amenorrhea is the absence of the menstrual cycle for more than 6 months. Normal hormonal cycles stop when body weight is too low. Normal estrogen levels are essential for bones to use calcium. A decrease in estrogen levels also interferes with the activity of bone-producing cells, which eventually causes the bones to become weak and increases the likelihood of stress fracture.

Osteoporosis includes not only bone loss but also new bone formation. Fractures can occur in the hip, spine, foot, or other sites without any visible evidence.

The effects of female athletic triad can be reversed by returning to normal exercise and eating patterns that allow for return of normal menstrual periods thus preventing further bone loss.

---

### 23-6    *Focus Box*

**Identifying a woman at risk for female athletic triad:**

- Compulsive exercise for more than 1 hour a day
- Cannot skip a day of exercise
- Restricts the amounts and kind of foods consumed
- Eats alone most of the time
- Thinks and talks a lot about food and body weight
- Seems depressed
- Has excessive injuries related to activity
- Irregular or absent menstrual periods

## Contraceptives

Female athletes have been known to take extra oral contraceptive pills to delay menstruation during competition. This practice is not recommended because the pills should be taken no more than 21 days, followed by a 7-day break. Side effects range from nausea, vomiting, fluid retention, and amenorrhea to the extreme effects of hypertension and double vision. Some oral contraceptives make women hypersensitive to the sun. Any use of oral contraceptives related to physical performance should be under the express direction and control of a physician. However, oral contraceptive use is acceptable for females with no medical problems who have coitus at least twice a week. New low-dose preparations, containing less than 50 mg of estrogen, add negligible risks for the healthy woman.[8]

## Exercise During Pregnancy

During pregnancy, athletes exhibit high levels of muscle tonicity. Women who suffer from a chronic disability after childbirth usually have a record of little or no physical exercise in the decade immediately preceding pregnancy. Generally, competition may be engaged in well into the third month of pregnancy unless bleeding or cramps are present and can frequently be continued until the seventh month if no handicapping or physiological complications arise. Such activity may make pregnancy, childbirth, and postparturition less stressful. Many athletes do not continue beyond the third month because of a drop in their performance that can result from a number of reasons, some related to their pregnancy, others perhaps psychological. It is during the first 3 months of pregnancy that the dangers of disturbing the pregnancy are greatest. After that period there is less danger to the mother and fetus because the pregnancy is stabilized. There is no indication that mild-to-moderate exercise during pregnancy is harmful to fetal growth and development or causes reduced fetal mass, increased perinatal or neonatal mortality, or physical or mental retardation.[8] It has been found, however, that extreme exercise may lower birth weight.

Many athletes compete during pregnancy with no ill effects. Most physicians, although advocating moderate activity during this period, believe that especially vigorous performance, particularly in activities in which there may be severe body contact or heavy jarring or falls, should be avoided.

## SEXUALLY TRANSMITTED INFECTIONS (STIs)

Sexually transmitted infections (STIs) are of major concern in sports because many athletes are at an age during which they are more sexually active than they will be at any other time in their lives. Sexually transmitted infections are infectious diseases that can be contracted through sexual contact. Any of the STIs can potentially be transmitted through sexual contact (including vaginal and anal intercourse and oral-genital

**TABLE 23-4** Sexually transmitted infections

| STI | Signs | Care | Possible Problems |
|---|---|---|---|
| Chlamydia | About 75% of infected people have no symptoms. However, there may be a mild mucuslike discharge from the genitals or stinging when urinating. Also, there may be pain in the testicles (men) or abdomen (women). | Infected persons and their sexual partners must be tested and treated with antibiotics. | Painful infections of the reproductive organs, which may lead to infertility in both men and women. |
| Genital herpes | Sores around genitals or anus, often with small, painful blisters. Some people have no symptoms but are still infected and contagious. | Infected persons should avoid intimate sexual contact while sores persist. Acyclovir capsules or ointment may be helpful but will not cure herpes. | May contribute to cervical cancer and be transmitted to infants during childbirth. |
| Crab lice | Visible, blood-sucking lice in pubic hair. Causes itching. Eggs (nits) attached to hair shafts. | Treatments to kill lice. Recent sexual partners, clothing, and bed linen should be treated. | None. |
| Genital warts | Usually painless growths around the genitals or anus occur about 1–3 months after contact. In rare cases, growths may itch, burn, or bleed, or may not appear for years. | Chemical treatment, liquid nitrogen, laser beam, or surgery. May return after treatment. | May obstruct the urethra or complicate vaginal delivery in childbirth; may be connected to cervical cancer. |
| Trichomoniasis | Among women, symptoms may include a vaginal discharge, discomfort during sexual intercourse, abdominal pain, pain when urinating, and itching in the genital area. Most men have no symptoms, but some men may experience a penile discharge, painful urinating, or a "tingly" feeling in the penis. | Infected persons and their partners are treated with antibiotics. | If untreated, may lead to bladder and urethral infections in men and women. |
| Gonorrhea | Men may have a creamy puslike penile discharge and pain when urinating, or they may have no symptoms. Women may have vaginal discharge and pain when urinating, but often have no symptoms. | Infected persons and their sexual partners must be tested and treated with antibiotics. | If untreated, can cause arthritis, dermatitis, heart problems, and reproductive problems in both men and women. Can be transmitted to infants at birth, causing blindness. |
| Syphilis | Painless ulcer (chancre) at point of contact, usually penile shaft, around vaginal opening, or anus. Secondary stage may include rash or swollen lymph nodes. | Infected persons and their sexual partners must be tested and treated with antibiotics. | If untreated, may affect brain or heart, or even be fatal. Pregnant women can transmit to unborn infant. |
| AIDS (Acquired immunodeficiency syndrome) | Increased susceptibility to common infections and unusual cancers. Most people infected with the virus may show no symptoms for many years but are still contagious. | No current proven treatment. Avoid sexual contact or practice safe sex. | Full-blown AIDs almost always is fatal. Outlook for carriers of the virus is uncertain. |

For more information on AIDS, see chapter 8.

contact) with an infected partner who may or may not show any signs or symptoms. STIs may be caused by bacteria or viruses. Bacterial infections such as gonorrhea, syphilis, and chlamydia may be cured with antibiotics in the majority of cases. Serious health problems are prevented if these infections are diagnosed and treated early. Viral infections such as herpes, genital warts, and HIV are much more difficult to treat, and in some cases no cure exists.

STIs do not go away by themselves, and in many cases, relatively quick, painless treatments are available. No one is immune to STIs. Everyone who is sexually active can get or transmit an STI. The current trend is to emphasize prevention through "safer sex" practices and treatment of STIs rather than focus on the ethics of sexual behavior. Most important, some of these diseases have the potential to cause serious, long-term health problems, even death.

Table 23-4 discusses the common STIs, their symptoms, treatment, and potential effects.

## SUMMARY

- The most common skin infections in athletes are caused by viruses, bacteria, and fungi. Viral infections include herpes simplex (e.g., the cold sore) and herpes zoster. The two most common types of bacterial infections are streptococcus and staphyloccus. Ringworm, or tinea, is the fungus infection commonly attacking all areas of the body; tinea pedis (athlete's foot) is the most common.

- The common cold, sinusitis, sore throat, hay fever, and asthma are respiratory tract illnesses that can adversely affect the athlete. Asthma can be chronic (e.g., bronchial) or induced by physical activity. Care of the athlete who is having an acute asthmatic attack requires understanding the early symptoms and signs and responding accordingly.

- A number of conditions of the digestive system, such as diarrhea, vomiting, constipation, and gastroenteritis, commonly affect the athletic population.

- Anemia is a problem for some athletes. Iron-deficiency anemia is a condition found most often in women. In an athlete with iron-deficiency anemia, the red blood cells are either too small or too large and hemoglobin is decreased. The athlete with sickle-cell anemia may have an adverse reaction at high altitudes at which the sickle-shaped red blood cell is unable to transport oxygen adequately.

- Diabetes mellitus is a complex hereditary or developmental disease of carbohydrate metabolism. Decreased effectiveness of insulin or an insufficient amount of insulin is responsible for most cases of diabetes. The diabetic athlete must carefully monitor his or her energy output to ensure a balance of food intake and the burning of sugars via insulin. If this balance is not maintained, diabetic coma or insulin shock may result.

- Epilepsy is defined as "a recurrent paroxysmal disorder of cerebral function characterized by sudden, brief attacks of altered consciousness, motor activity, sensory phenomena, or inappropriate behavior." A coach must recognize that an athlete is going into seizure and be able to provide proper immediate care.

- The athlete with high blood pressure may have to be carefully monitored by the physician. Hypertension may require the avoidance of heavy resistive activities.

- Because communicable viral diseases such as German measles, mumps, and infectious mononucleosis can infect many athletes on a team, early recognition is necessary. When such a disease is suspected, the athlete should be isolated from other athletes and immediately referred to a physician for diagnosis.

- Sexually transmitted disease has its highest incidence among younger, sexually active persons. Because most athletes are in this high-risk age group, coaches should be concerned about the spread of these diseases. Suggestions to avoid these infections are safe sex, which involves the use of a condom or the elimination of multiple partners, and complete abstinence from sexual intercourse.

- A major problem in sports participation is the extensive use of performance aids, consisting of drugs and blood doping. Certain performance-enhancing drugs, including stimulants, narcotic analgesics, diuretics, anabolic steroids, and human growth hormone, have been banned. Blood doping has also been placed in the banned category.

- Another area of concern is recreational drug abuse. This abuse is worldwide. It leads to serious psychological and physical health problems. The most prevalent substances that are abused are alcohol, nicotine, cocaine, and marijuana.

- The highly active female may have menstrual irregularities, including dysmenorrhea, amenorrhea, or oligomenorrhea. Female athlete triad is a combination of amenorrhea, disordered eating, and osteoporosis.

- Many female athletes compete during pregnancy with no ill effects. There is no indication that mild to moderate exercise during pregnancy is harmful to fetal development.

- The sexually transmitted infections with the highest incidence among the young athletic population are chlamydia, genital herpes, trichomoniasis, genital candidiasis, condyloma acuminata, gonorrhea, and syphilis.

---

### *Solutions to Critical Thinking* Exercises

**23–1** Tinea pedis causes severe itching underneath and between the toes and on the sole of the foot. A red, white, or grayish scaling appearance may also be present. Scratching can cause infection. Generally this condition can be prevented by wearing clean, dry socks and making certain that the foot and toes are dry following bathing.

**23–2** It appears that the athlete is exhibiting signs and symptoms associated with the flu. In general the flu is caused by a viral infection, and thus the illness must simply be allowed to run its course while dealing with it symptomatically.

**23–3** The coach should tell the athlete that creatine may help to enhance performance during high intensity resistance exercise, however, there is not sufficient definitive evidence to support its use.

**23–4** The female athlete triad includes some form of eating disorder, amenorrhea, and osteoporosis. The eating disorder causes amenorrhea, in which menstruation stops, thus reducing the production of estrogen, which ultimately causes a loss of calcium from the bone.

## REVIEW QUESTIONS AND CLASS ACTIVITIES

1. Describe the organisms underlying the common skin infections seen in athletes. Name a disease caused by each one.
2. Invite a dermatologist or other professional to speak to the class about skin conditions, skin disease, and their care. He or she may wish to discuss specific conditions that pose a serious threat to the athlete's health and to others.
3. Describe the anemias that most often affect the athlete. How should each be managed?
4. What are the most common conditions related to the digestive system?
5. What is diabetes mellitus? What is the difference between diabetic coma and insulin shock? How is each managed?
6. What is epilepsy? What should an athletic trainer do for the athlete during a seizure? After it?
7. What is hypertension and how should it be addressed in athletics?
8. In a sports setting, what is the indication that an athlete has a contagious disease?
9. Discuss the ethics of using drugs to improve sports performance.
10. How do stimulants enhance an athlete's performance? Do they, in fact, enhance it?
11. What are the deleterious effects of hormonal manipulation in sports?
12. Describe blood doping in sports. Why is it used? What are its dangers?
13. List the dangers of smokeless tobacco. List the effects of nicotine on the body.
14. Select a recreational drug to research. What are the physiological responses to it, and what dangers does it pose to the athlete?
15. How can an athlete who is abusing drugs be identified? Describe behavioral identification and drug testing.
16. Discuss menstrual irregularities that occur in highly active athletes. Why do they occur? How should they be managed? How do they relate to reproduction? What is the female athletic triad and how can it be prevented?

### REFERENCES

1. Browne A, Lachance V, Pipe A: The ethics of blood testing as an element of doping control in sport, *Med Sci Sports Exerc* 31(4):497, 1999.
2. Burkhart CG: Skin disorders of the foot in active patients, *Physician Sportsmed* 27(2):88, 1999.
3. Chatard JC, Mujika I, Guy C: Anemia and iron deficiency in ath-

letes: practical recommendations
for treatment, *Sports Med* 27(4):
229, 1999.

4. Colberg SR, Swain DP: Exercise
and diabetes control: a winning
combination, *Physician Sportsmed*
28(4):63, 2000.

5. Corbin L: How to steer clear of
seasonal allergies, *Running Times*
(249), June 1998, 14, 45.

6. Deakin V: Alcohol: the legal drug
in sport, *Sports Coach* 22(2):22,
1999.

7. Flowers L: Understanding sickle-
cell anemia, *First Aider* 69(1):2,
1998.

8. Frankovich RJ, Lebrun CM: Menstrual cycle, contraception, and
performance, *Clin Sports Med* 19(2):
25, 2000.

9. Hand JW, Wroble RR: Prevention
of tinea corporis in collegiate
wrestlers, *J Ath Train* 34(4):350,
1999.

10. Jones AR, Ipichot JT: Stimulant
use in sports, *Am J Addict* 7(4):243,
1998.

11. Locke RJ, Warren MP: Exercise
and primary dismenorrhoea, *Br J
Sports Med* 33(4):227, 1999.

12. MacKnight, JM: Hypertension in
athletes and active patients: tailor-
ing treatment to the patient, *Physician Sportsmed* 27(4):35, 1999.

13. Malkia E., Impivaara O: Intensity
of physical activity and respiratory
function in subjects with and
without bronchial asthma, *Scand J
Med Sci Sports* 8(1):27, 1998.

14. Mujika I, Padilla S, Ibanez J: Creatine supplementation and sprint
performance in soccer players,
*Med Sci Sports Exerc* 32(2):518,
2000.

15. Ramsey ML: Skin care for active
people, *Physician Sportsmed* 25:131,
1997.

16. Sallis R, Chassay CM: Recognizing and treating common cold–
induced injury in outdoor sports,
*Med Sci Sports Exerc* 31(10):1367,
1999.

17. Sanborn CF et al: Disordered eating and the female athlete triad,
*Clin Sports Med* 19(2):199, 2000.

18. Schnirring L: Growth hormone
doping: the search for a test, *Physician Sportsmed* 28(4):16, 2000.

19. Schnirring L: New drugs should
help fight influenza this winter,
*Physician Sportsmed* 27(12):15,
1999.

20. Smith C: Infectious mononucleosis and the athlete, *Sideline View*
20(7):1, 1999.

21. Stilger VG et al: Androstenedione
and anabolic-androgenic steroids:
what you need to know, *Ath Ther
Today* 5(1):56, 2000.

22. Terrel T et al: Identifying exercise
allergies, *Physician Sportsmed* 24:76,
1996.

23. Vantu RV: Epilepsy and athletics,
*Clin Sports Med* 17(1):61, 1998.

24. Weaver J, Denegar CR, Hertel J:
Exercise-induced asthma, *Ath Ther
Today* 5(3):38, 2000.

## ANNOTATED BIBLIOGRAPHY

Berkow R, Beers M, Fletcher A, editors: *The Merck manual of medical information: home edition*, New York,
1999, Pocket Books.

*This text book is one of the classical
medicine references available to the
health care professional. It covers most
medical conditions.*

Hamann B: *Diseases: identification, prevention, and control*, St Louis, 2000,
Mosby.

*An excellent reference guide for the
health professional on the most common
human diseases.*

*Tabor's cyclopedic medical dictionary*,
Philadelphia, 1997, FA Davis.

*Despite the dictionary format, there is
a wealth of valuable information on various health conditions contained in this
volume.*

## WEBSITES

American Academy of Dermatology: http://www.aad.org/

*The American Academy of Dermatology is committed to advancing the science promoting a lifetime of healthier skin, hair, and nails.*

Asthma and Allergy Foundation of America (AAFA): http://www.aafa.org/

*Asthma and Allergy Foundation of America (AAFA) is dedicated to helping people with asthma and allergic diseases through education and support for research.*

American Gastroenterological Association: http://www. gastro.org/

*Includes information for physicians and the public about digestive disease symptoms, treatments, and research.*

American Diabetes Association: http://www.diabetes.org/

*This site offers the latest information on diabetes and living with the disease.*

American Epilepsy Society: http://www.aesnet.org/

*The American Epilepsy Society promotes research and education for professionals dedicated to the prevention, treatment, and cure of epilepsy.*

Hypertension Network: BloodPressure.com: http://www.bloodpressure.com/

*Information for the consumer on hypertension (high blood pressure).*

Sexually Transmitted Infections: Index: http://www.plannedparenthood.org/STI-SAFESEX/stifacts.htm

Sexually Transmitted Infections: The Facts

Substance Abuse and Mental Health Service Administration: http://www.samhsa.gov/

American Board of Obstetrics and Gynecology: http"//www.abog.org/

# Young Athletes

*When you finish this chapter you will be able to:*

■ Explain the impact that sports have on young athletes.

■ Describe the advantages and disadvantages of training and conditioning of young athletes.

■ Explain the pros and cons of children competing in organized sports.

■ Explain the need for better trained coaches and for the certification of coaches.

■ Describe the child's potential for injury in sports activities.

Sports can promote:
• Responsible social behaviors
• Greater academic success
• Confidence in physical abilities
• Appreciation of health and fitness
• Positive ethical behaviors

Many parents and health professionals question the value of sports for the immature child.

Under the best of circumstances, sports programs for young participants promote responsible social behaviors, greater academic success, confidence in physical abilities, an appreciation of personal health and fitness, and the development of strong social bonds. Sports, when specifically planned for, can provide a venue for the learning of positive ethical behaviors.

## CULTURAL TRENDS

Organized competitive sports in North America continue to grow at a high rate although there is some concern by parents, educational professionals, and some physicians. In 1974 the American Academy of Pediatrics adopted a position stand against organized competitive athletics for children under the age of fourteen, primarily because of excessive emotional and physical stress that might be placed on the growing child. It is obvious that this stand has not been accepted by most individuals in our society, especially those who are deeply involved with youth sports.[4]

Parents and professionals in the areas of education, psychology, and medicine have long questioned whether vigorous physical training and competition are advisable for the immature child. Increasingly, children are engaging in intense programs of training that may require many hours of daily commitment extending over many years. Swimmers may practice 2 hours, two times a day, covering 6,000 to 10,000 meters each session; gymnasts may practice 3 to 5 hours per day; and runners may cover as many as 70 miles each week.

**TABLE 24-1** Estimated number of young people ages 5–17 enrolled in specific categories of youth sports.[3]

| Activities | Estimated number of participants |
|---|---|
| Agency-sponsored sports (Little League baseball, Pop Warner football) | 22 million |
| Club sports (Fee-based services such as gymnastics, ice skating, and swimming) | 2.4 million |
| Recreational sports programs (Everyone Plays, sponsored by recreational departments) | 14.5 million |
| Intramural sports (in middle, junior, senior high schools) | 0.5 million |
| Interscholastic sports (in middle, junior, senior high schools) | 7.5 million |

The number of young people between 5 and 17 years of age in the United States engaging in youth sports is estimated at more than 46 million. The National Youth Sports Safety Foundation estimates that between 20 and 30 million U.S. children are in organized out-of-school sports with another 25 million participating in competitive school sports (Table 24-1).[7]

## PHYSICAL IMMATURITY AND THE PROPER MATCHING OF ATHLETES

Many professionals concerned with the well-being of young athletes believe that highly competitive sports, especially collision sports, place great stresses on immature skeletal structures.[1] The skeleton is not completely mature until early adulthood. For example, the femur does not reach full maturity until approximately 9 years of age. The main concern of individuals against highly competitive contact or collision sports is that injuries can cause an immature cessation of growth in a particular bone. With this concern in mind, the following activities should be performed with caution:

- Falling, jumping, and landing with straight legs
- Excessive stress to the shoulder and elbow from repeated hard throwing motions
- Long duration exercise involving weight bearing, such as long distance running
- Heavy weight lifting

All youth sports participants should be matched by physical maturation, weight, size, and skill levels. Of major importance is that a physical examination should be given before the child enters organized competitive sports.[2]

Forty-six million young people between the ages of five and seventeen engage in sports.

24–1

*Critical Thinking* Exercise

The estimated number of youth participants between 5 and 17 years of age in the United States is more than 46 million.

? What are the predominant injuries sustained by this age group?

Young athletes should be matched by:
- Physical maturation
- Weight
- Size
- Skill level
- Extent of experience in the sport

**Fig. 24-1**

Unsupervised play is
generally more dangerous
than organized sports
activities.

Loose-jointed children appear to be more susceptible to injuries in contact and collision sports and should be directed to other sports until their bodies can withstand the rigors of falling and of physical contact. In contrast the child whose muscular system is very tight is more prone to muscle strains with an increased risk of injury to extremities and spinal region.[4]

## PHYSICAL CONDITIONING AND TRAINING

According to current data, youngsters adapt well to the same type of training routines used to train the mature athlete.[9] Coaches and parents should note, however, that children do not relate to the same motivation to work as adults do. Until about 12 years of age, children are not usually aware of the different levels of effort that they can expend and do not understand that they can increase their ability in the sport by increasing their effort.

Extreme training intensity can increase a child's chance of sustaining an overuse injury. Even though Wolff's law is at work when the growing child is experiencing intensive physical training, close supervision by coaches is necessary to avoid a risk of injury (Figure 24-1).

## GENDER CONSIDERATIONS

There is no need to separate preadolescent girls and boys in competitive sports.

The American Academy of Pediatrics indicates that there is no physical reason to separate preadolescent girls and boys by gender in recreational or competitive sports activities. Separation of genders should occur in collision-type sports once boys have attained greater muscle mass in proportion to their body weight.

## PSYCHOLOGICAL AND LEARNING CONCERNS

Of even more concern than the physical aspects of sports are the psychological stresses that may be placed on children by overzealous parents and coaches. Children must not be considered to be miniature adults. Although children can mimic adult skills, they often cannot understand sports concepts such as playing fair unless specifically taught.

Children usually are eager to please adults, making them vulnerable to coercion and manipulation. A coach must use a positive approach by giving children frequent encouragement with positive reinforcements followed by corrective feedback. With this method the young athlete has the opportunity to develop a sense of self-worth and positive self-esteem.

Sports should allow boys and girls to develop positive self-esteem.

Not all children are equal in ability. Some children respond well to competition, others respond poorly, as usually demonstrated by their level of performance. A child must be shown that there are benefits in experiencing a loss and that trying to the best of his or her ability is the most important factor in competition. Parents and coaches must realize that children are not good at making performance corrections unless instructions are given instantly at the time of the situation. In other words, half-time performance suggestions given a half-hour later may have little effect on the child.

Enjoyment of an activity, rather than winning at all costs, should be the focus of a child's training, conditioning, and competition. Too often parents who were fine athletes or who wanted to be great athletes coerce their young children to the point of anxiety and a dislike for the sport.

## COACHING QUALIFICATIONS

No federal laws require coaching education at any level of competition. Currently, the way to become trained as a coach in the United States is to complete a university degree program, a National Body of Sports certification program, and/or a youth sports coaching education program.[7] Up until 1996 no coaching standards had been developed.[5] The National Association for Sport and Physical Education (NASPE) is now in the process of developing an accreditation program.[5] The United States Olympic Committee (USOC) has mandated that all coaches participating under the governance of USOC receive certification in the safety training course developed by the American Red Cross/USOC.[9]

Often coaches of youth sports have little or no background in providing safe and positive sports experiences. It is estimated that 2.5 million volunteer coaches lack formal preparation.[3] Every youth sport coach should be certified and dedicated to the highest ideals of coaching. One organization that promotes such ideals is the National Youth Sports Coaches Association (NYSCA).[5] Currently the NYSCA has a membership of more than 143,000 that serves more than 2 million boys and girls in the United States. This association offers three levels of certification

| TABLE 24-2 Youth Sports Injuries Treated in Hospital Emergency Rooms in 1998[6] | | | |
|---|---|---|---|
| **Sport** | **Estimated # of Cases** | **Sport** | **Estimated # of Cases** |
| Archery | 3,110 | Ice Skating | 33,741 |
| Ball Sports | 41,534 | In-Line Skating | 110,783 |
| Baseball | 180,582 | Martial Arts | 23,018 |
| Basketball | 631,186 | Roller Skating | 53,681 |
| Bicycles | 577,621 | Rugby | 8,361 |
| Bleachers | 19,161 | Skateboards | 54,532 |
| Bowling | 23,130 | Skating (not specified) | 27,481 |
| Boxing | 9,183 | Snow Skiing | 81,787 |
| Cheerleading | 18,858 | Soccer | 169,734 |
| Dancing | 38,427 | Softball | 132,625 |
| Diving or Diving Boards | 11,124 | Squash, Racquet Ball, or Paddle | 8,984 |
| Exercise w/o Equipment | 123,177 | | |
| Exercise Equipment | 33,320 | Swimming | 49,331 |
| Field Hockey | 4,666 | Tennis | 22,665 |
| Football | 355,247 | Track & Field | 15,560 |
| Golf | 46,019 | Trampolines | 95,239 |
| Gymnastics | 31,446 | Volleyball | 66,191 |
| Hockey (not specified) | 42,285 | Water Skiing | 14,487 |
| Horseback Riding | 64,692 | Weight Lifting | 60,039 |
| Ice Hockey | 22,231 | Wrestling | 43,917 |

consisting of the fundamentals of coaching, first aid and safety, and common sports injuries; it also offers instruction in the psychological aspects of losing and in discipline. All youth sport coaches must also have a good understanding of normal child development—physical, emotional, and psychological.

## INCIDENCE OF INJURIES IN YOUTH SPORTS

Of the 30 million young athletes involved in organized sports in the United States, 10 percent will sustain a sports-related injury. Each year more than 775,000 young athletes under the age of fifteen are treated in hospital emergency rooms for sports-related injuries, reports the National Electronic Injury Surveillance of the U.S. Consumer Product Safety Commission. Table 24-2 shows the number of sports-related injuries involving children between 8 and 14 years of age.[6]

## INJURY CONCERNS

The coach and parent must realize why the young athlete is vulnerable to sports injuries. Three sites on the long bones characterize a child's

Youth coach sports must be
certified and educated in:
• Techniques of coaching
• Supervising conditioning
• Sport safety
• First aid
• Child development

10 percent of youth in
organized sports sustain
an injury.

growth. These sites are at the ends of the bones, and include the joint surfaces, the growth plates, and the sites of major muscle-tendon insertions. Because this growth tissue is cartilage, it is softer than mature cartilage and bone, and it has a greater chance of injury. Contact sports are of particular concern for growth plate injuries. In noncontact sports such as throwing sports, gymnastics, or distance running, high-velocity trauma is not likely, but intense repetitive training can produce recurrent microtraumas.

Many pediatric physicians are concerned about these repeated microtraumas that can occur to the young athlete over time. Such small traumas can compound and produce chronic and, in some cases, degenerative conditions within the immature musculoskeletal system.

Children are susceptible to many of the same sport injuries that the physically mature athlete is, including joint sprains, muscle and tendon strains, and skeletal fractures. In addition, children can sustain a pulling away of soft tissue from bones (avulsion).[2]

## SPORTS INJURY PREVENTION

The simplest way to prevent serious sports injuries in the young athlete is to give close attention to the complaints of pain and/or dysfunction, especially about the major joints. With early first aid and treatment and with proper rest, healing is enhanced.[4]

Many injuries can be prevented when children are matched to the sport instead of the sport to the child. The physical matchup is important to the child's safety, but a proper emotional matchup is also important. In other words, the child should want to play the sport and at the same time have the type of personality that fits the sport.

Another way to reduce children's sports injuries is to assess the rules and tactics of the game. Every organized sport in the United States was initially designed to be played by the older and more mature athlete. Good examples of positive changes are the Little League pitchers' limit of six innings per week and the Pop Warner football limit of cross-body blocking and spearing.[3]

It is now evident that children are capable of cardiovascular training similar to that of adults with little risk of injury.[8] In addition, weight training can strengthen bones, joints, and ligaments and thereby decrease trauma to the musculoskeletal system, if the weight training is properly performed and supervised.

The role of protective equipment in preventing injury in the young has frequently been overemphasized. It is faulty thinking that youngsters who use protective equipment are safely protected when participating in adult-style games.

Young athletes must practice good basic health principles. They must avoid rapid weight loss to wrestle at a lower weight or to increase performance in gymnastics or diving. Excessive concern with thinness can lead to anorexia and/or bulimia.

24-2

*Critical Thinking* Exercise

Young athletes can be characterized as physically immature.

? What implications does this have for the prevention of injuries?

Youth athletes must practice good hygiene and other health habits.

**COACH'S CORNER**

The following is a checklist of things for a coach to guard against that can result in youth sports injuries.

- ☐ Inadequate preparticipation exams
- ☐ Improper, poorly fitted, or lack of protective equipment
- ☐ Grouping teams by age instead of size
- ☐ Hazardous playing fields and other environmental hazards
- ☐ Training errors
- ☐ Undue fatigue or overtraining
- ☐ Lack of coaching education
- ☐ Insufficient or incorrect instruction
- ☐ Failure to do proper warm-up stretching and cooldown
- ☐ Allowing the athlete to play when injured
- ☐ Delated or insufficient medical care
- ☐ Poor nutrition
- ☐ Poor health habits

## SUMMARY

- The extent to which young athletes train and compete must be carefully monitored to avoid physical and emotional injuries.
- The estimated number of young people engaging in some sport in the United States is 46 million.
- A major concern to some parents and professionals is the stress placed on the young body from intense sports competition and training.
- All youth sport participants should be matched by physical maturation, weight, size, skill level, and experience.
- Young athletes can positively respond to some types of conditioning exercises, if the exercises are properly supervised and conducted.
- Activities such as falling, jumping, landing on straight legs, repeated hard throwing motions, running very long distances, and lifting heavy weights may produce injuries to the immature musculoskeletal system.
- Children are not miniature adults; coaching must be based on their emotional and cognitive level.
- Separation of genders in sport activities needs to occur only when boys have attained greater muscle mass in proportion to their body weight.
- Enjoyment of an activity, rather than winning at all costs, must be stressed to children as the most important factor in sports participation.
- An overzealous coach can cause the young athlete great emotional stress.

- Coaches participating in youth sports must be trained in techniques and skills, safety and injury prevention, first aid, and growth and development.
- Coaches should be certified.
- Each year more than 775,000 young athletes under 15 years of age are treated for sports-related injuries.
- Young athletes are prone to the same injuries that the mature athlete is, but they must also contend with injuries to their skeletal growth centers.
- Injuries to young athletes can be avoided through proper conditioning and supervision, proper matching, use of proper equipment, and competing under appropriate rules of competition.
- Young athletes must be encouraged to practice good health habits.

---

*Solutions to Critical Thinking* Exercises

**24-1** Injuries are predominantly to lower and upper limbs, respectively.

**24-2** All athletes must be matched according to maturation and size.

## REVIEW QUESTIONS AND CLASS ACTIVITIES

1. Discuss the advantages and disadvantages of training and conditioning the physically immature athlete.
2. Discuss the pros and cons of the young athlete engaging in intense competition.
3. Observe a Little League or Pop Warner game, assessing the coaches' activities and conduct that might be harmful to the children.
4. Develop a conditioning and training program for young athletes engaging in tackle football, taking into consideration their immature physical and emotional nature.

**REFERENCES**

1. American Academy of Orthopedic Surgeons, P.O. Box 1998, Des Plaines, IL 60017.
2. Arnheim D, Prentice B: *Principles of athletic training*, ed 10, 2000, McGraw-Hill. Dubuque, IA.
3. Carnegie Corporation of New York, 437 Madison Ave, New York, NY 10022.
4. Michelli U: Safe state, injury prevention in Massachusetts. Presentation by Massachusetts Dept. of Public Health, Bureau of Family and Community Health, Division of Prevention, Injury Prevention and Control Program, Boston, September 18, 1996.
5. National Association for Sports and Physical Education (NASPE), 1900 Association Dr., Reston, VA 22091.
6. National Electronic Injury Surveillance System, US Consumer Product Safety Commission, National Injury Information Clearinghouse, 1998.
7. National Youth Sports Safety Foundation, 333 Longwood Ave, Suite 202, Boston, MA 02115.
8. Prentice W: *Fitness for college and college life*, ed 5, St Louis, 1997, Mosby.

9. United States Olympic Committee (USOC), National Governing Bodies of Sports, One Olympic Plaza, Colorado Springs, CO 80909.

## ANNOTATED BIBLIOGRAPHY

American Academy of Pediatrics: *Sports medicine: health care for young athletes,* Elk Grove Village, IL, 1991, American Academy of Pediatrics.

*A comprehensive guide to training, conditioning, and injury care of the young athlete.*

Appenzeller H: *Youth sports and the law: a guide to legal issues,* Chapel Hill, NC, 2000, Carolina Academic Press.

*Studies various court cases to understand the legal principles involved in sport participation. The objective of the book is to provide better and safer sporting experiences for today's children.*

Duff JF: *Youth sports: a medical handbook for parents and coaches,* New York, 1992, Collier Books.

*Designed to bring a medical understanding of sports injuries to both the parent and coach.*

Flegel M: *Sport first aid,* Champaign, Ill, 1996, Human Kinetics.

*Provides excellent coverage of the immediate care of sports injuries.*

Michelli U, Jenkins MD: *Sportwise: an essential guide for young athletes, parents and coaches,* Boston, 1990, Houghton Mifflin.

*Addresses sports injuries and their prevention and care.*

*Sidelines,* National Youth Sports Safety Foundation, 333 Longwood Ave, Suite 202, Boston, MA 02115.

*Low-cost fact sheets on coaching topics and selected sports injuries.*

## WEBSITES

National Youth Sports Safety Foundation: http://www.nyssf.org

American Academy of Pediatrics: http://www.aap.org

National Association for Sport and Physical Education: http://www.aahperd.org/naspc

KidsHealth: http://www.kidshealth.com

National Safe Kids Campaign: http://www.safekids.org

# Appendix A

# Recognition of the Athletic Trainer as an Allied Health Professional

In June 1991 the American Medical Association officially recognized athletic training as an allied health profession. The primary purpose of this recognition was for accrediting educational programs. The AMA's Committee on Allied Health Education and Accreditation (CAHEA) was charged with the responsibility of developing essentials and guidelines for academic programs to use in preparation of individuals for initial entry into the profession through the Joint Review Committee on Athletic Training (JRC-AT). As of 1993, all entry-level athletic training education programs became subject to the CAHEA accreditation process.[1]

In June 1994 CAHEA was dissolved and was replaced immediately by the Commission on Accreditation of Allied Health Education Programs (CAAHEP). Currently seventeen professional review committees are sponsored by the forty-nine separate organizations that make up CAAHEP. The NATA is one of those organizations. CAAHEP is recognized as an accreditation agency for allied health education programs by the U.S. Department of Education. Entry-level college and university based athletic training education programs at both the undergraduate and graduate level that were at one time approved by the NATA and subsequently by CAHEA must now be accredited by CAAHEP. The JRC-AT currently includes representatives from the NATA, the American Academy of Pediatrics, the American Association for Sports Medicine, and the American Academy of Family Practice.

The effects of CAAHEP accreditation are not limited to the educational aspects. In the future, this recognition may affect regulatory legislation, the practice of athletic training in nontraditional settings, and insurance considerations. This recognition will continue to be a positive step in the development of the athletic training profession.

1. Committee on Allied Health Education and Accreditation: *Essentials and guidelines for an accredited educational program for athletic trainers,* Chicago, 1992, American Medical Association.

# Employment Settings for the Athletic Trainer

## SECONDARY SCHOOLS

It would be ideal to have certified athletic trainers serve every secondary school in the United States.[1] Many of the physical problems that occur later from improperly managed sports injuries could be avoided if proper care from an athletic trainer is provided initially. Many times a coach does all of his or her own athletic training, although in some cases a coach is assigned additional athletic training responsibilities and is assisted by a student athletic trainer. If a secondary school hires an athletic trainer, it is commonly in a faculty-trainer capacity. This individual is usually employed as a teacher in one of the school's classroom disciplines and performs athletic training duties on a part-time or extracurricular basis.[2] In this instance, compensation usually is on the basis of released time from teaching and/or a stipend as a coach.[3]

Another means of obtaining high school or community college athletic training coverage is by using a certified graduate student from a nearby college or university. The graduate student receives a graduate assistantship with a stipend paid by the secondary school or community college. In this situation both the graduate student and the school benefit.[4] However, this practice may prevent a school from employing an athletic trainer on a full-time basis.

## SCHOOL DISTRICTS

Some school districts have found it effective to employ a centrally placed certified athletic trainer. In this case the athletic trainer, who may be full- or part-time, is a nonteacher who serves a number of schools. The advantage is savings; the disadvantage is that one individual cannot provide the level of service usually required by a typical school.

## COLLEGES OR UNIVERSITIES

At the college or university level, the athletic training position varies considerably from institution to institution. In smaller institutions, the athletic trainer may be a half-time professor in physical education and a half-time athletic trainer. In some cases, if the athletic trainer is a physical therapist rather than a teacher, he or she may spend part of the time in the school health center and part of the time in athletic training. Increasingly at the college level, athletic training services are being offered to members of the general student body who participate in intramural and club sports. In most colleges and universities the athletic trainer is full-time, does not teach, works in the department of athletics, and is paid by the state or from student union or alumni funds.

## PROFESSIONAL TEAMS

The athletic trainer for professional sports teams usually performs specific team training duties for 6 months out of the year; the other 6 months are spent in off-season conditioning and individual rehabilitation. The athletic trainer working with a professional team is involved with only one sport and is paid according to contract, much like a player. Playoff and championship money can add substantially to the yearly income.

## SPORTS MEDICINE CLINICS

For years, sports medicine clinics were considered a nontraditional setting for employment as an athletic trainer. Today, more athletic trainers are employed in sports medicine clinics than in any other employment setting. The role of the athletic trainer can vary greatly from one clinic to the next. Most clinical athletic trainers see patients with sports-related injuries during the morning hours in the clinic. In the afternoons, trainers' services are contracted out to local high schools or small colleges for game and/or practice coverage. For the most part, private clinics have well-equipped facilities in which to work, and salaries for their trainers are generally somewhat higher than in the more traditional settings.

## INDUSTRIAL SETTING

It is becoming more common for corporations or industries to employ athletic trainers to oversee fitness and injury rehabilitation programs for their employees. In addition to these responsibilities, trainers may be assigned to conduct wellness programs and provide education and individual counseling. It is likely that many job opportunities will exist for the athletic trainer in industry in the next few years.

1. Knight K: Athletic trainers for secondary schools, *Ath Train* 23(4):313, 1988.
2. Prentice W, Mischler B: A national survey of employment opportunities for athletic trainers in the public schools, *Ath Train* 21(3):215, 1986.
3. Lephart S, Metz K: Financial and appointment trends of the athletic trainer clinician/educator, *Ath Train* 25(2):118, 1990.
4. Hossler P: How to acquire athletic trainers on the high school level, *Ath Train* 20(3):199, 1985.

# Appendix C

# Requirements for Certification as an Athletic Trainer

An athletic trainer who is certified by the NATA Board of Certification is a highly qualified paramedical professional educated and experienced in dealing with the injuries that occur with participation in sports. Candidates for certification are required to have an extensive background of both formal academic preparation and supervised practical experience in a clinical setting, according to CAAHEP guidelines. The guidelines listed in Focus Box A-1 have been established by the National Athletic Trainers' Association Board of Certification.[1]

A-1 ▷ **Focus Box**

### NATA Certification

#### Purpose of certification

The National Athletic Trainers' Association Board of Certification (NATABOC) was established in 1970 to implement a program of certification for entry-level athletic trainers. The purpose of the certification program is to establish standards for entry into the profession of athletic training.

To attain certification as an athletic trainer, an applicant must fulfill the following core requirements and must either complete a CAAHEP-accredited entry-level program or an internship program.

#### Core requirements

Note: If one or more of the core requirements are not fulfilled at the time of application, the application will be returned.

1. The athletic training student must have a high school diploma to begin accumulating directly supervised clinical hours that are to be used to meet requirements for NATABOC certification.

2. Proof of graduation (an official transcript) at the baccalaureate level from an accredited college or university located in the United States of America. Foreign-degreed applicants who wish to credit this degree toward a bachelor's degree requirement will be evaluated, at the candidate's expense, by an independent consultant selected by the NATABOC. Students who have begun their last semester or quarter of college are eligible to take the certification examination before graduation, provided the other core and section requirements have been fulfilled at the time of application. Verification of intent to graduate must be provided to the Board of Certification by the dean or department chairperson of the college or university the applicant is attending. Certification will not be issued until an official transcript indicating date of degree is received by the Board of Certification.

3. Proof of current American National Red Cross Standard First Aid Certification and current Basic CPR (American Red Cross or American Heart Association); EMT equivalent instead of First Aid and CPR will be accepted. Both cards must be current at the time of application.

4. At the time of application, all candidates for certification (curriculum and internship) must verify that at least 25 percent of their athletic training experience hours credited in fulfilling the certification requirements were attained in actual (on location) practice or game coverage with one or more of the following sports:

*continued*

## NATA Certification—cont'd

football, soccer, hockey, wrestling, basketball, gymnastics, lacrosse, volleyball, and rugby.

5. Endorsement of certification application by a NATA-certified athletic trainer.

6. Subsequent passing of the certification examination (written, oral-practical, and written-simulation sections).

### Section Requirements

#### CAAHEP *accredited program*

The candidate must graduate from an undergraduate or graduate program accredited by the Commission on Accreditation of Allied Health Education Programs (CAAHEP). Students applying to take the certification exam must complete formal instruction in the following core curriculum subject areas:

Human anatomy
Human physiology
Psychology
Kinesiology/biomechanics
Exercise physiology
Prevention of athletic injuries/illness
Evaluation of athletic injuries/ illness
First aid and emergency care
Therapeutic modalities
Therapeutic exercise
Personal community health
Nutrition
Administration of athletic training programs

It is recommended that students complete course work in physics, chemistry, pharmacology, research design, and statistics. In addition, students are required to complete a minimum of 800 clinical hours under the direct supervision of a NATA-certified athletic trainer at that college or an affiliated site. Applicants who are applying for NATA certification from a CAAHEP-accredited undergraduate or graduate program must receive their degree from that college or university.

#### Internship programs*

If a student does not attend a CAAHEP-accredited program, he or she may still be eligible for certification by completing an internship. At the time of application, each internship candidate must present documentation of attaining at least 1,500 hours of athletic training experience under direct supervision of a NATA-certified athletic trainer. These hours must have been attained over a minimum of two calendar years and not more than five years. Of these 1,500 hours, at least 1,000 hours must be attained in a traditional athletic setting at the interscholastic, intercollegiate, or professional sports level. The additional 500 hours may be attained from an allied clinical setting and/or sport camp setting under the direct supervision of a NATA-certified athletic trainer. Each candidate must present, via official transcript, proof of completion of formal course work no more than seven years before the date of application, with at least one course in each of the following areas:

Health (i.e., nutrition, drugs/substance abuse, health education)
Human anatomy
Kinesiology/biomechanics
Human physiology
Physiology of exercise
Basic athletic training
Advanced athletic training (a course in therapeutic modalies or rehabilitation may satisfy the advanced course requirement)

Basic and advanced athletic training courses must be successfully completed in a college or university in the United States or taught by a NATA-certified athletic trainer in a foreign college or university for credit. The remaining core courses may be accepted from foreign universities as deemed acceptable by the NATABOC.

*As of January 2004, completion of an internship program will no longer be recognized or accepted as a means of becoming NATABOC certified. After that date, to be eligible for certification you must complete a CAAHEP-accredited program.*

## THE CERTIFICATION EXAMINATION

Once the requirements have been fulfilled, applicants are eligible to sit for the certification examination. The certification examination has been developed by the National Athletic Trainers' Association Board of Certification in conjunction with Columbia Assessment Services, Inc., and is administered four times each year at various locations throughout the United States.[1] The examination consists of three sections: a written portion, an oral-practical portion, and a written-simulation portion. The examination tests for knowledge and skill in six major domains: (1) athletic injury prevention and risk management, (2) recognition, evaluation, and assessment of injuries, (3) immediate care of injuries and illnesses, (4) rehabilitation and reconditioning of athletic injuries, (5) health care organization and administration, and (6) professional development and responsibility. Successful performance on the certification exam leads to certification as an athletic trainer.

## CONTINUING EDUCATION REQUIREMENTS

To ensure ongoing professional growth and involvement by the certified athletic trainer, the NATABOC has established requirements for continuing education.[2] To maintain certification, all certified trainers must document a minimum of eighty CEUs* attained during each 3-year recertification term. CEUs may be awarded for attending symposiums, seminars, workshops, or conferences; serving as a speaker, panelist, or certification exam model; participating in the USOC program; authoring a research article in a professional journal; completing an NATA journal quiz; completing postgraduate course work; and obtaining CPR, first aid, or EMT certification. All certified athletic trainers must also demonstrate proof of CPR certification at least once during the 3-year term.

### REFERENCES

1. National Athletic Trainers' Association Board of Certification, Inc: *Study guide for the NATABOC entry-level athletic trainer certification examination*, Philadelphia, 1993, Davis.

2. National Athletic Trasiners' Association Board of Certification, Inc, Continuing Education Office: *Continuing education file 2000–2001*, Dallas, 2000, NATABOC.

---

*1 ceu = 1 contact hour

# Glossary

**abduction**  A movement of a body part away from the midline of the body

**accident**  An act that occurs by chance or without intention

**accommodating resistance**  Form of isokinetic exercises in which speed is an element

**act of commission**  Where an individual commits an act that is not legally theirs to perform

**act of omission**  Where an individual fails to perform a legal duty

**acute injury**  An injury with sudden onset and short duration

**ad libitum**  In the amount desired

**adduction**  A movement of a body part toward the midline of the body

**afferent nerve fibers**  Nerve fibers that carry messages toward the brain

**agonist muscles**  Muscles directly engaged in contraction as related to muscles that relax at the same time

**ambulation**  Move or walk from place to place

**ameboid action**  A leukocyte moving through a capillary wall through the process of diapedisis

**amenorrhea**  Absence or suppression of menstruation

**amnesia**  Loss of memory

**analgesia**  Pain inhibition

**anemia**  Lack of iron

**anesthesia**  Partial or complete loss of sensation

**anomaly**  Deviation from the norm

**anorexia**  Lack or loss of appetite; aversion to food

**anorexia nervosa**  Eating disorder characterized by a distorted body image

**anoxia**  Lack of oxygen

**antagonist muscles**  Muscles that counteract the action of the agonist muscles

**anterior**  Before or in front of

**anterior cruciate ligament**  Stops external rotation

**anteroposterior**  Refers to the position of front to back

**anxiety**  A feeling of uncertainty or apprehension

**apophysis**  A bone outgrowth to which muscles attach

**arrhythmical movement**  Irregular movement

**arthroscopic examination**  Viewing the inside of a joint via the arthroscope, which utilizes a small camera lens

**articulation**  A joint

**assumption of risk**  The individual, through expressed or implied agreement, assumes some risk or danger will be involved in a particular undertaking

**asymmetries (body)**  A lack of symmetry of sides of the body

**atrophic necrosis**  Death of an area due to lack of circulation

**atrophy**  Wasting away of tissue or of an organ; diminution of the size of a body part

**automatism**  Automatic behavior before consciousness or full awareness has been achieved following a brain concussion

**avascular necrosis**  Death of tissue resulting from a lack of blood supply

**avulsion**  A tearing away

**axial loading**  A blow to the top of the athlete's head while in flexion

**axilla**  Armpit

**ballistic stretching**  Older stretching technique that uses repetitive bouncing motions

**bandage**  A strip of cloth or other material used to hold a dressing in place

**bilateral**  Pertaining to both sides

**biomechanics**  Branch of study that applies the laws of mechanics to living organisms and biological tissues

**bipedal**  Having two feet or moving on two feet

**body composition**  Percent body fat plus lean body weight

**bowlegged**  Bending outward of the lower joint

**bradykinin**  Peptide chemical that causes pain in an injured area

**bulimia**  Binge-purge eating disorder

**bursae**  Pieces of synovial membrane that contain a small amount of fluid

**bursitis**  Inflammation of a bursa, especially those bursae located between bony prominences and a muscle or tendon, such as those of the shoulder or knee

**calcific tendinitis**  Deposition of calcium in a chronically inflamed tendon, especially the tendons of the shoulder

**calisthenic**  Exercise involving free movement without the aid of equipment

**callus** New bone formation over a fracture

**calorie (large)** Amount of heat required to raise 1 kg of water 1° C; term used to express the fuel or energy value of food or the heat output of the organism; the amount of heat required to heat 1 lb of water to 4° F

**cardiorespiratory endurance** Ability to perform activities for extended periods of time

**catastrophic injury** A permanent injury to the spinal cord that leaves the athlete quadriplegic or paraplegic

**cauterization** A purposeful destruction of tissue

**cerebrovascular accident** Stroke

**chondromalacia** A degeneration of a joint's articular surface, leading to softening

**chronic injury** An injury with long onset and long duration

**circuit training** Exercise stations that consist of various combinations of weight training, flexibility, calisthenics, and aerobic exercises

**circumduct** Act of moving a limb such as the arm or hip in a circular motion

**clavus durum** Hard corn

**clavus molle** Soft corn

**clonic muscle cramp** Involuntary muscle contraction marked by alternate contraction and relaxation in rapid succession

**closed fracture** Fracture that does not penetrate superficial tissue

**collagenous tissue** The white fibrous substance composing connective tissue

**collision sport** Athletes use their bodies to deter or punish opponents

**commission (legal liability)** Performing an act outside of an individual's legal jurisdiction

**communicable disease** A disease that may be transmitted directly or indirectly from one individual to another

**concentric (positive) contraction** The muscle shortens while contracting against resistance

**conduction** Heating by direct contact with a hot medium

**conjunctivae** Mucous membrane that lines the eyes

**contact sport** Athletes make physical contact, but not with the intent to produce bodily injury

**contrecoup brain injury** After head is struck, brain continues to move within the skull and becomes injured opposite the force

**convection** Heating indirectly through another medium, such as air or liquid

**conversion** Heating by other forms of energy (e.g., electricity)

**convulsions** Paroxysms of involuntary muscular contractions and relaxations

**core temperature** Internal, or deep body, temperature monitored by cells in the hypothalamus, as opposed to shell, or peripheral, temperature, which is registered by the layer of insulation provided by the skin, subcutaneous tissues, and superficial portions of the muscle masses

**corticosteroid** A steroid produced by the adrenal cortex

**coryza** Profuse nasal discharge

**counterirritant** An agent that produces a mild inflammation and in turn acts as an analgesic when applied locally to the skin (e.g., liniment)

**crepitus** A crackling feel or sound

**cryokinetics** Cold application combined with exercise

**cryotherapy** Cold therapy

**cubital fossa** Triangular area on the anterior aspect of the forearm directly opposite the elbow joint (the bend of the elbow)

**cutaneous** Of or pertaining to the skin

**cyanosis** Slightly bluish, grayish, slatelike, or dark purple discoloration of the skin due to a reduced amount of blood hemaglobin

**debride** Removal of dirt and dead tissue from a wound

**deconditioning** A state in which the athlete's body loses its competitive fitness

**degeneration** Deterioration of tissue

**dermatome** A segmental skin area innervated by various spinal cord segments

**diapedisis** Passage of blood cells by ameboid action through the intact capillary wall

**diaphragm** A musculomembranous wall separating the abdomen from the thoracic cavity

**diarthrodial joint** Ball and socket joint

**diastolic blood pressure** The residual pressure when the heart is between beats

**diplopia** Seeing double

**dislocation** A bone is forced out and stays out until surgically or manually replaced or reduced

**distal** Farthest away from a point of reference

**doping** The administration of a drug that is designed to improve the competitor's performance

**dorsiflexion** Bending toward the dorsum or rear, opposite of plantar flexion

**dorsum** The back of a body part

**dressing** A material, such as gauze, applied to a wound

**duration**   Length of time that an athlete works during a bout of exercise

**dysmenorrhea**   Painful or difficult menstruation

**dyspepsia**   Imperfect digestion

**dyspnea**   Difficulty in breathing

**eccentric (negative) contraction**   The muscle lengthens while contracting against resistance

**ecchymosis**   Black and blue skin discoloration due to hemorrhage

**ectopic**   Located in a place different from normal

**ectopic bone formation**   Bone formation occurring in an abnormal place

**edema**   Swelling as a result of the collection of fluid in connective tissue

**electrolyte**   Solution that is a conductor of electricity

**electrotherapy**   Treating disease by electrical devices

**embolus**   Fat or plaque that migrates through the vascular system

**encephalon**   The brain

**endurance**   The ability of the body to undergo prolonged activity

**entrapment**   Organ becomes compressed by nearby tissue

**epidemiological approach**   The study of sports injuries involving the relationship of as many injury factors as possible

**epilepsy**   Recurrent paroxysmal disorder characterized by sudden attacks of altered consciousness, motor activity, and sensory perception

**epiphysis**   The cartilagenous growth region of a bone

**epistaxis**   Nosebleed

**etiology**   Pertaining to the cause of a condition

**eversion of the foot**   To turn the foot outward

**exostoses**   Benign bony outgrowths that protrude from the surface of a bone and are usually capped by cartilage; callus formations

**extraoral mouth guard**   A protective device that fits outside the mouth

**extravasation**   Escape of a fluid from its vessels into the surrounding tissues

**exudates**   Accumulation of a fluid in an area

**fascia**   Fibrous membrane that covers, supports, and separates muscles

**fasciitis**   Fascia inflammation

**fibrinogen**   A protein present in blood plasma that is converted into a fibrin clot

**fibroblast**   Any cell component from which fibers are developed

**fibrocartilage**   A type of cartilage in which the matrix contains thick bundles of collagenous fibers (e.g., intervertebral disks)

**fibrosis**   Development of excessive fibrous connective tissue; fibroid degeneration

**flash-to-bang method**   Provides an estimation of how far away lightning is occurring

**foot pronation**   Combined foot movements of eversion and abduction

**foot supination**   Combined foot movements of inversion and abduction

**frequency**   Number of times per week that an athlete exercises

**genitourinary**   Pertaining to the reproductive and urinary organs

**genu recurvatus**   Hyperextension at the knee joint

**genu valgum**   Knock knees

**genu varum**   Bow legs

**glycogen supercompensation**   High carbohydrate diet

**hemarthrosis**   Blood in a joint cavity

**hematoma**   Blood tumor

**hematuria**   Blood in the urine

**hemoglobin**   Molecules that carry oxygen in the blood

**hemoglobinuria**   Hemoglobin in the urine

**hemophilia**   A hereditary blood disease in which coagulation is greatly prolonged

**hemorrhage**   Discharge of blood

**hemothorax**   Bloody fluid in the pleural cavity

**hirsutism**   Excessive hair growth and/or the presence of hair in unusual places

**homeostasis**   Maintenance of a steady state in the body's internal environment

**hyperemia**   An unusual amount of blood in a body part

**hyperextension**   Extreme stretching out of a body part

**hyperflexibility**   Flexibility beyond a joint's normal range

**hyperhidrosis**   Excessive sweating; excessive foot perspiration

**hypermobility**   Mobility of a joint that is extreme

**hypertension**   High blood pressure; abnormally high tension

**hypertonic**   Having a higher osmotic pressure than a compared solution

**hypertrophy**   Enlargement of a part caused by an increase in the size of its cells

**hyperventilation**   Abnormally deep breathing that is prolonged, causing a depletion of carbon dioxide, a fall in blood pressure, and fainting

**hypoallergenic**   Low allergy producing

**hypoxia**   Lack of an adequate amount of oxygen

**idiopathic**   Of unknown cause

**iliotibial band friction syndrome**   Runner's knee

**injury**   An act that damages or hurts

**innervation**   Nerve stimulation of a muscle

**integument**   A covering or skin

**intensity**   Increasing the workload

**interosseous membrane**   Connective tissue membrane between bones

**interval training**   Alternating periods of work with active recovery

**intervertebral**   Between two vertebrae

**intramuscular bleeding**   Bleeding within a muscle

**intraoral mouth guard**   A protective device that fits within the mouth and covers the teeth

**intravenous**   Substances administered to a patient via a vein

**inversion of the foot**   To turn the foot inward. Inner border of the foot lifts

**ions**   Electrically charged atoms

**ipsilateral**   Situated on the same side

**ischemia**   Local anemia

**isokinetic exercise**   Resistance is given at a fixed velocity of movement with accommodating resistance

**isokinetic muscle resistance**   Accommodating and variable resistance

**isometric exercise**   Contracts the muscle statically without changing its length

**isometric muscle contraction**   Muscle contracts statically without a change in its length

**isosceles triangle**   Triangle with two sides equal in length

**isotonic exercise**   Form of exercise that shortens and lengthens the muscle through a complete range of motion

**isotonic muscle contraction**   Shortens and lengthens the muscle through a complete range of motion

**joint**   Point at which two bones join together

**joint capsule**   Saclike structure that encloses the ends of bones in a diarthrodial joint

**keloid**   An overgrowth of collagenous scar tissue at the site of a wound of the skin

**keratolytic**   Pertaining to loosening the horny layer of skin

**knock knee**   Bending inward of the lower joint

**kyphosis**   Exaggeration of the normal thoracic spine

**labile**   Unsteady; not fixed; easily changed

**lactase deficiency**   Difficulty digesting dairy products

**lateral**   Pertaining to point of reference away from the midline of the body

**liability**   Legal responsibility for the harm one causes to another person

**lordosis**   Abnormal lumbar vertebral convexity

**luxation**   Total dislocation

**lysis**   Breakdown

**macerated skin**   Skin softened by soaking

**malaise**   Discomfort and uneasiness caused by an illness

**managed care**   Costs of health care is monitored closely by insurance carriers

**margination**   Accumulation of leukocytes on blood vessel walls at the site of injury during early stages of inflammation

**mechanoreceptors**   Located in muscles, tendons, ligaments, and joints; provide information on position of a joint

**medial**   Pertaining to point of reference closest to the midline of the body

**menarche**   Onset of menses

**meninges**   Any one of the three membranes that enclose the brain and the spinal cord, comprising the dura mater, the pia mater, and the arachnoid

**menorrhagia**   Abnormally heavy or long menstrual periods

**metabolites**   Products left after metabolism has taken place

**metatarsalgia**   Pain in the metatarsal

**metatarsophalangeal joint**   Joint at which the phalanges meet the metatarsal bones

**microtrauma**   Small musculoskeletal traumas that are accumulative

**mononucleosis (infectious)**   A disease, usually of young adults, causing fever, sore throat, and lymph gland swelling

**muscle**   Tissue that when stimulated contracts and produces motion

**muscle contracture**   Abnormal shortening of muscle tissue in which there is a great deal of resistance to passive stretch

**muscle cramps**   Involuntary muscle contraction

**muscle guarding**   Muscle contraction in response to pain

**muscular endurance**   The ability to perform repetitive muscular contractions against some resistance

**muscular strength**   The maximum force that can be applied by a muscle during a single maximum contraction

**musculoskeletal**   Pertaining to muscles and the skeleton

**myoglobin**   A respiratory pigment in muscle tissue that is an oxygen carrier

**myositis**   Inflammation of muscle

**myositis ossificans**   Calcium deposits that result from repeated trauma

**myotatic reflex**   Stretch reflex

**necrosis**   Death of tissue

**negative resistance**   Slow eccentric muscle contraction against resistance with muscle lengthening

**negligence**   The failure to use ordinary or reasonable care

**nerve entrapment**   A nerve that is compressed between bone or soft tissue

**neuritis**   Chronic nerve irritation

**neuroma**   Enlargement of a nerve

**NOCSAE**   National Operating Committee on Standards for Athletic Equipment

**noncontact sport**   Athletes are not involved in any physical contact

**nystagmus**   A constant involuntary back and forth, up and down, or rotary movement of the eyeball

**occlusion**   Alignment of the teeth; malocclusion means that the upper and lower teeth do not line up.

**omission (legal)**   Person fails to perform a legal duty

**open fracture**   Overlying skin has been lacerated by protruding bone fragments

**orthosis**   Used in sports as an appliance or apparatus to support, align, prevent, or correct deformities, or to improve function of a movable body part

**osteoarthritis**   A wearing down of hyaline cartilage

**osteoblasts**   Bone-forming cells

**osteochondral**   Refers to relationship of bone and cartilage

**osteochondritis**   Inflammation of bone and cartilage

**osteochondritis dissecans**   Fragment of cartilage and underlying bone is detached from the articular surface

**osteochondrosis**   A disease state of a bone and its articular cartilage

**osteoclasts**   Cells that absorb and remove osseous tissue

**osteoporosis**   A decrease in bone density

**palpate**   To use the hands or fingers to examine

**palpation**   Feeling an injury with the fingers

**papule**   Pimple

**paraplegia**   Paralysis of lower portion of the body and of both legs

**paresthesia**   Abnormal sensation such as numbness, prickling, and tingling

**patellar tendinitis**   Jumper's knee

**pathology**   Study of the nature and cause of disease

**pediatrician**   A specialist in the treatment of children's diseases

**periodization**   Varying training techniques during different seasons

**periosteum**   The fibrous covering of a bone

**peristalis**   A progressive, wavelike movement that occurs in the alimentary canal

**pes planus**   Flat feet

**phagocytosis**   Process of ingesting microorganisms, other cells, or foreign particles, commonly by monocytes, or white blood cells

**phalanges**   Bones of the fingers and toes

**phalanx**   Any one of the bones of the fingers and toes

**photophobia**   An intense intolerance of light

**plantarflexion**   The forepart of the foot is depressed relative to the ankle

**plica**   A fold of tissue within the body

**plyometric exercise**   An exercise that maximizes the myotatic, or stretch, reflex

**pneumothorax**   A collapse of a lung due to air in the pleural cavity

**point tenderness**   Pain is produced when the site of injury is palpated

**polymers**   Natural or synthetic substances formed by the combination of two or more molecules of the same substance

**positive resistance**   Slow concentric muscle contraction against resistance with muscle shortening

**posterior**   Toward the rear or back

**posterior cruciate ligament**   A ligament that stops internal rotation

**posttraumatic amnesia**   Inability of athlete to recall events since injury

**power**   Ability to accelerate a load, depending on the level of strength and velocity of a muscle contraction

**primary assessment**   Initial first aid evaluation

**prophylactic**   Pertaining to prevention, preservation, or protection

**prophylaxis**   Guarding against injury or disease

**proprioceptive neuromuscular facilitation (PNF)**   Stretching techniques that involve combinations of alternating contractions and stretches

**proprioceptors**   Organs within the body that provide the athlete with an awareness of where the body is in space (kinesthesis)

**prostaglandin**   Acidic lipids widely distributed in the body; in musculoskeletal conditions it is concerned with vasodilation, histaminelike effect; it is inhibited by aspirin

**prothrombin**   Interacts with calcium to produce thrombin

**proximal**   Nearest to the point of reference

**psychogenic**   Of psychic origin; that which originates in the mind

**psychophysiological**   Involving the mind and the body

**psychosomatic** Showing effects of mind-body relationship; physical disorder caused or influenced by the mind (i.e., by the emotions)

**quadriplegia** Paralysis affecting all four limbs

**referred pain** Pain that is felt at a point of the body other than its actual origin

**regeneration** Repair, regrowth, or restoration of a part such as tissue

**residual** That which remains; often used to describe a permanent condition resulting from injury or disease (e.g., a limp or a paralysis)

**resorption** Act of removal by absorption

**retrograde amnesia** Memory loss for events occurring immediately before trauma

**revascularize** Restoration of blood circulation to an injured area

**rhinitis** Inflammation of the nasal mucus lining

**RICE** *R*est, *i*ce, *c*ompression, and *e*levation

**rotation** Turning around an axis in an angular motion

**SAID principle** *S*pecific *a*daptations to *i*mposed *d*emands

**Scheuermann's disease (osteochondrosis)** A degeneration of the vertebral epiphyseal endplates

**sciatica** Inflammatory condition of the sciatic nerve; commonly associated with peripheral nerve root compression

**sclera** White outer coating of the eye

**scoliosis** A lateral deviation curve of the spine

**secondary assessment** Follow up; a more detailed examination

**seizure** Sudden attack

**shin splints** Medial tibial stress syndrome; anterior lower leg pain

**sign** Objective evidence of an abnormal situation within the body

**sling psychrometer** Instrument for establishing the wet-bulb, globe temperature index

**spasm** A sudden, involuntary muscle contraction

**spica** A figure-eight, with one of the two loops being larger

**spondylolisthesis** Forward slipping of a vertebral body, usually a lumbar vertebrae

**spondylolysis** A degeneration of the vertebrae and a defect in the pars intermedia of the articular processes of the vertebrae

**sprain** Injury to a ligament that connects bone to bone

**staleness** Deterioration in the usual standard of performance; chronic fatigue, apathy, loss of appetite, indigestion, weight loss, and inability to sleep or rest properly

**standard of reasonable care** Assumes that an individual is a person of reasonable and ordinary prudence

**staplylococcus** A genus of micrococci, some of which are pathogenic, causing pus and tissue destruction

**static stretching** Passively stretching an antagonist muscle by placing it in a maximal stretch position and holding it there

**statute of limitation** A specific length of time to sue for damages from negligence

**strain** A stretch tear, or rip in the muscle or its tendon

**strength** Ability of a muscular contraction to exert force to move an object (dynamic) or to perform work against a fixed object (static)

**streptococcus** Oval bacteria that appear in a chain

**stress** The positive and negative forces that can disrupt the body's equilibrium

**stress fracture** Spot of irritation on the bone

**stressor** Anything that affects the body's physiological or psychological condition

**stroke volume** The heart's capacity to pump blood

**subcutaneous** Beneath the skin

**subluxation** A bone is forced out but goes back into place

**subthreshold** Below the point at which a physiological effect begins to be produced

**symptom** Subjective evidence of an abnormal situation within the body

**syndrome** Group of typical symptoms or conditions that characterize an injury, a deficiency, or a disease

**synergy** To work in cooperation with

**synovia** A transparent lubricating fluid found in joints, bursae, and tendons

**synovitis** Inflammation of a synovial membrane

**synthesis** Buildup

**systolic blood pressure** The pressure caused by the heart's pumping

**tendinitis** Inflammation of the tendon

**tendon** Tough band of connective tissue that attaches muscle to bone

**tennis leg** Strain of the gastrocnemius muscle

**tenosynovitis** Inflammation of a tendon and its synovial sheath

**tetanus toxoid** Tetanus toxin modified to produce active immunity against *Clostridium tetani*

**thrombi** Plural of thrombus

**thromboplastin** Substance within the body's tissues that accelerates blood clotting

**thrombus** Blood clot that blocks small blood vessels or a cavity of the heart

**time-loss injuries** Injuries that require the player to suspend activity within a day of an injury's onset

**tinea** Ringworm; skin fungus disease

**tonic muscle cramp** Continuous muscle contraction that is long in duration

**tonic muscle spasm** Rigid muscle contraction that lasts over a period of time

**tonus (muscle)** Residual state of muscle contraction

**torque** A twisting force produced by contraction of the medial femoral muscles that tends to rotate the thigh medially

**torsional** Rotating or twisting of a body part

**tort** Legal wrongs committed against another

**training effect** Stroke volume increases while heart rate is reduced at a given exercise load

**transitory paralysis** Temporary inability to move

**traumatic** Pertaining to the course of an injury or wound

**traumatic arthritis** Arthritis stemming from repeated joint injury

**traumatic asphyxia** Result of a violent blow to, or compression of, the rib cage, causing cessation of breathing

**trigger point** Area of tenderness in a tight band of muscle

**valgus** Bent outward

**variable resistance** Resistance is varied throughout the range of motion

**varus** Bent inward

**vasoconstriction** Decrease in the diameter of a blood vessel

**vasodilation** Increase in the diameter of a blood vessel

**vasospasm** Blood vessel spasm

**venule** Tiny vein fed by a capillary

**verruca** Virus causing a wart

**viscera** Internal organs

**viscus (organs)** Any internal organ enclosed within a cavity

**volar** Referring to the palm or the sole

**water ad libitum** Unlimited access to water

**xerostomia** Having a dry mouth

**xiphoid process** Smallest of three parts of the sternum

# Credits

## Chapter 2
**Figs. 2-3, 2-4, pp. 25, 26,** Courtesy, The University of North Carolina at Chapel Hill; **Fig. 2-5, p. 28,** Courtesy, D Bailey, California State University at Long Beach.

## Chapter 3
**Fig. 3-2, p. 41,** Courtesy, The University of North Carolina at Chapel Hill.

## Chapter 4
**Figs. 4-3 through 4-16, Figs. 4-18 through 4-44, Figs. 4-46 through 4-59, pp. 59-95,** From Prentice, WE: *Fitness for college and life,* ed. 5, Dubuque, IA: WCB/McGraw-Hill, 1997.

## Chapter 5
**Figs. 5-1, 5-4, pp. 105, 119, & Tables 5-1, 5-2, pp. 107, 109,** From Prentice, WE: *Fitness for college and life,* ed. 5, Dubuque, IA: WCB/McGraw-Hill, 1997; **Fig. 5-2, p. 113,** From Prentice, WE: *Get fit stay fit,* Dubuque, IA: McGraw-Hill, 2001; **Fig. 5-3, p. 114,** US Dept of Agriculture/US Dept of Health & Human Services, August, 1992.

## Chapter 6
**Fig. 6-1, p. 135,** Courtesy, Robert Freligh, California State University at Long Beach; **Figs. 6-12, 6-13, pp. 143, 144,** From Nicholas, JA, Hershman, EB: *The lower extremity and spine in sports medicine,* ed. 2, St. Louis: Mosby, 1995; **Figs. 6-21, 6-24, (middle), pp. 150, 152,** Courtesy, Mueller Sports Medicine; **Fig. 6-18, p. 146,** From Prentice, WE: *Fitness for college and life,* ed. 5, Dubuque, IA: WCB/McGraw-Hill, 1997.

## Chapter 7
**Fig. 7-16, p. 183,** Courtesy, Hartwell Medical Corporation, Carlsbad, CA.

## Chapter 8
**Focus box, p. 197,** From Payne, WA, Hahn, DB: *Understanding your health,* ed. 5, Dubuque, IA: WCB/McGraw-Hill, 1998.

## Chapter 10
**Table 10-2, p. 226,** Modified from Berkow, R: *The Merck manual of diagnosis and therapy,* ed. 14, Rahway, NJ: Merck & Co., 1982.

## Chapter 13
**Figs. 13-5, 13-6, 13-8, pp. 282-285,** From Prentice, WE: *Rehabilitation techniques in sports medicine,* Dubuque, IA: WCB/McGraw-Hill, 1999.

## Chapter 15
**Fig. 15-7, p. 321,** Courtesy, Cramer Products, Gardner, KS; **Figs. 15-17, 15-20, pp. 330, 348,** From Williams, JGP: *Color atlas of injury in sport,* ed. 2, Chicago: Year Book Medical Publishers, 1990.

## Chapter 16
**Fig. 16-10C, p. 349,** Courtesy, Robert Barclay and Renee Reavis Shingles, Central Michigan University.

## Chapter 17
**Fig. 17-7, p. 369,** Courtesy, Ken Bartlett, California State University at Long Beach; **Figs. 17-9, 17-21 (right), pp. 370, 379,** From Williams, JGP: *Color atlas of injury in sport,* ed. 2, Chicago: Year Book Medical Publishers, 1990; **Figs. 17-16, 17-20, pp. 376, 379,** Courtesy, Robert Barclay and Renee Reavis Shingles, Central Michigan University; **Fig. 17-17, p. 377,** Courtesy BRACE International, Phoenix, AZ.

## Chapter 18
**Figs. 18-2, 18-5, pp. 385, 388,** From Nicholas, JA, Hershman, EB: *The upper extremity in sports medicine,* ed. 2, St. Louis: Mosby, 1995; **Fig. 18-17, p. 397,** art by Don O'Connor.

## Chapter 19
**Figs. 19-3, 19-4, pp. 406, 407,** Courtesy Ken Bartlett, California State University at Long Beach; **Figs. 19-5, 19-21, 19-24, pp. 407, 422, 424,** From Nicholas, JA, Hershman, EB: *The upper extremity in sports medicine,* ed. 2, St. Louis: Mosby, 1995; **Fig. 19-12, p. 415,** From Booher, JM, Thibodeau, GA: *Athletic injury assessment,* ed. 3, Dubuque, IA: WCB/McGraw-Hill, 1994; **Figs. 19-22 (left), p. 422, 19-23, p. 423,** From Nicholas, JA and Hershman, EB: *The upper extremity in sports medicine,* ed. 2, St. Louis: Mosby, 1995.

## Chapter 20
**Fig. 20-5, p. 433,** art by Don O'Connor; **Fig. 20-16B, p. 447,** From Williams, JGP: *Color atlas of injury in sport,* ed. 2, Chicago: Year Book Medical Publishers, 1990.

## Chapter 22
**Figs. 22-22, pp. 484, 503,** Allsport; **Table 22-3, p. 483,** Adapted from Cantu, RC: Guidelines for return to contact sports after a cerebral concussion, *The physician in sportsmedicine* 14 (10): 79, 1986; **Figs. 22-10 (top), 22-11, 22-14, pp. 488, 490, 492,** From Williams,

JGP: *Color atlas of injury in sport,* ed. 2, Chicago: Year Book Medical Publishers, 1990.

## Chapter 23
**Figs. 23-1, 23-2, pp. 504, 505,** From Habif, TP: *Clinical dermatology,* ed. 3, St. Louis: Mosby, 1996; **Fig. 23-4, p. 506,** From Stewart, WD, Danto, JL, Madden, S: *Dermatology: diagnosis and treatment of cutaneous disorders,* ed. 4, St. Louis, 1978; **Table 23-4, p. 531,** Modified from American College Health Association: *Making sex safer,* Baltimore: American College Health Association, 1990.

## Chapter 24
**Fig. 24-1, p. 540,** From Coakley, J: *Sport in society,* ed. 7, McGraw-Hill, 2001, photo by James Bryant.

# Index